J.V. Byrne · G. Guglielmi

Endovascular Treatment of Intracranial Aneurysms

Foreword by Charles G. Drake

With 98 Illustrations in 188 Parts

Springer

Dr. James V. Byrne, MD, FRCS, FRCR
Radcliffe Infirmary
Woodstock Road
Oxford OX2 6HE, GB

Guido Guglielmi, MD
Professor
Division of Interventional Neuroradiology
U.C.L.A. Medical Centre
Los Angeles, CA 90095-1721, USA

ISBN-13: 978-3-642-80383-3 e-ISBN-13: 978-3-642-80381-9
DOI: 10.1007/978-3-642-80381-9

Library of Congress Cataloging-in-Publication Data
Byrne, J.V. (James V.), 1950–. Endovascular treatment of intracranial aneurysms / J.V. Byrne, G. Guglielmi. p. cm. Includes bibliographical references and index.

1. Intracranial aneurysms – Endoscopic surgery. I. Guglielmi, G. (Guido), 1948–. II. Title. [DNLM: 1. Cerebral Aneurysm – therapy. 2. Cerebral Aneurysm – diagnosis. 3. Embolization, Therapeutic – methods. WL 355 B995e 1998]. RD594.2.B95 1998. 617.4'81-dc21. DNLM/DLC for Library of Congress. 97-28768 CIP

Softcover reprint of the hardcover 1st edition 1998

Cover design: Anna Deus, Heidelberg
Typesetting: K+V Fotosatz, Beerfelden

SPIN 10523000 21/3135-5 4 3 2 1 0 – Printed on acid-free paper

Endovascular Treatment of Intracranial Aneurysms

Springer
Berlin
Heidelberg
New York
Barcelona
Budapest
Hong Kong
London
Milan
Paris
Santa Clara
Singapore
Tokyo

Dedication

To Nella, Marta, Silvia,
To my brother, Nick Byrne
and Juliet, Rowena, Tom, George, and Henry

Foreword

This is the story of endovascular treatment of brain aneurysms whose recent rapid evolution from detachable balloons to packing with detachable coils is extraordinary. It prompted a look back over 40 years of my attempts, and those of others, to find the ideal safe treatment of intracranial aneurysms by surgical (extravascular) means, which for me came to an end with retirement in 1992 and experience with over 4000 aneurysms.

Although carotid occlusion had been used even in the last century, intracranial surgery for aneurysm, while beginning in the 1930s, was not widely attempted until after WWII. Those operations done early after bleeding using only small unremovable silver clips or ligatures resulted in high morbidity. Then with the safety of delayed operation there was appalling loss of life with rebleeding while waiting, and measures to prevent early rebleeding were only modestly successful. That many postoperative catastrophes were associated with vasospasm was not recognized until the early 1960s, and even today this phenomenon remains a major cause of morbidity.

Surgeons concentrated on techniques to dissect a slack aneurysm from its branches and perforators and prevent inadvertent rupture using varying degrees of systemic hypotension and even hypothermia for a time. Only gradually did operative morbidity decline in these trying early years, until microneurosurgery began. Magnified vision first with loupes in the 1960s and then under the surgical microscope in the 1970s provided a new operative world for the surgeon, revealing the most intimate details of the origin and relations of the aneurysm to its neighbourhood of nervous structures and vessels.

Aneurysm clip design improved rapidly with removable spring clips of many sizes and shapes. The fenestrated clip solved the problem of the bulbous neck and could be used in tandem or in parallel to occlude even the widest aneurysm necks. After 1980, the use of gentle temporary clipping of the parent vessel came into wider use so that the surgeon had a slack or even collapsed aneurysm with which to deal. Coupled with new microsurgical tools most aneurysm necks could be clipped with exquisite accuracy. Today in experienced hands most nongiant aneurysms in good condition patients can be obliterated with morbidities under 10% even on the basilar circulation.

The first use of an endovascular embolus may have been that of Brooks of Nashville, who in 1931 introduced a long thin strip of muscle into the carotid artery for treatment of a CC fistula; the patient had a good result but a blind eye. Russian surgeons later used a muscle embolus tethered with a suture so that it could be retrieved if the bruit persisted or weakness resulted. In the excellent historical review herein, it is evident that it was not until 1974 when Serbinenko's use of flow-directed detachable balloons in aneurysms, AVMs and CC fistulas ignited wide interest and sent a tremor through the neurosurgical world. We had occasionally used the Luessenhop technique since the mid 1970s but it was the arrival on our unit of Gerard Debrun, who had introduced these balloon techniques in Paris, which galvanized our interest and collaborative participation in endovascular approaches. Not surprising was the decline of enthusiasm for balloon occlusion of the aneurysm sac itself, which produced high morbidity from premature detachment and embolization, rupture of the aneurysm or the balloon with its contents. Seldom was obliteration of the aneurysm complete since a balloon could not usually conform to the shape of the sac. Detachable balloons have found their niche in proximal parent artery occlusion for inoperable aneurysms and in closing CC fistulae.

The evolution of treatment with wire coils was rapid after the development of wire-guided catheters. It was the ingenuity of Guglielmi and his engineer Sepetka that led to tethering the coil to the wire so that it could be detached electrically only after its placement in the aneurysm seemed appropriate and safe; multiple coil placements are usual.

The ease with which catheters could be guided into virtually all intracranial arteries was astonishing. But technical failure to enter aneurysms, due to tortuosity of atherosclerotic vessels or the take off angle of the aneurysm, may occur in up to 10% of cases. Coil placement is not without morbidity – mostly thromboembolism and occasional rupture of the aneurysm. Surgeons have sympathy for radiologists who are faced with these potentially catastrophic events, in having to deal with them at the end of a catheter instead of directly. The authors conclude that the endovascular technique carries less morbidity than conventional craniotomy. However it should be noted that the overall good outcome in the largest series of coiling for acute aneurysms (85%) is about the same as early craniotomy for ruptured basilar aneurysms. The disappointment is that complete obliteration is seldom possible except in small necked aneurysms which are so straightforward for surgeons. Even small remnants of an incompletely clipped neck are known to enlarge into a new and dangerous aneurysm. One wonders what will happen over the years with wholly open ostia or those merely plugged with wire. Yet medium follow-up over the first few years in small series has shown little recurrence except in aneurysms with necks over 4 mm in diameter.

It is predictable that advances with coil techniques for the complete obliteration of larger aneurysms will occur, perhaps with the assistance of balloon packing, stents, or even endosaccular plastic.

The endovascular approach to the coiling of aneurysms has an appealing simplicity and will be widely adopted outside major centres even though plagued with incompleteness. If this can be rectified it may become the preferred primary treatment for most intracranial aneurysms if its morbidity remains low. Until then and in response to the authors' plea for collaborative management, I have suggested that in units where few endovascular procedures are done that only the fundus of acutely ruptured aneurysms be packed with coils down to the waist leaving the neck open, which could be done with little morbidity. The patients now safe from early rebleeding could be tided over their hemorrhagic brain injury even using hypertension and angioplasty for vasospasm. Then a month or so later an operation for clipping completely the remaining neck could be carried out under a slack healed brain also with very low morbidity. Such an approach should accomplish the desirable; prevent rebleeding, and complete the obliteration of the aneurysm with a combined long-term morbidity far less than either technique alone. Patients with wide necked aneurysms would not have to face the risk of thromboembolism again when the enlarging residual sac had to be repacked every few months or years. This approach would not preclude those few investigating new techniques from continuing their attempts for more complete endosaccular occlusions. However, I suspect it will be difficult to stay the hands of many endovascular radiologists or surgeons who will want to try for completeness on their own.

Charles G. Drake, O.C., M.D., FRCSC

Preface

The collaboration between the two authors that has resulted in the production of this book began 8 years ago. Dr. Byrne visited the University of California at Los Angeles at a time when clinical trials of the Guglielmi detachable coil were just beginning, and he subsequently imported the technology to the United Kingdom, performing the first clinical treatment there in 1992. The authors have worked together since to establish training programmes for the propagation of the techniques involved in coil embolisation. As a result, regular GDC Training Courses have been held in Oxford and Los Angeles over the last 4 years, and many of the principles described here owe their origins to the intellectual discipline needed in such teaching. Because the technology involves the development and practice of new skills, the timing of a book such as this is critical. We now feel that the technology is mature enough for didactic description but are sensitive to its youth and the need for its continued critical evaluation.

The authors are however bound by more than a thin piece of platinum wire. In producing this text we have drawn on surgical principles learnt in the neurosurgical training both of us experienced before practising interventional neuroradiology. It was obvious to us that a text book based on a single technology, such as the Guglielmi detachable coil, would simply be a technical manual. We have therefore attempted to present the technology in the context of its role in the management of patients with intracranial aneurysms. Such management has been practised by neurosurgeons for the last 60 years and that experience is vital to endovascular therapists coming lately to the bedside of patients with subarachnoid haemorrhage. We simply cannot afford not to build on the neurosurgical heritage. Inevitably, the technical aspects of what we have written will date, but the principles of operative surgery which we have tried to bring to the work are virtually timeless.

We would like to acknowledge the assistance of Mrs. Min-Joo Sohn in the preparation of the manuscript, the medical illustration departments of UCLA Medical Centre and Oxford University and our respective colleagues for their help and advice. The hand-drawn illustrations are the work of Juliet Bailey, who happens to be married to the English author. We are also most grateful to Dr. Charles Drake for providing a foreword to the book.

J. V. Byrne
G. Guglielmi

Contents

CHAPTER 1

Introduction to Intracranial Aneurysms

1.1 Introduction

An aneurysm is a localised persistent dilatation of the wall of a blood vessel or the heart. The term is derived from the Greek word *aneurysma*; *ana* meaning across and *eurys* broad. This definition allows for venous and cardiac aneurysms, but since we are primarily concerned with aneurysms arising on arteries, the term will be used to mean arterial aneurysms. Intracranial aneurysms are traditionally classified by aetiology and morphology. The majority are idiopathic and saccular. They occur at arterial branch points around the circle of Willis and have thin walls comprising adventitia and intima only. Saccular aneurysms involve part of the circumference of the artery from which they arise and with which they communicate at a single opening or neck. Fusiform aneurysms involve the entire artery wall, without a neck. Rarely can a specific cause be identified and most saccular intracranial aneurysms are thought to be the result of a combination of structural and haemodynamic factors.

1.2 History

It has been claimed that the ancient Egyptians knew of aneurysms and that the earliest description was by Galen [120]. In 1761 Morgagni described a case of bilateral posterior cerebral artery aneurysms [85], and Biumi in 1765 reported a ruptured aneurysm found at post mortem examination [18]. The first clinical description of aneurysmal subarachnoid haemorrhage (SAH) was by Blackhall in 1813 [19], and in 1850 Brinton [24] published a series of 52 cases. His conclusions from study of this small series make interesting reading: rupture could occur from birth to old age, the average age being 40 years; the sex ratio was two males to one female; the commonest aneurysm site was the basilar artery which accounted for a third of cases; and aneurysms were equally common on the anterior, middle and internal carotid arteries. One can only speculate about whether the variation from current dermography is due to differences in pathophysiology or the size of his sample.

The clinical features of ruptured and unruptured aneurysms were described by several physicians [13, 40, 54]. In 1907, Beadles [15] divided the presenting features of intracranial aneurysms into those that presented with: (a) apoplexy, (b) symptoms of cerebral tumour prior to fatal apoplexy, (c) symptoms of cerebral tumour without aploplexy and (d) as incidental findings at post mortem examination. Symonds produced a modern description of clinical signs in 1923 [129] and was the first to recognise early rebleeding after aneurysmal SAH [130]. The clinical diagnosis of SAH was put on a firmer footing with the introduction of lumbar puncture [103] in 1891 and Froin's description of the findings in cerebrospinal fluid after SAH in 1904 [49]. Not until the introduction of cerebral angiography by Moniz in 1927

[83] was it possible to diagnose and localise ruptured and smaller unruptured aneurysms in vivo – a landmark in diagnosis not repeated until the advent of computed tomography (CT) in 1973 [3, 61].

Clinicopathological descriptions were made by several early authors, notably Bramwell in 1886 [21] and Eppinger in 1887 [37]. The latter suggested that noninfective aneurysms were due to congenital weakness in the elastic properties of the arterial wall. In 1918, Turnbull [136] separated aneurysms on the basis of their pathology into those of infective, congenital and degenerative aetiologies. The decline of infectious desease has decreased the incidence of infectious aneurysms. The relative importance of congenital and degenerative factors in the causation of intracranial aneurysm has been debated for much of this century [23].

1.3 Aetiology of Intracranial Aneurysms

1.3.1 Structural Causes

The walls of intradural arteries are different from those of peripheral vessels because the adventitia is thin, there is no external elastic lamina and the media is thin and absent at bifurcations. They are more prone to develop aneurysms and this tendency may be increased by wall degeneration due to atherosclerosis or injury caused by trauma or inflammation. Saccular aneurysms were originally described as "congenital" by Eppinger in 1887 [37], but as doubts emerged about their aetiology, the more neutral term "berry aneurysm" was proposed by Collier in 1931 [28], based simply on their macroscopic appearance.

Early authors, recognising that the walls of intradural cerebral arteries are thinner than those of their extradural counterparts, suggested that aneurysms were due to "congenital" weakness of the unsupported arterial wall in the subarachnoid space [37, 54]. Forbus [44] demonstrated that the muscle of the media at the crotch of cerebral arterial divisions was deficient in infants and adults and suggested that these defects in the wall represented points of weakness. Several authors supported the suggestion that aneurysms were caused by herniation of the intima through these defects in the overlying muscle layer [23, 45]. Medial defects appeared to explain the characteristic of saccular aneurysms to develop at arterial branch points (Fig. 1.1).

However, the concept that aneurysms and the medial defects described by Forbus represented congenitally determined lesions has been challenged [51, 125]. Stehbens [125] showed that the defects were more frequent in older people and that pre-aneurysmal arterial dilatations may arise adjacent to, rather than at the site of, medial defects. They occurred in all the animal species he studied, but in only one (a chimpanzee) was he able to demonstrate an aneurysm [122]. He also pointed out that, in other parts of the body, when muscle fibres diverge and are forced to pull against each other in contraction (as at the acute angle formed by arterial bifurcations) there is usual-

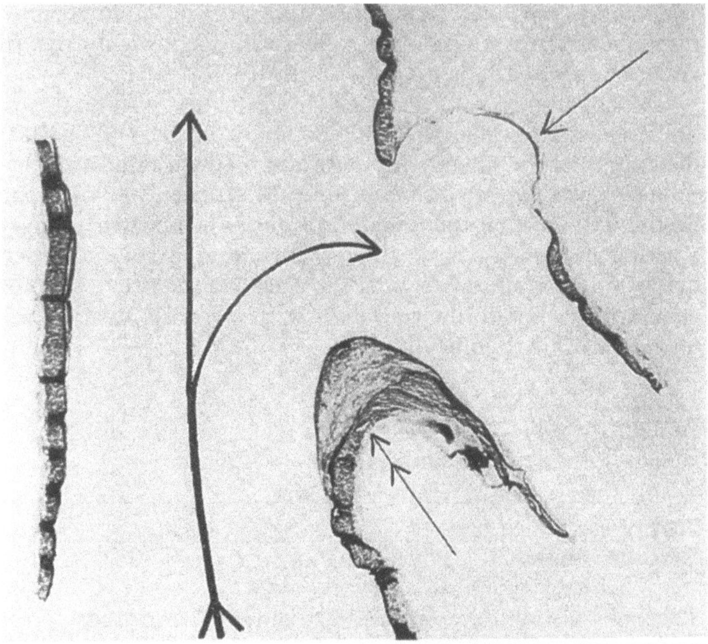

a

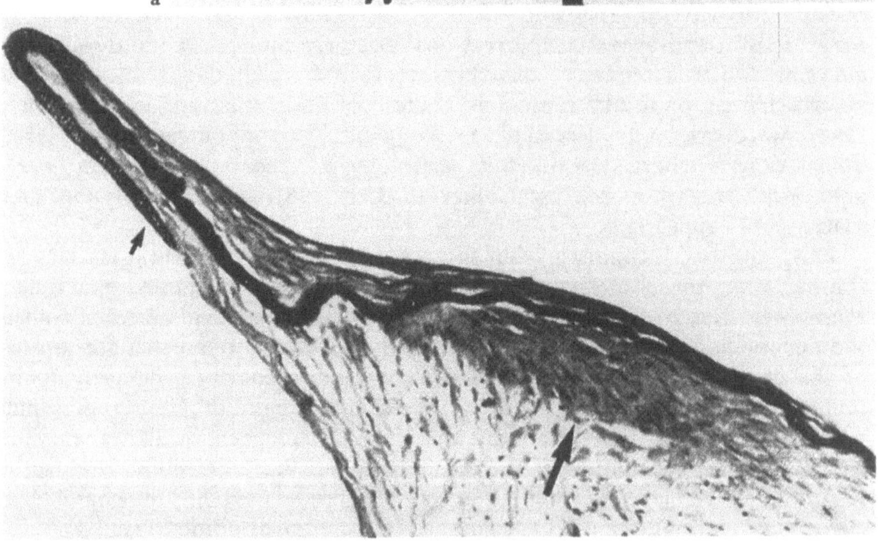

b

Fig. 1.1. a An aneurysm developing at the branch point of two arteries. This histological section shows the direction of blood flow (*large arrows*), a very small aneurysm (*single arrow*) and the intimal cushion at the angle between main and branch arteries (*double arrow*). **b** Magnified section of the boundary between the wall of an intracranial artery and aneurysm. The media of the parent artery (*large arrow*) does not extend into the aneurysm neck, whilst the internal elastic lamina extends for a short distance into the aneurysm (*small arrow*). (After [59])

ly a separating support such as bone or ligament. He suggested that the divergence of longitudinal muscle fibres forming medial defects should be renamed "medial raphe". Medial defects, therefore, arise as a consequence of cerebral artery design and, although they may contribute to aneurysm formation, they are neither pathological entities nor necessarily their initiating cause.

1.3.2 Haemodynamic Causes

Turbulence of blood flow at arterial bifurcations was suggested as the cause by Hassler [59]. Turbulence is more frequent at arterial branch points, bifurcations and fenestrations, as well as in high-flow arteries and may cause structural fatigue and degeneration of elastic fibres, as occurs in post-stenotic dilatation [106]. Stehbens considered that haemodynamically induced degenerative changes initiated aneurysm formation [122], but Ferguson [42] showed that at normal flow rates there is little turbulence at bifurcations and that, when it does occur (at abnormally high flow rates), it does so proximal to the apex of the bifurcation and therefore not at the site of most saccular aneurysms. However, haemodynamic stress is maximal in the wall of the artery at the apex of a bifurcation, and Ferguson suggested that these stresses cause local degeneration of the internal elastic lamina initiating the formation of a sac [105]. Once a sac has formed, turbulence of blood flow within the sac causes its enlargement and possible rupture [41, 42].

Intracranial aneurysms occur in several conditions and situations which result in alterations of cerebral arterial haemodynamics (Table 1.1). Aneurysms develop on hypertrophied vessels (arteries and veins) supplying cerebral arteriovenous malformations [14, 33, 47]. Arterial aneurysms related to arteriovenous malformations (AVM) may develop on a feeding pedicle, within the nidus or on unrelated arteries. Those that develop on a feeding pedicle are, like the hypertrophy of such vessels, due to increased blood flow [33, 71, 128] rather than part of an underlying developmental abnormality responsible for the malformation. Since aneurysms have been reported to develop de novo on afferent arteries of arteriovenous shunts within 3 years [8] and successful treatment of the shunt can cause their regression [142]. The frequency of aneurysms on arteries other than those feeding an AVM, which are therefore not subjected to increased blood flow is similar to that in the general population [95], i.e. they are probaby incidentally associated. The reported prevalence of associated aneurysms depends on whether patients are studied by selective or superselective angiography and if intranidal aneurysms are included. Turjman et al. [135] reported aneurysms in 58% of patients with brain arteriovenous malformations studied by superselective angiography, whereas a prevalence of only 1%–5% was reported in earlier non-superselective studies [47, 98, 112].

Alterations in local haemodynamics are assumed to occur with anatomical variations of the circle of Willis. Aneurysms are associated with asymmetry in the size or development of arteries forming the circle [69, 145], carotid ar-

Table 1.1. Causes of intracranial aneurysms

- Haemodynamic causes
  - Flow aneurysms associated with arteriovenous malformations
  - Nishimoto-Takahashi-Kodo disease (moyamoya)
  - Persistent carotid-basilar anastomoses
  - Asymmetries of the circle of Willis (aplasia, hypoplasia or occlusions of contralateral arteries)
- Hypertension
  - Polycystic renal disease
  - Co-arctation of aorta
  - Essential hypertension
  - Fibromuscular dysplasia
- Genetic causes
  - Familial aneurysms
  - Hereditary mesenchymal disorders
  - Ehlers-Danlos syndrome, Marfan's syndrome
    - Pseudoxanthoma elasticum, Rendu-Osler-Weber syndrome
    - Klippel-Trenaunay-Weber syndrome
  - Type III collagen deficiency
- Traumatic causes
  - Penetrating and non-penetrating head injury
  - Surgical trauma
  - Radiation
- Inflammatory
  - Infections (embolic or local)
  - Associated with intravenous drug abuse
  - Giant cell arteritis
  - Wegener's granulomatosis
- Degenerative
  - Atherosclerosis (fusiform aneurysms)
- Neoplastic
  - Atrial myxoma
  - Choriocarcinoma
  - Anaplastic carcinoma

tery agenesis or ligation [87, 113, 114] and persistent primitive carotid–basilar anastomoses [145]. Servo [118] reported a 23% incidence of aneurysm associated with carotid artery agenesis and Salar and Mingrino [114] estimated that after carotid artery ligation the risk of developing contralateral aneurysms increased by 2%. Increased collateral flow in response to arterial stenosis in moyamoya disease presumably causes the majority of aneurysms that occur in this condition, since they develop on unaffected arteries, usually in the posterior cerebral circulation [137]. The incidence of aneurysms of all types in moyamoya has been estimated at 5%–15% [5, 59]. Aneurysms have been reported in association with persistent trigeminal [50] (Fig. 6.1) and hypoglossal arteries [35, 70, 74], though the relationship with alterations in flow dynamics is not clear cut. Fenestrations [132] and duplications [145] of intracranial arteries are also associated with aneurysms (Fig. 1.2). In the former, aneurysms typically occur at the proximal point of a fenestration which may be due to a combination of turbulent flow and inherent weakness of the wall [132]. The reason for their association with arterial duplications is unknown.

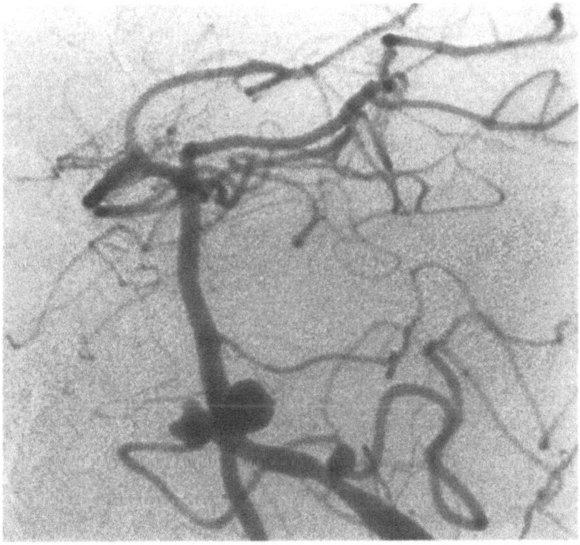

Fig. 1.2.
Vertebral intra-arterial digital subtraction angiogram with reflux filling of the contralateral vertebral artery (VA). The proximal basilar artery is fenestrated; two aneurysms are present at the site of the fenestration. They point away from the direction of blood flow in the opposite VA. A third aneurysm is present at the origin of the left posterior inferior cerebellar artery. Aneurysms associated with fenestrations occur at the proximal end of the lesion

1.3.3 Associated Pathology

The role of primary systemic hypertension in the genesis of aneurysms is uncertain. Both are common conditions and likely to co-exist; Redekop and Ferguson [105], in a review of the subject, stated that hypertension alone does not appear to be a major factor in the origin of aneurysms, but might be expected to contribute to the development and rupture of aneurysms once formed. The association between intracranial aneurysms and polycystic renal disease or coarctation of the aorta, has been attributed to the effect of chronic hypertension and vascular degenerative disease [125]. Aneurysms occur in 2.5%–10.6% of patients with coarctation [131] and SAH occurs at a younger age than in unaffected aneurysm patients [115]. The presence of chronic hypertension probably contributes to the development of intracranial aneurysms in this condition since the incidence of SAH is reduced if effective treatment is performed before the age of 20 years. At autopsies of patients with polycystic renal disease, intracranial aneurysms are present in 7%–16% [17, 111]. Fox [46] found a strong correlation between aneurysms and hypertension in reports of patients with polycystic renal disease. However, no correlation was found by Wakabayashi et al. [138] who reported aneurysms in 63% of normotensive and in only 22% of hypertensive patients. In polycystic renal disease genetic factors are therefore relevant. Aneurysms occur in up to 50% of patients with fibromuscular dysplasia [48, 80], but the majority of patients with aneurysms are normotensive [81]. However, hypertension was correlated with the occurrence of SAH in patients with fibromuscular dysplasia by Mettinger [80]; a finding which supports the concept that it acts as an aggravating factor (Fig. 1.3).

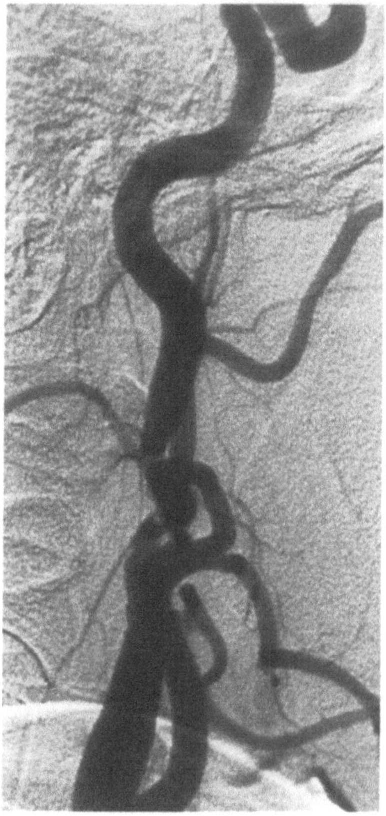

Fig. 1.3.
Common carotid intra-arterial digital subtraction angiogram showing segmental narrowing of the internal carotid artery (ICA) due to fibromuscular dysplasia. This patient was treated by coil embolisation for a ruptured intracranial aneurysm after a guide-catheter had been placed across the carotid lesion. Note that the intracranial ICA and external carotid artery are unaffected

A genetic cause for intracranial aneurysms has been proposed on the basis of an increased incidence amongst members of some families [56, 58] and in patients with hereditary connective tissue disorders. Lozano [76], reviewing the literature in 1987, noted that patients with a family history of intracranial aneurysm presented younger than those without. A dominant inheritance was suggested by Evans [39] but others, notably Bannerman et al. [10] and Pakarinen [97], were unable to demonstrate any hereditary tendency. An, as yet, unrecognised mesenchymal defect may be responsible for some cases. Ter Berg et al. [134] reported aneurysms in seven members of a family in which two other members were diagnosed with Marfan's syndrome. Diseases affecting arterial collagen or elastin are likely to weaken the wall since these proteins are responsible for most of its tensile strength. Ehlers-Danlos syndrome is a heterogeneous group of disorders of which type IV is associated with a deficiency of type III collagen. In this form of the syndrome, intracranial aneurysms and carotico-cavernous fistulae may occur [109]. Type III collagen is involved in intimal proliferation and repair [11] and its deficiency has been reported in patients with saccular aneurysms without other features of Ehlers-Danlos syndrome [91, 101]. Aneurysms have been reported in other hereditary mesenchymal disorders including Marfan's syndrome [43]

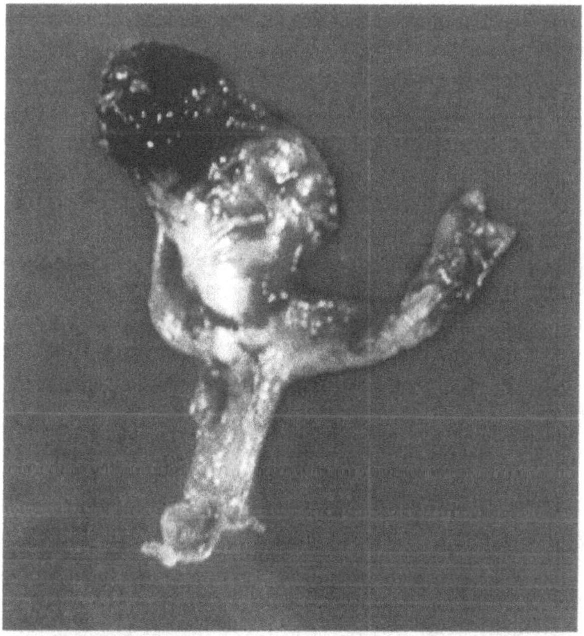

a

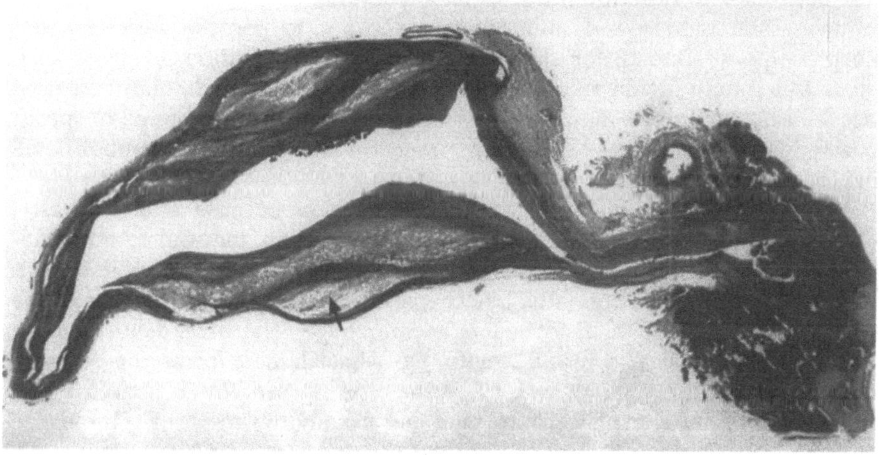

b

Fig. 1.4. **a** Post-mortem specimen of a ruptured intracranial aneurysm. This macroscopic specimen has a well defined neck arising in the crotch of an arterial bifurcation. The fundus is stained by thrombosis at the rupture point. The sac is lobulated in outline, presumably due to intramural haematoma at the fundus. **b** Microscopic appearance of the same specimen. The aneurysm wall is atherosclerotic (*arrow*) and the fundal haemorrhage is clearly seen. Subsequent reorganisation of such thrombus will extend the lumen which can be identified as a "pimple" on angiography. (Courtesy of Dr J. Morris)

pseudoxanthoma elastica [34, 88] and Rendu-Osler-Weber syndrome [142]. In these conditions the walls of blood vessels are inherently fragile and therefore liable to develop aneurysms. It is likely that this tendency is exacerbated by abnormal local haemodynamics.

The role of atherosclerosis in the aetiology of fusiform aneurysms is generally accepted (Fig. 1.4). Atheromatous plaques thicken the wall and disrupt the internal elastic lamina over a wide area, reducing its ability to withstand intraluminal pressure and causing the vessel to elongate and dilate [124]. Atheroma of cerebral arteries and saccular aneurysms frequently coexist in angiographic [36] and histopathological [123] studies. In 1966, Crompton [31] found evidence of atherosclerosis in 52% of patients with aneurysms, but considered that this incidence was to be expected based on the prevalence of hypertension in the study cohort. He suggested that the frequent association of hypertension with atherosclerosis caused aneurysms and that it would be virtually impossible to separate the effects of the two conditions. It can therefore be concluded that intracranial aneurysms are caused by a combination of factors and a single responsible agent is, at the moment, rarely identifiable in any particular patient.

1.4 Morbid Anatomy: Macroscopic and Microscopic Appearances

Various terms based on morphology, aetiology and pathology have in the past been used to describe intracranial aneurysms. These include berry, congenital, atheromatous and miliary. In order not to confuse aetiology and morphology, we intend, for the first part of this description, to avoid such terms and simply divide aneurysms into saccular and non-saccular, accepting that the same aetiology may be the cause of both types. Aneurysms of specific aetiology (i.e. trauma, dissection, infection and malignant emboli) will then be discussed.

Both saccular and fusiform aneurysms develop because a blood vessel wall, weakened by disease, stretches and thereby forms the wall to the aneurysm sac. Such aneurysms are termed true aneurysms to distinguish them from false aneurysms. The latter are the result of complete disruption of the vessel wall, usually with perivascular haemorrhage. The breakdown of perivascular hematoma in continuity with the vessel lumen forms the sac of a false aneurysm, the walls of which are therefore formed by organised blood clot. Intradural false aneurysms are rare and usually the result of trauma.

1.4.1 Saccular Aneurysms

Saccular aneurysms are characteristically sited on the circle of Willis or its major branches and develop at bifurcations or at the origins of branch arteries (Fig. 1.5). They are typically spherical in shape and described as comprising a neck, body and fundus. Flowing blood enters the lumen at the neck or ostium and the body and fundus are usually in line with the direction of dominant flow in the parent artery. Two or more locules may develop and recently ruptured aneurysms often have a small locule or pimple at the point where rupture occurred [127] (Fig. 1.6).

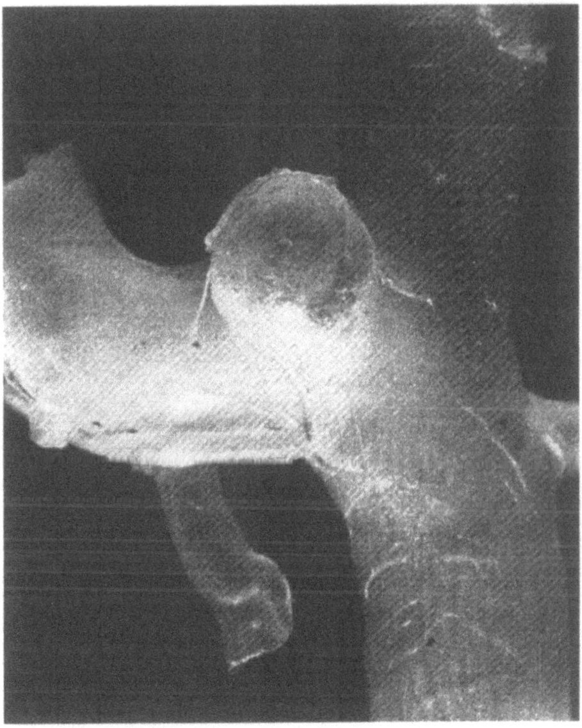

Fig. 1.5.
A small saccular aneurysm (pre-aneurysm) developing in the crotch of two vessels. (From [124])

The dimensions of an aneurysm determined by angiography depend on radiographic contrast medium filling the lumen which tends to underestimate the lumen size and does not take account of wall thickness. Planar scanning provides a better assessment of external dimensions and overall aneurysm size. Despite this shortcoming, aneurysms are usually measured from angiograms and described as small or large when the maximum diameter is less than 25 mm and giant when it is greater than 25 mm. The neck enlarges in proportion with lumen size; necks with a width greater than 4 mm are described as wide. The origins of adjacent arteries, especially at bifurcations, may be incorporated into the neck so that branches of the parent artery issue directly from the base of the aneurysm sac near the neck, and not from the fundal region. Enlargement greater than 10–15 mm is variably associated with the formation of laminated thrombi within the lumen which may thicken the walls. The walls of giant aneurysms are generally thick and often calcified.

Microscopic Anatomy. The walls of intradural arteries are thinner than those of peripheral arteries with three definable layers: adventitia, media and intima. The intima comprises an inner endothelial layer, a thin collagen layer and a conspicuous internal elastic lamina [110]. The media is devoid of an external elastic lamina and is thin or absent at bifurcations [59, 110]. The adventitia is thinner than that of an extradural artery of equivalent size and there are no normal vasa vasorum beyond the most proximal part of the intradural arteries[147].

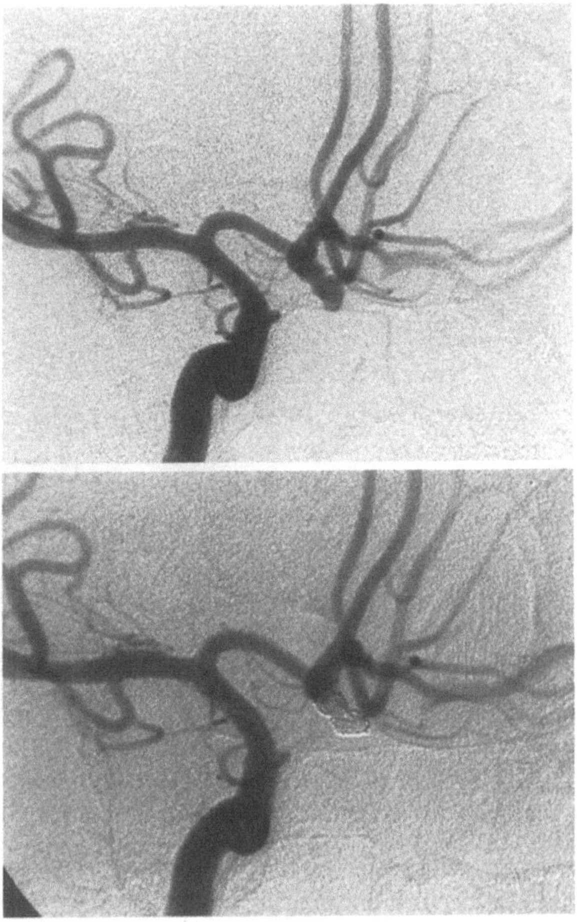

Fig. 1.6a,b. Oblique frontal intra-arterial digital subtraction angiograms of a lobulated aneurysm of the anterior communicating artery **a** before and **b** after coil embolisation. The aneurysm has a lobulated outline with a fundal lobule which is the likely site of rupture

The walls of saccular aneurysms do not have a media or internal elastic lamina. Muscle fibres of the media cease abruptly at the neck and elastic tissue tapers and ceases in the neck wall (Fig. 1.1b). The integrity of the endothelial layer is variable; it is complete only in small aneurysms [127]. The wall is therefore principally composed of loose fibrous tissue continuous with the adventitia of the parent artery. Atherosclerotic changes may be present in the parent artery and around the neck where foam cells, lipophages and cholesterol clefts may be found (Fig. 1.4b).

The interior of an intracranial aneurysm is smooth or irregular due to areas of intimal thickening or organised thrombus. Thickening of the walls of small aneurysms may be a reparative response to mechanical trauma possible with mural haemorrhages or degeneration secondary to atheroma [93]. Suzuki and Ohara [127] demonstrated thickening in the dome of 1- to 2-mm aneurysms containing endothelial cells, fibroblasts and elastic fibres. The domes of larger unruptured aneurysms (4–10 mm) were irregular in thick-

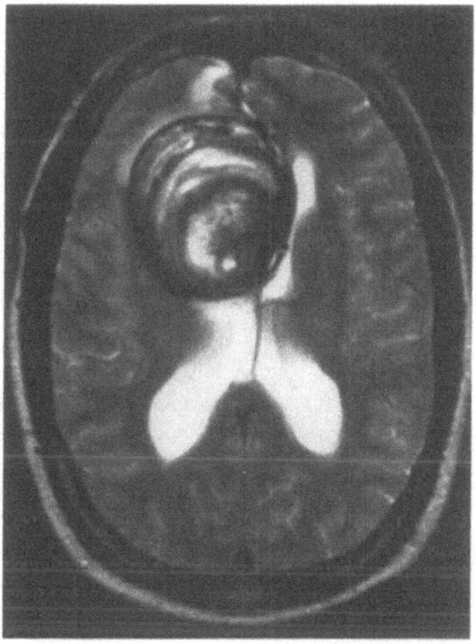

Fig. 1.7.
Axial T2-weighted magnetic resonance imaging (MRI) at the level of the foramen of Munro. A giant aneurysm of the anterior communication artery region is distorting the ventricles and causing moderately severe hydrocephalus. The walls of the aneurysm return low signal due to calcification and the lumen is virtually filled (at this level) by laminated thrombus of heterogeneous signal

ness and composed of collagen with few cells. In places the wall may be infiltrated by inflammatory cells with red cells and haemosiderin [32]. Thinning of the wall, presumably secondary to mechanical pressures determined by local blood flow dynamics, is usual at the fundus, the most common site of rupture [30].

The site of acute rupture may be identified by the presence of a lobule or nipple shaped protuberance at or near the fundus on angiograms (Fig. 1.6). This may subsequently thrombose or act as a focus for growth. The absence of an aneurysm wall, since the acute defect is closed by clot, lead Stehbens to describe this situation as a "false" aneurysm [124]. He considered that tearing of the wall, whether this resulted in mild leakage or serious haemorrhage, was the most likely cause of mural thrombosis within the aneurysm sac. The formation of fibrin from the clot and its subsequent organisation into the sac wall may cause small aneurysms to enlarge [127]. The histological finding of haemosiderin laden macrophages within the wall suggests that mural haemorrhage, with or without rupture, is part of the process of wall thickening associated with growth. Enlargement of the sac is probably due to a cycle of wall thinning, injury and repair, although the factor or factors that initiate and sustain the cycle are less well defined (Fig. 1.4).

In large and giant aneurysms layers of fibrous tissue, patches of haemosiderin and cholesterol deposits and foci of calcification thicken the wall (Fig. 1.7). Such changes may be the result of mural damage or the formation of intra-luminal thrombosis. The latter, frequently found in giant aneurysms, is caused by the slower circulation of blood within large aneurysms. Its subsequent organisation results in a wall thickened by laminated thrombi which may reduce the risk of rupture but provides a soft lining into which endosaccular coils tend to migrate.

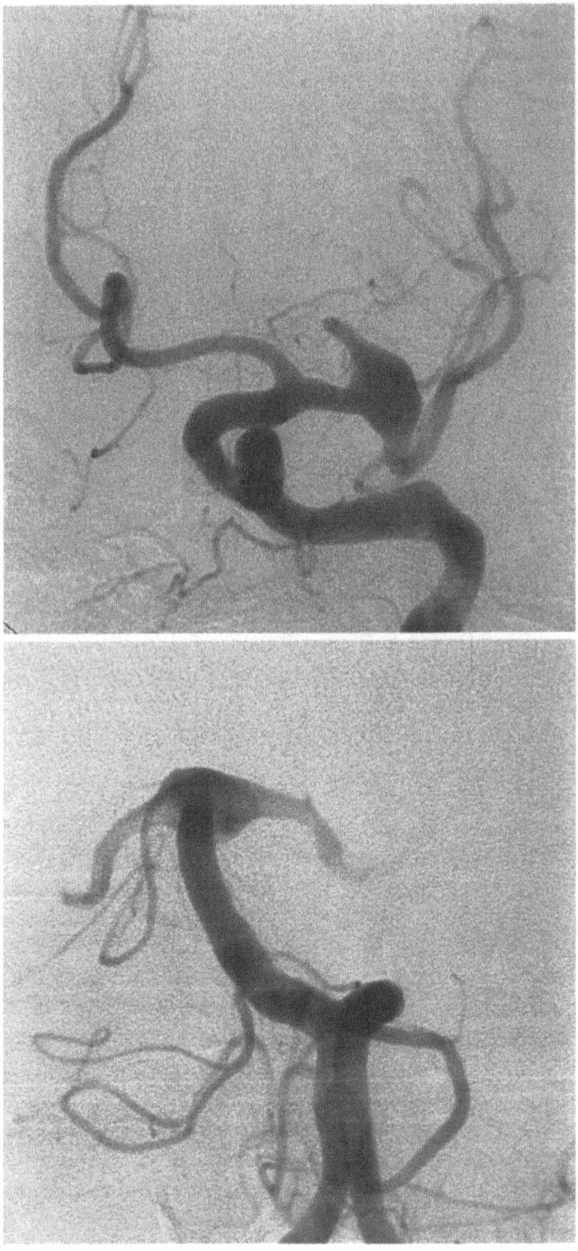

Fig. 1.8.
a Carotid and **b** vertebral intra-arterial digital subtraction angiograms. **a** The middle cerebral artery bifurcation and **b** the basilar artery termination are ectactic and dilated. Elsewhere mural irregularity is present due to extensive atherosclerosis

1.4.2 Non-saccular Aneurysms

Fusiform aneurysms are most commonly the result of arterial enlargement due to severe atheroma but may result from focal arterial injury. Ectatic dilatation of larger intradural arteries is caused by loss of normal mural elasticity (Fig. 1.8). The vertebral, basilar and internal carotid arteries are most commonly affected [4, 86, 146]. The progression from ectatic artery to fusiform aneurysm is presumably initiated by degeneration of the wall and exacerbated by pulsatile blood flow. In addition, intra-luminal thrombosis may develop secondary to slowed blood flow within parts of the resulting tortuous channel. Intimal haemorrhage may also occur, compounding the loss of normal wall structure and possibly causing dissection (see Sect. 1.4.4).

They affect men more commonly than women and occur in middle and old age [52]. They vary in shape from a simple fusiform pattern to complicated distortions of the parent artery (Fig. 1.9). In the former the aneurysm clearly separates blood in-flow and out-flow, whereas arterial ectasia in the latter type may result in the proximal and distal portion of the parent artery lying close together and simulating a saccular lumen.

Microscopic Anatomy. Histological examination shows fibrosis of the elastic membrane with hyaline degeneration, and deposition of cholesterol, inflammatory cells and intimal haemorrhage in the wall and intra-luminal thrombosis [117]. Rarely, fusiform aneurysms may occur in children and young adults in whom the underlying pathology is often uncertain. In this situation, histological examination has demonstrated loss of the internal elastic and medial muscle layers without degenerative feature [104].

1.4.3 Traumatic Intracranial Aneurysms

Traumatic intracranial aneurysms may be true, false or mixed types of aneurysms depending on the extent of wall injury. If all the wall layers are breached there is, at least initially, no arterial wall to the sac resulting in a false aneurysm. If the adventitia is preserved and the other layers breached a true or dissecting aneurysm may form. The common feature, however, is that the artery is not completely severed since that would cause the two ends to retract and clot. They are rare lesions; in 1983, Fox [46] reviewed the world literature and found only 232 reported cases. He found that 75% of cases occurred after closed head injury, 14% after penetrating trauma and 11% after craniotomy and transphenoidal or other paranasal sinus surgical procedures. They principally involve longitudinal sections of larger arteries but may rarely occur on small peripheral arteries [26]. The petrous and cavernous portions of the internal carotid artery are at risk when fractures involve the skull base because of their fixed positions and the anterior cerebral artery (ACA) from acceleration/ deceleration forces because of its proximity to the falx. Traumatic aneurysms caused by penetrating head injury should

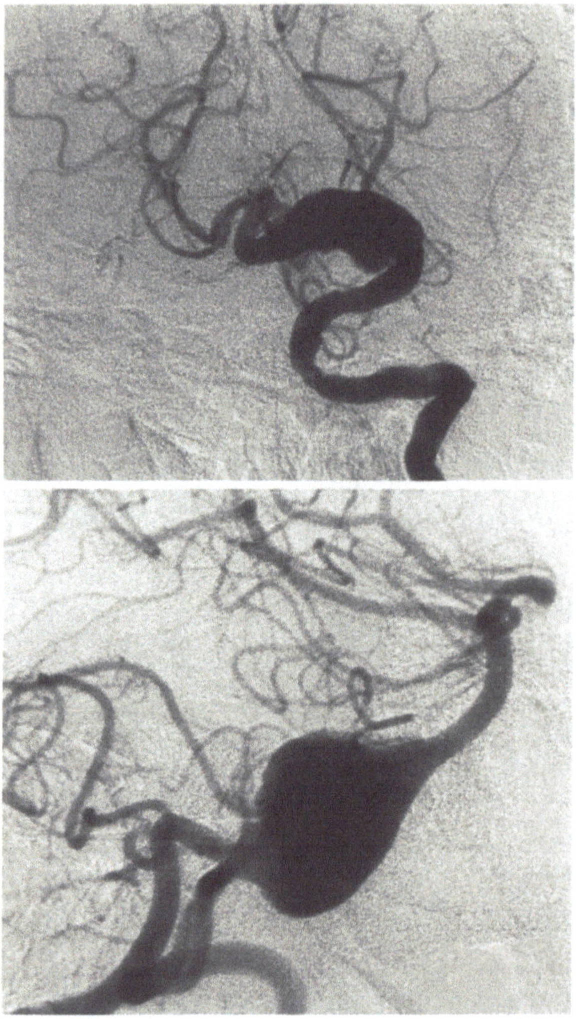

Fig. 1.9 a, b.
Fusiform aneurysms of the basilar artery. **a** The trunk is distorted and enlarged (dolichoectactic) due to atheroma. The proximal artery is also diseased. **b** Isolated fusiform aneurysm of the proximal basilar artery in a young man, without evidence of atherosclerosis. One vertebral artery has a duplicated distal segment

be distinguished from shear injury [1]. Haddad et al. [55] found 30 cases of traumatic intracranial aneurysms caused by missiles in the world literature and added 15 of their own. Their cases were overwhelming due to shrapnel and involved the middle cerebral artery (MCA). Most traumatic aneurysms caused by penetrating or non-penetrating injury are supratentorial, although posterior fossa aneurysms have been described [84]. The natural history is unpredictable; they may rupture, enlarge or thrombose spontaneously and it is well recognised that they may not be evident on initial angiography.

Microscopic Anatomy. The microscopic findings are variable. Partial breakdown within peri-arterial haematoma forms the lumen and the formation of a fibrin wall creates the aneurysm. The histological findings are therefore similar to those at the rupture point of a saccular aneurysm. Incomplete disruption of the arterial wall with some layers surviving may result in a saccular aneurysm of mixed true and false types [102]. The absence of a supporting wall in false aneurysms is a contra-indication to endovascular treatment by endosaccular packing and their management often requires occlusion of the parent artery.

1.4.4 Dissecting Intracranial Aneurysms

Arterial dissection is characterised by penetration of circulating blood into the substance of the wall and its subsequent extension, for a varying distance, between the layers of the wall. Dissection may cause cerebral ischaemia when extradural or intradural cranial arteries are affected. It occurs more commonly in extradural arteries, either spontaneously or following trauma. Closed or penetrating injuries can cause dissection and direct carotid puncture for angiography was, in the past, the commonest cause of iatrogenic trauma [29]. Intradural dissections are rare; Stehbens [46] reviewed 55 cases in which the mean age was 27 years, two thirds of the patients were men and 40% of the dissections involved the MCA, 23% vertebro-basilar arteries and 13% the ACA. The cause was usually unknown though trauma was a factor in 34% and arteritis in 10%.

Dissection of intradural arteries occurs deep to the internal elastic layer rather than in the external portion of the media or between media and adventitia, as is usual in extradural arteries [119], presumably because of the different wall structure or possibly because atheromatous degeneration implicated in extradural arterial dissections occurs in the medial layer [100]. The torn intima may act as an obstructing flap and occlude the true lumen or a distal tear allow re-entry to the true lumen and re-establish flow. Rarely, the dissecting channel penetrates the adventitia causing SAH [2]. Dissections may cause sudden death and are associated with mortality rates of over 50% [90]; if the patient survives the findings at angiography are variable. The lumen is generally narrowed but may taper to complete occlusion or narrow and then dilate in sequence resulting in angiographic appearances with a variety of descriptions, e.g. string sign or pearl and string sign. Macroscopically the vessel is dilated and distended with clot, something angiography underestimates and planar scanning, in particular magnetic resonance imaging (MRI), is often best at imaging.

Microscopic Anatomy. On microscopy the tear usually involves the majority of the vessel circumference. The over-lying intima is thickened and convoluted with thrombus in the false lumen. Acutely thrombus will be present in the true lumen if the artery has occluded and is often evident in distal arteries either in continuity or following embolism.

Surgical treatment is based on the principle that isolation of the involved segment will prevent distal progression of the lesion and wall rupture. Anticoagulants are generally not employed because of the risk of SAH [2, 16].

Endovascular parent artery occlusion may be possible in the proximal circulation, alone or combined with surgical trapping, but is more difficult in the circulation distal to the circle of Willis. Preliminary balloon occlusion tests may also be employed to assess the consequences of arterial occlusion and the need for collateral support by surgical by-pass.

1.4.5
Infectious Intracranial Aneurysms

Infectious intracranial aneurysms has replaced the term "mycotic" aneurysms, since most of these lesions are caused by non-fungal arteritis. Furthermore the term "mycotic", which is ascribed to Osler and has been used for any intracranial aneurysms with an infectious aetiology, was not used by him to describe intracranial aneurysms; he used it in regard to debris found in an aortic arch aneurysm [96]. Possible causes can be separated into three groups: (1) septic emboli classically associated with bacterial endocarditis, (2) fungal and other non-bacterial infections, possibly associated with an impaired immune system and (3) extension of an extravascular infection such as meningitis, osteomyelitis, paranasal sinusitis or cavernous sinus thrombophlebitis.

Estimates of the prevalence of aneurysms in patients with bacterial endocarditis range from 4% to 15% [67] with 18% having multiple aneurysms [20] (Fig. 1.10). Stehbens (see p 357 in [124]) reviewed 133 bacterial aneurysms and found that the majority involved arteries distal to the circle of Willis and that the commonest site was peripheral branches of the MCA (47% of all aneurysms). The finding of aneurysms distal to the circle of Willis should raise the possibility of bacterial endocarditis even in the absence of a cardiac murmur [107]. Infectious aneurysms due to causes other than endocarditis, e.g. local extravascular sepsis or fungal infections, are more often sited proximally [12]. The high mortality associated with bacterial infectious aneurysms was emphasised by Bohmfalk et al. [20] who collected 85 cases and reported mortality rates of 30% without rupture and 80% following rupture. The situation is even more dire for aneurysms due to fungal infection, with 100% mortality amongst the three patients reported by Barrow and Prats [12]. Furthermore, these authors could find no reports in the literature of any patients surviving such lesions. In bacterial infections, the responsible organism is most commonly a species of *Streptococcus* or *Staphylococcus*, and for fungal aneurysms species of *Aspergillus*, *Candida* and *Phycomycetes*, although aneurysms associated with other types of bacteria, fungi, and amoebae have been reported.

The pathogenesis of infectious aneurysms is via two routes. In patients with bacterial endocarditis and after intravenous drug abuse, septic emboli are assumed to impact in end-arteries or at arterial branch point where they initiate a local arteritis and transient thrombosis of the artery. Alternatively, the inflammatory process affects the adventitia first, as occurs in cavernous sinus thrombophlebitis and other extra-vascular sepsis, as well as experimen-

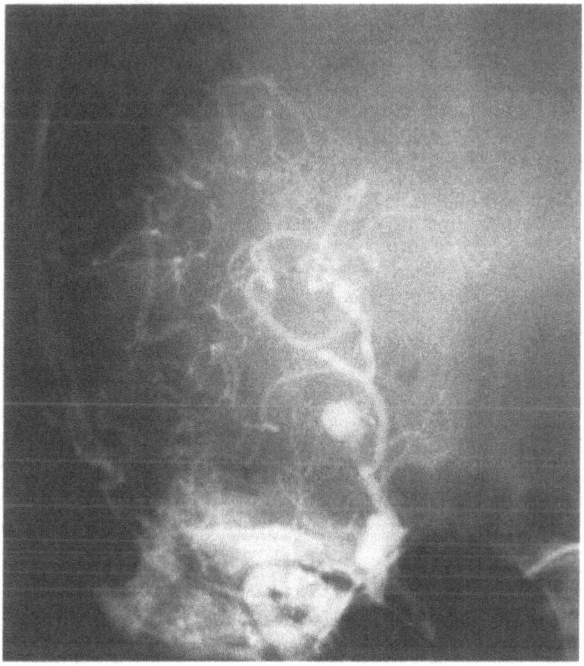

Fig. 1.10.
Infective aneurysm. Frontal carotid angiogram of an aneurysm of the terminal portion of the internal carotid artery with focal stenosis of the adjacent middle and anterior cerebral arteries. This patient presented with subacute bacterial endocarditis; blood cultures were positive for *Staphylococcus*

tal aneurysms induced by adventitial infection [82]. Either way, the end result is an arteritis which damages and weakens the wall (Fig. 1.11).

Microscopic Anatomy. Histological examination shows changes of an acute and severe arteritis with subendothelial exudate and destruction of the normal wall architecture. In the sac wall remnants of media and internal elastic lamina may be found with polymorpholeukocytes and colonies of bacteria. Subacute changes exhibit evidence of healing by the formation of intimal loose connective tissue and spindle cells with an infiltration of inflammatory cells [124]. The characteristic findings are therefore loss of elastic tissue and the presence of an acute inflammatory response.

Management of patients with infectious aneurysms depends on identification and management of the underlying cause and treatment with the appropriate antibiotics. Although only 5% of patients with bacterial endocarditis suffer intracranial haemorrhages and only a small proportion will be due to aneurysms [57], diagnosis of the latter requires careful consideration of additional surgical treatment because of the high mortality associated with rupture [20]. Resolution of infectious aneurysms on antibiotic treatment is well recognised, although they have been reported to occur even after successful treatment of endocarditis [9]. When diagnosed without rupture, appropriate antibiotic treatment is imperative with frequent interval angiography to assess response if conservative management is pursued. As the aneurysm is often inaccessible and the sac friable and difficult to clip, surgery has been reserved for ruptured and enlarging aneurysms [60]. Endovascular treatment

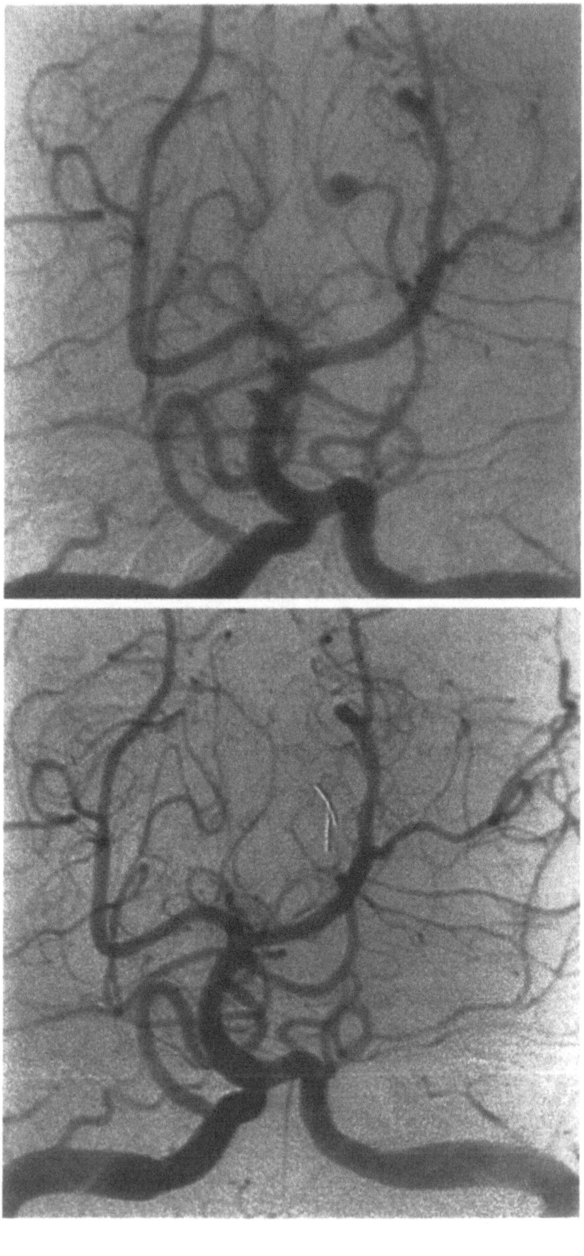

Fig. 1.11a, b.
Distal aneurysm of the superior cerebellar artery associated with intravenous drug abuse. Vertebral intra-arterial digital subtraction angiograms of a small saccular aneurysm before (**a**) and after (**b**) endovascular occlusion of the superior cerebellar artery using thrombogenic (fibre) coils. This patient presented following spontaneous intracranial haemorrhage with predominantly subarachnoid haemorrhage

now offers a simpler method of treating peripheral aneurysms by parent artery occlusion with cyanoacrylate [116]. Endosaccular packing with coils is probably not advisable with septicaemia, but coils have been used to perform parent artery occlusions after active infection has been excluded.

1.4.6 Neoplastic Aneurysms

Very rarely aneurysms develop because of arterial wall invasion by tumour emboli. The commonest cause of this lesion is cardiac myxoma, because this tumour usually involves the left atrium and embolises to cranial arteries. Branches of the MCA are the commonest vessel to be affected and multiple and bilateral lesions are described. Tumour deposits invade the wall causing fusiform or lobulated aneurysms arising in terminal branch arteries, frequently at or near bifurcations [124]. Choriocarcinoma metastases may also invade intracranial arteries, penetrating and disrupting the internal elastic lamina and media; this tumour may cause the vessel to rupture or occlude [141].

Microscopic Anatomy. Macroscopically aneurysms due to cardiac myxoma are small grey-white arterial swellings, less than 5 mm in size, but lesions of up to 25 mm have been recorded [92]. Microscopic examination shows myxoma deposits in wall and lumen, which are responsible for the angiographic findings in this condition of vessel dilatation, narrowing or even occlusion. At sites of aneurysmal dilation the wall is thickened by tumour deposits with loss of its normal structure [25].

Resection of tumour aneurysms has been performed with little success [22] and endovascular therapy has no current role except possibly to deliver experimental chemotherapeutic agents.

1.5 Natural History

Since most aneurysms are diagnosed after rupture our understanding of the natural history of these lesions is largely based on studies conducted in patients following subarachnoid haemorrhage. The incidence of subarachnoid haemorrhage and the associated clinical features will be discussed in Chap. 2, but it is worth considering some features here because they are relevant to our understanding of the aetiology of intracranial aneurysms.
Aneurysms occur in all racial groups. The prevalence is slightly higher in Caucasian than African Americans [79, 94, 133]; Taylor et al. [133] found rates of unruptured aneurysms of 60.3 per 100000 for Caucasians versus 51.8 per 100000 for African Americans in a population of elderly patients. However, national variations in reporting, given the current worldwide disparities in health care, are of uncertain value. Aneurysmal SAH is rare in children

and its frequency increases with age. In the cooperative study, only seven of 2627 patients were under 10 years [75]. Stebhens (see p 357 in [124]) reviewed eight reports, including the cooperative study [75], and found only 6.6% of patients were under 30 years and 1.9% under 20 years. Pakarinen [97] found the incidence peaked in the sixth decade and Fox [46] in the fifth decade. The annual incidence determined by Philips et al. [99] was less than 1 per 100000 of the population under 25 years and 40 per 100000 over 75 years. Overall aneurysms are more common in women; the male to female ratio is 1:1.5 [72]. This female preponderance is not apparent until the fifth decade [105]. There is a modest increased frequency in males up to about 40 years [36, 75].

The prevalence of intracranial aneurysms amongst the general population is difficult to assess since no non-invasive means of diagnosis has been available in the past. Estimates of the prevalence of unruptured cerebral aneurysm made from autopsy studies range from 0.8% to 8.1% of the population [27, 62, 77–79, 121, 126]. However, autopsy populations are to a greater or lesser extent selected and unlikely to reproduce the entire population at risk. In addition, there is an element of subjectivity about what constitutes an aneurysm and how diligently they are sought. These problems are exemplified by Hassler [59], who reported an incidence of 17% but included aneurysms as small as 2 mm (which others presumably ignore) and excluded subjects under 30 years. The largest series was described by Jellinger [66] and included data from 87772 autopsies. He reported a prevalence of 1.6% [66]. Bannerman et al. also reviewed a large series, collecting 51360 cases, and reported a prevalence of 1.43%, of which 0.34% were ruptured and 1.09% unruptured [10]. Their findings were quoted by Weir [142], who, summarising the available data, wrote: "less than 2% of the entire population will have an aneurysm; such an intracranial aneurysm will rupture in less than 1% of the population and will be the cause of death in 0.5%."

The prevalence estimated from angiographic studies range from 0.2% to 6.5% [7, 36, 63, 64, 89, 139], but the figures are subject to shortcomings similar to those of autopsy studies. The highest rate was reported by Nakagawa et al. [89] who performed cerebral angiograms in 400 volunteers and found 27 (6.75%) asymptomatic unruptured aneurysms measuring 5–15 mm. However, many of the volunteers gave histories of headache or a family history of subarachnoid haemorrhage. Improvements in magnetic resonance angiography (MRA) techniques may provide more data about aneurysm prevalence since there is little doubt that unruptured aneurysms are currently underdiagnosed in vivo. Taylor et al. [133] calculated from the medical records of hospitalised patients over 65 years of age that unruptured aneurysms were diagnosed in only 58.4 per 100000 of this population in the U.S.A.

The above data suggest that that only a proportion of intracranial aneurysms, perhaps a third, rupture and are diagnosed in life. This estimate is based on the following calculation: if the prevalence of unruptured aneurysms is 1.6% at autopsy and the incidence of aneurysmal subarachnoid haemorrhage is 13 per 100000 per annum and allowing 30 years for an aneurysm to develop and rupture then 0.39% is the prevalence (i.e. 30×13 per 100000 or 390 per 100000). This estimate is supported by the finding of

Table 1.2. Observation studies of unruptured intracranial aneurysms

Reference	Patients (*n*)	Aneurysms (*n*)	Age Mean	Age Range	Follow-up (years)	Annual rupture rate (%)
Graf 1971 [53]	52	–	–	–	5	0.8
Weibers et al. 1981 [140]	65	81	54.4	17–79	8.2	1 .2
Winn et al. 1983 [144]	38	–	47	–	10	1.0–2.2
Rosenørn et al. 1986 [108]	40	54	–	–	8	1.6–2.8
Weibers et al. 1987 [143]	130	161	56.2	17–79	8.3	1.1
Eskesen et al. 1987 [38]	48	53	–	–	2	4
Juvela et al. 1993 [68]	142	181	41.9	15–61	13.7	1.4
Asari et al. 1993 [6]	54	72	60.5	34–74	3.6	1.92

McCormick and Acosta-Rua [78] who found that 40% of the aneurysms in their study of 178 autopsies, had ruptured.

There have been several observational studies of patients with unruptured aneurysms (Table 1.2). Jane et al. [65] estimated the risk of rupture in unruptured aneurysms discovered incidentally or coincidental to a ruptured aneurysm in patients with multiple aneurysms, to be 1% per annum. Amongst the eight series listed in Table 1.2 the annual rupture rate ranges from 0.8% to 4%. There have been several attempts to identify features of the patients and aneurysms which correlate with subsequent rupture. Asari and Ohmoto [6] followed 54 patients with 72 aneurysms and found hypertension, aneurysm shape and location were risk factors. The features of aneurysms associated with rupture were lobulated shapes and vertebro-basilar locations, whereas Juvela et al. [68] and Weibers et al. [143], who followed 142 and 130 patients respectively, found only aneurysm size to be relevant. In the report by Wiebers et al., none of the aneurysms under 10 mm in size ruptured and they suggested that, although rupture probably occurs after a period of rapid expansion, a small but stable aneurysm has a lower chance of rupture. Contrary to a widely held view that larger aneurysms (because of thick walls) are less likely to rupture, Juvelta et al. [68] concluded that a size limit with a negligible potential for rupture could not be established. The annual risk of rupture of a previously unruptured aneurysm is about 1%–2%. This compares with rerupture rates of up to 30% in the first 3 weeks after aneurysmal subarachnoid haemorrhage, falling to 3% per annum after 6 months [68].

References

1. Achram M, Rizk G, Haddad FS (1980) Angiographic aspects of traumatic intracranial aneurysms following war injuries. Br J Radiol 53:1144–1149
2. Adams HP, Aschenbrener CA, Kassell NF et al (1982) Intracranial hemorrhage produced by spontaneous dissecting intracranial aneurysms. Arch Neurol 39:773–775
3. Ambrose J (1973) Computerised transaxial scanning (tomography) II Clinical application. Br J Radiol 46:1023–1047
4. Anson JA, Lawton MT, Spetzler RF (1996) Characteristics and surgical treatment of dolichoectatic and fusiform aneurysm. J Neurosurg 84:185–193

5. Aoki N, Mizutani H (1984) Does moyamoya disease cause subarachnoid hemorrhage: review of 54 cases with intracranial hemorrhage confirmed by computerized tomography. J Neurosurg 60:348–353
6. Asari S, Ohmoto T (1993) Natural history and risk factors of unruptured cerebral aneurysm. Clin Neurol Neurosurg. 95:205–214
7. Atkinson JLD, Sundt TM Jr, Houser OW et al (1989) Angiographic frequency of anterior circulation intracranial aneurysms. J Neurosurg 70:551–555
8. Azzam CJ (1987) Growth of multiple peripheral high flow aneurysms of the posterior inferior cerebellar artery associated with a cerebellar arteriovenous malformation. Neurosurgery 21:934–939
9. Bamford J, Hodges J, Warlow C (1986) Late rupture of a mycotic aneurysm after "cure" of bacterial endocarditis. J Neurol 233:51–53
10. Bannerman RM, Ingall GB, Graf CJ (1970) The familial occurrence of intracranial aneurysms. Neurology 20:283–292
11. Barnes MJ (1985) Collagens in atherosclerosis. Coll Relat Res 5:65–97
12. Barrow DL, Prats AR (1990) Infectious intracranial aneurysms: comparison of groups with and without endocarditis. Neurosurgery 27:562–572
13. Bartholow R (1872) Aneurisms of the arteries at the base of the brain: their symptomatology, diagnosis and treatment. Am J Med Sci 64:373
14. Batjer H, Suss RA, Samson D (1986) Intracranial arteriovenous malformations associated with aneurysms. Neurosurgery 18:29–35
15. Beadles CF (1907) Aneurisms of the larger cerebral arteries. Brain 30:285
16. Berger MS, Wilson CB (1984) Intracranial dissecting aneurysms of the posterior circulation. J Neurosurg 61:882–894
17. Bigelow NH (1953) The association of polycystic kigney with intracranial aneurysms and other related disorders. Am J Med Sci 225:485
18. Biumi F (1778) Observations antomicae. Observatio V. In: Sandifort E (ed) Thesaurus dessertatiorum, vol 3. Milan, S&J Luchmans (reprinted 1778), pp 373–379
19. Blackhall L (1813) Observations on the nature and cure of dropsies. Longman, London, p 126
20. Bohmfalk GL, Story JL, Wissinger JP, Brown WE (1978) Bacterial intracranial aneurysm. J Neurosurg 48:369–382
21. Bramwell B (1886) Clinical and pathological memoranda illustrated. Edinb Med J 32(2):97–108
22. Branch CL, Laster DW, Kelly DL (1985) Left atrial myxoma with cerebral emboli. Neurosurgery 16:675–680
23. Bremer JL (1943) Congenital aneurysms of the cerebral arteries. Arch Pathol 35:819–831
24. Brinton W (1850/1851) Report on cases of cerebral aneurysms. Trans Pathol Soc Lond 3:47–49
25. Burton C, Johnston J (1970) Multiple cerebral aneurysms and cardiac myxoma. N Engl J Med 282:35–36
26. Burton C, Velasco F, Dorman J (1968) Traumatic aneurysm of a peripheral cerebral artery. Review and case report. J Neurosurg 28:468–474
27. Cohen MM (1955) Cerebrovascular accidents. A study of two hundred one cases. Arch Pathol 60:296–307
28. Collier J (1931) Cerebral haemorrhage due to other causes than arteriosclerosis. Br Med J 2:519
29. Crawford T (1956) The pathological effects of cerebral arteriography. J Neurol Neurosurg Psychiatry 19:217
30. Crompton MR (1966) Mechanism of growth and rupture in cerebral berry aneurysms. Br Med J 1:1138–1142
31. Crompton MR (1966) The comparative pathology of cerebral aneurysms. Brain 89:789–796
32. Crompton MR (1966) The pathogenesis of cerebral aneurysms. Brain 89:797–814
33. Cronqvist S, Troupp H (1966) Intracranial arteriovenous malformation and arterial aneurysms in the same patient. Arch Neurol Scand 42:307–316
34. Dixon JM (1951) Angioid streaks and pseudoxanthoma elasticum with aneurysm of the internal carotid artery. Am J Ophthalmol 34:1322–1323
35. Drake CG (1979) The treatment of aneurysms of the posterior circulation. Clin Neurosurg 26:96–144
36. Du Boulay GH (1965) Some observations on the natural history of intracranial aneurysms. Br J Radiol 38:721–757

37. Eppinger H (1887) Pathogenesis (Histogenesis und Aetiologie) der Aneurysmen einschliesslich des Aneurysma equi verminosum. Arch Klin Chir 35 [Suppl]:1–563
38. Eskesen V, Rosenøren J, Schmidt K et al (1987) Clinical features and outcome in 48 patients with unruptured intracranial saccular aneurysms: a prospective consecutive study. Br J Neurosurg 1:47–52
39. Evans TW, Venning MC, Strang FA et al (1981) Dominant inheritance of intracranial berry aneurysm. Br Med J 283:824–825
40. Fearnsides EG (1916) Intracranial aneurysms. Brain 39:224
41. Ferguson GG (1970) Turbulence in human intracranial saccular aneurysms. J Neurosurg 33:485–497
42. Ferguson GG (1972) Physical factors in the initiation, growth, and rupture of human intracranial saccular aneurysms. J Neurosurg 37:666–677
43. Finney HL, Roberts TS, Anderson RE (1976) Giant intracranial aneurysm associated with Marfan's syndrome. Case report. J Neurosurg 45:342–347
44. Forbus WD (1930) On the origin of miliary aneurysms of the superficial cerebral arteries. Johns Hopkins Hosp Bull 47:239
45. Forster FM, Alpers BJ (1945) Anatomical defects and pathological changes in congenital cerebral aneurysms. J Neuropathol Exp Neurol 4:146–154
46. Fox JL (1983) Intracranial aneurysms, vol 1. Springer, Berlin Heidelberg New York
47. Fox JL (1991) Concurrent intracranial aneurysm and arteriovenous malformation. In: Wilkins RH, Rengachary SS (eds) Neurosurgery update II. McGraw-Hill, New York, pp 126–128
48. Frens DB, Petajan JH, Anderson R, Deblanc HJ (1974) Fibromuscular dysplasia of the posterior cerebral artery: report of a case and review of the literature. Stroke 5:161–166
49. Froin G (1904) Les hémorrhagies sous-arachnoidiennes et le mécanisme de l'hématolyse en général. Thèse de Paris. Steinher, Paris
50. George AE, Lin JP, Morantz RA (1971) Intracranial aneurysms on a persistent primitive trigeminal artery: case report. J Neurosurg 35:601–604
51. Glynn LE (1940) Medial defects in the circle of Willis and their relation to aneurysm formation. J Pathol Bacteriol 51:213–222
52. Goldstein SJ, Tibbs PA (1981) Recurrent subarachnoid hemorrhage complicating cerebral arterial ectasia: case report. J Neurosurg 55:139–142
53. Graf C (1971) Prognosis for patients with non-surgically treated aneurysms. Analysis of the co-operative study of intracranial aneurysms and subarachnoid hemorrhage. J Neurosurg 35:438–443
54. Gull W (1859) Cases of aneurism of the cerebral vessels. Guy's Hosp Rep 3rd Ser 5:281–304
55. Haddad FS, Haddad GF, Taha J (1991) Traumatic intracranial aneurysms caused by missiles: their presentation and management. Neurosurgery 28:1–7
56. Halal F, Mohr G, Toussi T et al (1983) Intracranial aneurysms: a report of a large pedigree. Am J Med Genet 15:89–95
57. Hart RG, Kagan-Hallet K, Joerns SE (1987) Mechanisms of intracranial hemorrhage in infective endocarditis. Stroke 18:1048–1056
58. Hashimoto I (1977) Familial intracranial aneurysms and cerebral vascular anomalies. J Neurosurg 46:419–427
59. Hassler O (1961) Morphological studies of the large cerebral arteries with reference to the aetiology of subarachnoid hemorrhage. Acta Psychiatr Neurol Scand 36 [Suppl 154]:1
60. Heros RC (1990) Comment. Neurosurgery 27:572–573
61. Hounsfield GN (1973) Computerised transverse axial scanning (tomography) I. Description of system. Br J Radiol 46:1016–1022
62. Inagawa T, Hirano A (1990) Autopsy study of unruptured incidental aneurysms. Surg Neurol 34:361–365
63. Iwata K, Misu N, Terada K et al (1991) Screening for unruptured asymptomatic intracranial aneurysms in patients undergoing coronary angiography. J Neurosurg 75:52–55
64. Jakubowski J, Kendall B (1978) Coincidental aneurysms with tumours of pituitary origin. J Neurol Neurosurg Psychiatry 41:972–979
65. Jane JA, Winn HR, Richardson AE (1977) The natural history of intracranial aneurysm. Rebleeding rate during the acute and long-tern period and implication for surgical management. Clin Neurosurg 24:176–184
66. Jellinger K (1979) Pathology and aetiology of intracranial aneurysms. In: Pia HW, Langmaid C, Zierski J (eds) Cerebral aneurysms: advances in diagnosis and therapy. Springer, Berlin Heidelberg New York, pp 5–19

67. Jones HR Jr, Siekert RG, Geraci JE (1969) Neurologic manifestations of bacterial endocarditis. Ann Intern Med 71:21–28
68. Juvela S, Porras M, Heiskanen O (1993) Natural history of unruptured intracranial aneurysms: a long-term follow-up study. J Neurosurg 79:174–182
69. Kayembe KNT, Sasahara M, Hazama F (1984) Cerebral aneurysms and variations in the circle of Willis. Stroke 15:846–850
70. Kodama N, Ohara H, Suzuki J (1976) Persistent hypoglossal artery associated with aneurysms: report of two cases. J Neurosurg 45:449–451
71. Kondziolka D, Nixon BJ, Lasjaunias P et al (1988) Cerebral arteriovenous malformations with associated arterial aneurysms: hemodynamic and therapeutic considerations. Can J Neurol Sci 15:130–134
72. Kongable GL, Lanzino G, Germanson TP et al (1996) Gender-related differences in aneurysmal subarachnoid haemorrhage. J Neurosurg 84:43–48
73. Kudo T (1968) Spontaneous occlusion of circle of Willis: disease apparently confined to Japanese. Neurology 18:485–496
74. Lie TA (1968) Congenital anomalies of the carotid arteries. Williams and Wilkins, Baltimore
75. Locksley HB (1966) Natural history of subarachnoid hemorrhage, intracranial aneurysms and arteriovenous malformations. Based on 6368 cases in the cooperative study. J Neurosurg 25:219–239
76. Lozano AM, Leblanc R (1987) Familial intracranial aneurysms. J Neurosurg 66: 522–528
77. McCormick WF (1978) The natural history of intracranial saccular aneurysms. Neurol Neurosurg 1:1–8
78. McCormick WF, Acosta-Rua GJ (1970) The size of intracranial saccular aneurysms. An autopsy study. J Neurosurg 33:422–427
79. McCormick WF, Nofzinger JD (1965) Saccular intracranial aneurysms. An autopsy study. J Neurosurg 22:155–159
80. Mettinger KL (1982) Fibromuscular dysplasia and the brain. II. Current concept of the disease. Stroke 13:53–58
81. Mettinger KL, Ericson K (1982) Fibromuscular dysplasia and the brain. I Observations on angiographic, clinical, and genetic characteristics. Stroke 13:46–52
82. Molinari GF, Smith L Goldstein MN et al (1973) Pathogenesis of cerebral mycotic aneurysms. Neurology 23:325–332
83. Moniz E (1927) L'encéphalographie arterielle, son importance dans la localisation des tumeurs cérébrales. Rev Neurol 2:72–90
84. Morard M, de Tribolet N (1991) Traumatic aneurysm of the posterior inferior cerebellar artery: case report. Neurosurgery 29:438–441
85. Morgagni JB (1769) De sedibus et causis morborum per anatomen indagatis, book 1, letter 4. Venetiis, ex typog. Remodiniana. [Translated by Alexander B (1960) The seats and causes of diseases investigated by anatomy. Hafner, New York, pp 42–43, 77–78.]
86. Moseley IF, Holland IM (1979) Ectasia of the basilar artery: the breadth of the clinical spectrum and the diagnostic value of computed tomography. Neuroradiology 18:83–91
87. Moyes PD (1969) Basilar aneurysm associated with agenesis of the left internal carotid artery: case report. J Neurosurg 30:608–611
88. Munyer TP, Margulis AR (1981) Pseudoxanthoma elasticum with internal carotid artery aneurysm. AJR 136:1023–1024
89. Nakagawa T, Hashi K (1994) The incidence and treatment of asymptomatic, unruptured cerebral aneurysms. J Neurosurg 88: 217–223
90. Nass R, Hays A, Chutorian A (1982) Intracranial dissecting aneurysms in childhood. Stroke 13:204–207
91. Neil-Dwyer G, Bartlett JR, Nicholls AC et al (1983) Collagen deficiency and ruptured cerebral aneurysms: a clinical and biochemical study. J Neurosurg 59:16–19
92. New PFJ, Price DL, Carter B (1970) Cerebral angiography in cardiac myxoma. Correlation of angiographic and histopathological findings. Radiology 96:335–345
93. Northfield DWC (1973) The surgery of the central nervous system. Blackwells Scientific, Oxford, pp 346–401
94. Ohaegbulam SC, Dujovny M, Ausman JI et al (1990) Ethnic distribution of intracranial aneurysms. Acta Neurochir (Wien) 106:132–135
95. Okamoto S, Handa H, Hashimoto N (1984) Location of intracranial aneurysms associated with cerebral arteriovenous malformation: statistical analysis. Surg Neurol 22: 335–340
96. Osler W (1885) Gulstonian lectures on malignant endocarditis. Lancet 1:415–418

97. Pakarinen S (1967) Incidence, aetiology and prognosis of primary subarachnoid haemorrhage. Acta Neurol Scand [Suppl] 29:1–128
98. Paterson JH, McKissock WA (1956) A clinical survey of intracranial angiomas with special reference to their mode of progression and surgical treatment: a report of 110 cases. Brain 70:233–266
99. Philips LH, Whisnant JP, O'Fallon WM, Sundt TM Jr (1980) The unchanging pattern of subarachnoid hemorrhage in a community. Neurology 30:1034–1040
100. Pilz P, Hartjes HJ (1976) Fibromuscular dysplasia and multiple dissecting aneurysms of intracranial arteries. A further cause of moyamoya syndrome. Stroke 7:393–398
101. Pope FM, Nicholls AC, Narcisi P et al (1981) Some patients with cerebral aneurysms are deficient in type III collagen. Lancet 1:973–975
102. Pozzati E, Gaist G, Servadei F (1982) Traumatic aneurysms of the supraclinoid internal carotid artery: report of two cases. J Neurosurg 57:418–422
103. Quincke H (1891) Die Lumbarpunction des Hydrocephalus. Berl Klin Wochenschr 28:929–965
104. Read D, Esiri MM (1979) Fusiform basilar artery aneurysm in a child. Neurology 29:1045–1049
105. Redekop G, Ferguson G (1994) Intracranial aneurysms. In: Carter LH, Spetzler RI (eds) Neurovascular neurosurgery. McGraw-Hill, New York, pp 625–648
106. Roach MR (1963) Changes in arterial distensibility as a cause of post-stenotic dilation. Am J Cardiol 12:802
107. Roach MR, Drake CG (1965) Ruptured cerebral aneurysms caused by micro-organisms. N Engl J Med 273:240–244
108. Rosenørn J, Astrup J, Duel P et al (1986) Risko for blødning fra ikkerumperede intrakraniale sakkulate aneurysmer. Ugeskr Laeger 48:3363–3365
109. Rubinstein MK, Cohen NH (1964) Ehlers-Danlos syndrome associated with multiple intracranial aneurysms. Neurology 14:125–132
110. Sahs AL (1966) Observations on the pathology of saccular aneurysms. J Neurosurg 24:792–806
111. Sahs AL, Meyers R (1951) The coexistence of intracranial aneurysms and polycystic renal disease. Trans Am Neurol Assoc 76:147
112. Sahs AL, Perret GE, Locksley GB, Nishioka H (eds) (1969) Intracranial aneurysms and subarachnoid hemorrhage: a cooperative study. Lippincott, Philadelphia
113. Sakurai Y, Kowada M, Fukazawa H (1972) Agenesis of the internal carotid artery with an intracranial aneurysm: report of a case. Brain Nerve 24:1661
114. Salar G, Mingrino S (1977) Ligature of the cervical carotid artery for the treatment of intracranial carotid aneurysms: complications and late results. Acta Neurochir (Wien) 36:152
115. Schwartz MJ, Baronofsky ID (1960) Ruptured intracranial aneurysm associated with coarctation of the aorta. Am J Cardiol 6:983
116. Scotti G, Li MH, Righi C, Simionato F, Rocca A (1996) Endovascular treatment of bacterial intracranial aneurysms. Neuroradiology 38:186–189
117. Sengupta RP, McAllister VL (1986) Subarachnoid haemorrhage. Springer, Berlin Heidelberg New York, pp 46–53
118. Servo A (1977) Agenesis of the left internal carotid artery associated with an aneurysm on the right carotid syphon: case report. J Neurosurg 46:677–680
119. Sinclair W (1953) Dissecting aneurysm of the middle cerebral artery associated with migraine sydnrome. Am J Pathol 29:1083
120. Stehbens WE (1958) History of aneurysms. Med Hist 2:274
121. Stehbens WE (1963) Aneurysms and anatomical variation of cerebral arteries. Arch Pathol 75:45–64
122. Stehbens WE (1963) Cerebral aneurysms of animals other than man. J Pathol Bacteriol 86:161–168
123. Stehbens WE (1963) Histopathology of cerebral aneurysms. Arch Neurol 8:272
124. Stehbens WE (1972) Pathology of the cerebral blood vessels. Mosby, St Louis, pp356–357 and 446–449
125. Stehbens WE (1989) Etiology of intracranial berry aneurysms. J Neurosurg 70:823–831
126. Sugai M, Shoji M (1968) Pathogenesis of so-called congenital aneurysms of the brain. Acta Pathol 18:139–160
127. Suzuki J, Ohara H (1978) Clinicopathological study of cerebral aneurysms. Origins, rupture, repair and growth. J Neurosurg 48:505–514
128. Suzuki J, Onuma T (1979) Intracranial aneurysms associated with arteriovenous malformations. J Neurosurg 50:742–746

129. Symonds CP (1923) Contribution to the clinical study of intracranial aneurysm. Guy's Hosp Rep 4th Ser 73:139–158
130. Symonds CP (1924) Spontaneous subarachnoid haemorrhage. Q J Med 18:93
131. Takakura K, Saito I, Sasaki T (1991) Special problems associated with subarachnoid hemorrhage. In: Youmans JR (ed) Neurological surgery, vol 3, 3rd edn. Philadelphia, Saunders, pp 1864–1889
132. Tasker AD, Byrne JV (1997) Basilar artery fenestration in association with aneurysms of the posterior cerebral circulation. Neuroradiology 39:185–189
133. Taylor CL, Yuan Z, Selman WR et al (1995) Cerebral arterial aneurysm formation and rupture in 20767 elderley patients: hypertension and other risk factors. J Neurosurg 83:812–819
134. Ter Berg HWM, Bijlsma JB, Veiga Pires JA et al (1986) Familial association of intracranial aneurysms and multiple congenital anomalies. Arch Neurol 43:30–33
135. Turjman F, Massoud TF, Vinuela F et al (1994) Aneurysms related to cerebral arteriovenous malformations: superselective angiographic assessment in 58 patients. Am J Neuroradiol 15:1601–1605
136. Turnbull HM (1918) Intracranial aneurysms. Brain 41:50–56
137. Waga S, Tochio H (1985) Intracranial aneurysm associated with moyamoya disease in childhood. Surg Neurol 23:237–243
138. Wakabayashi T, Fujita S, Ohbora Y et al (1983) Polycystic kidney disease and intracranial aneurysms: early angiographic diagnosis and early operation for the unruptured aneurysm. J Neurosurg 58:488–491
139. Wakai S, Fukushima T, Furihata T et al (1979) Association of cerebral aneurysm with pituitary adenoma. Surg Neurol 12:503–507
140. Weibers DO, Whisnant JP, O'Fallon WM (1981) The natural history of unruptured intracranial aneurysms. N Engl J Med 304:696–698
141. Weir B, MacDonald N, Mielke B (1978) Intracranial vascular complications of choriocarcinoma. Neurosurgery 2:138–142
142. Weir BK (1985) Intracranial aneurysms and subarachnoid hemorrhage: an overview. In: Wilkins RH, Rengachary SS (eds) Neurosurgery. McGraw-Hill, New York, pp 1308–1329
143. Wiebers DO, Whisnant JP, Sundt TM Jr et al (1987) The significance of unruptured intracranial saccular aneurysms. J Neurosurg 6:23–29
144. Winn HR, Almaani WS, Berga SL et al (1983) The long-term outcome in patients with multiple aneurysms: incidence of late hemorrhage and implications for treatment of incidental aneurysms. J Neurosurg 59:642–651
145. Yasargil MG (1984) Microneurosurgery, vols 1 and 2. Thieme, Stuttgart
146. Yu YL, Moseley IF, Pullicino P et al (1982) The clinical picture of ectasia of the intracranial arteries. J Neurol Neurosurg Psychiatry 45:29–36
147. Zervas T, Liszizak TM, Mayberg MR et al (1982) Cerebrospinal fluid may nourish cerebral vessels through pathways in the adventitia that may be analagous to systemic vasa vasorum. J Neurosurg 56:475–481

CHAPTER 2

Symptomatology

2.1 Introduction

It is probable that a proportion of intracranial aneurysms are never discovered in life since, as discussed in Chap. 1, the prevalence at autopsy is considerably higher than the incidence of in vivo diagnosis. By far the commonest mode of presentation is spontaneous intracranial haemorrhage following aneurysm rupture. Less often, patients present with symptoms caused by pressure on local neural structures or ischaemia due to dissection or thromboembolism, the specific symptoms being determined by the site and size of the responsible aneurysm. Unruptured asymptomatic intracranial aneurysms are discovered either incidentally, i.e. during investigation of an unrelated condition, or coincidental to the diagnosis of a symptomatic aneurysm or aneurysms – the latter in patients with multiple aneurysm. This chapter will describe the clinical features of these three situations; namely ruptured, symptomatic unruptured and asymptomatic aneurysms. Asymptomatic aneurysms are generally termed incidental aneurysms whether they are solitary or not. Since the majority of patients present with spontaneous subarachnoid haemorrhage (SAH) much of this chapter will be devoted to considering the consequences of such bleeding.

2.2 Aneurysmal Subarachnoid Haemorrhage

Rupture of an intracranial aneurysm causes SAH with associated intracerebral haematoma in 20%, intraventricular haemorrhage in 20% and subdural haemorrhage in approximately 3% of patients [9, 99]. Extension of haemorrhage into the cerebral parenchyma or subdural space is the result of forceful bleeding causing disruption of the pia and arachnoid membranes. Intraventricular haemorrhage may be primary or secondary. The former because of direct bleeding into a ventricle and the latter via normal communications between the intraventricular and extraventricular subarachnoid spaces.

Spontaneous subarachnoid haemorrhage is due to aneurysm rupture in approximately 75% of patients. Aneurysms were discovered in 51% of 5836 SAH patients in the cooperative study performed in the 1960s [161], but angiographic diagnosis has since improved and aneurysms were found in

73.4% of the more recent Newcastle series [167]. Consequently, the incidence of normal angiography after SAH fell to 15%–20%; other vascular malformations were discovered in the remaining 6%–10% of patients.

The basal cerebral arteries are most vulnerable to aneurysm formation and rupture as they traverse the subarachnoid space. The space, lined by arachnoid and pia mater contains approximately 150 ml of cerebrospinal fluid (CSF), cranial nerves, arteries and veins, and fibrous bands between the meninges. In places, these fibrous bands or trabeculae, form sheets of connective tissue which separate the space, defining the supratentorial and infratentorial cisterns. The subarachnoid space extends into cerebral sulci and for a variable distance around those cerebral arteries and veins as they penetrate the cerebral substance. Cerebrospinal fluid percolates through the space, with the prevailing extraventricular flow from posterior fossa through the basal cisterns to parasagittal arachnoid villi. Haemorrhage into the subarachnoid space (Fig. 2.1) causes an immediate rise in the intracranial pressure because of the increased volume of CSF/blood within the space. Rises in intracranial pressure usually resolve rapidly within minutes or hours, but as with the severity of subsequent responses to SAH, the rate and completeness of recovery depend on how well blood is cleared from the space and whether CSF circulation and cerebral blood flow are disturbed in the process. The overall severity of the resulting illness thus depends to a large extent on the volume of haemorrhage.

2.2.1 Historical Background to the Diagnosis

The recognition of SAH as a clinical entity distinct from other types of cerebral haemorrhage and the understanding that in most patients it is due to intracranial aneurysm rupture gradually emerged in the literature of the last 200 years. Descriptions of apoplexy can be found in ancient medical and non-medical writings – a subject which has been extensively reviewed by Walton [203], who credited the first description of intracranial aneurysm as a cause for cerebral haemorrhage to Morgagni in *De sedibus et causis morborum per anatomen indagatis*, published in 1761 [131]. Walton considered the work to include the report of a patient with bilateral unruptured posterior communicating artery aneurysms (Book 1, Letter IV, Art. 19). However, Bull [20] concluded that Morgagni speculated rather than conclusively demonstrated that intracranial aneurysms existed and that only two autopsy descriptions of intracranial aneurysms were made in the whole of the eighteenth century, the first by Biumi in 1765 [11]. In *Observationes Anatomicae*, Biumi described the case of a woman who died in 1763 following rupture of what was probably an intracavernous aneurysm. The second report concerned the autopsy of a 65-year-old woman performed by John Hunter in 1792, at which he discovered bilateral parasellar aneurysms of the carotid arteries. This case was reported by Blane in 1800 [13].

The earliest clinical description of proven aneurysmal SAH was made in 1813 by Blackall [12]. He treated a 20-year-old woman who died several days

Fig. 2.1.
a Frontal intra-arterial digital subtraction angiography of the vertebral and basilar arteries. There is a bilobed aneurysm pointing laterally between the right posterior cerebral and superior cerebellar arteries. This patient was treated 3 days after presentation with subarachnoid haemorrhage and during coil embolisation the aneurysm has reruptured. **b** Contrast staining the subarachnoid space is evident, and the proximal portions of both posterior cerebral arteries (*arrows*) no longer fill due to acute vasospasm. Embolisation was completed and the patient survived to make a complete recovery

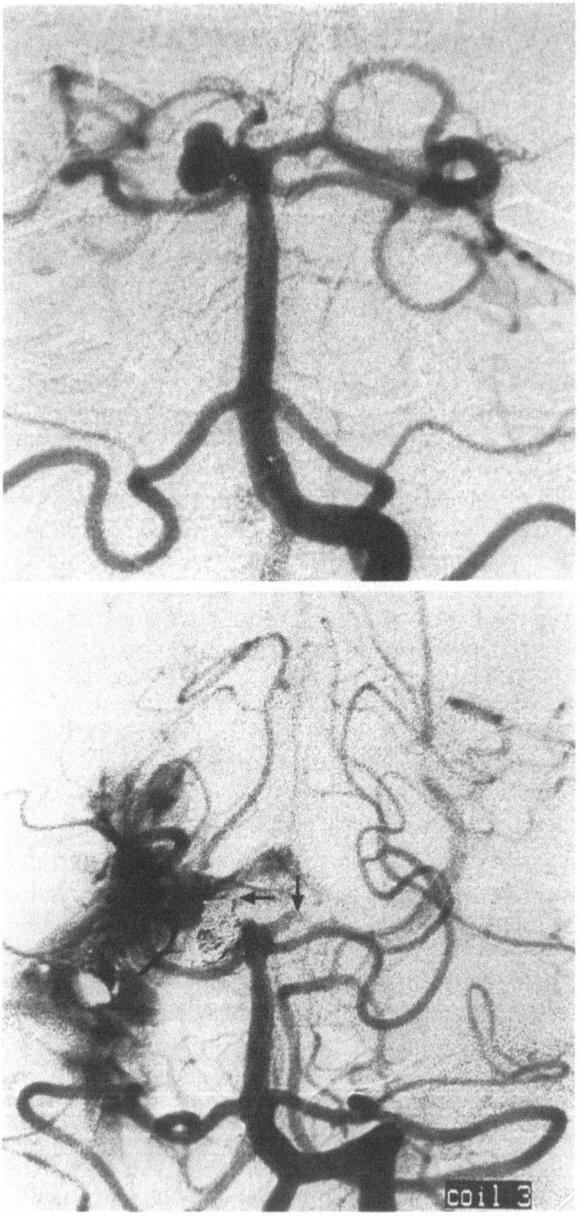

a

b

after the sudden onset of headache and vomiting which at post mortem examination was found to be due to rupture of a basilar artery aneurysm. During the nineteenth century there followed several case reports of patients presenting with spontaneous intracranial haemorrhage and aneurysms, but the causal link was not generally recognised. Brinton in 1850 [19] published a systematic study of 52 cases collected from the literature and Gull in 1859

[71] added 11 more cases. The latter stressed the importance of headache as a presenting symptom and that aneurysm rupture was the probable cause of apoplexy in young patients. This view was supported by Bramwell [17], Bartholomew [8] and Osler [142], but others, notably Gintac [62], Hayem [78] and Foin [60], appear to have regarded aetiologies such as intracranial infection, primary cerebral haemorrhage, sagittal sinus thrombosis and sunstroke to be equally important.

However by the end of the nineteenth century the clinical syndrome of SAH was well established; Quinke introduced the technique of lumbar puncture in 1891 [152] and Widal [210] and Froin [60] described the sequential changes that occur in CSF following SAH. Fearnside in 1916 [51] and Turnbull [195] 2 years later published descriptions of the effects of SAH. Fearnsides [51] described, in detail, the clinical effects of intracranial aneurysm rupture, but recognition of primary SAH as a clinical syndrome distinct from other causes of spontaneous intracranial haemorrhage was not generally made until the definitive papers by Collier [26] and Symonds [185, 186] between 1922 and 1924. Their descriptions of its clinical symptomatology have stood the test of time. Collier [26] described five types of presentation: apoplectic, meningitic, lumbarsacral, recurrent coma and migrainous. The following year Symonds published a series of five cases [185], and in 1924 [186] a detailed review of 124 cases collected from the literature, to which he added three cases of his own. He recognised that the commonest cause of primary SAH was rupture of an intracranial aneurysms and wrote: "the extravasation of any large quantity of blood into the subarachnoid space produces results which are in the main due to mechanical effects, but are partly derived from the inflammatory reaction which accompanies the presence of free blood in a serious cavity" [186]. He recognised that the consequences of aneurysm rupture were related to the amount of haemorrhage and that recurrent bleeding occurred in patients presenting with aneurysmal SAH.

The clinical syndromes associated with SAH were therefore recognised some time before reliable in vivo diagnosis or effective treatment of intracranial aneurysms was possible. In both respects, imaging has played a major role in the development of current patient management. Cerebral angiography and computerised tomography introduced in 1927 [129] and 1973 [85], respectively, have revolutionised our ability to diagnose SAH and its causes and complications. Intracranial aneurysms were first demonstrated in vivo by cerebral angiography in 1933 [39, 130] and post-SAH cerebral vasospasm first described in 1951 [47]. The contribution of imaging has been not only to identify structural vascular causes of spontaneous SAH, but also to distinguish complications such as ischaemia and rebleeding, which may not be possible on physical examination alone. Recent developments in imaging and treatment of SAH tend to obscure the diagnostic achievements of the past. Neuroradiological examinations can generally identify causes of haemorrhagic stroke and distinguish SAH from other forms of apoplexy. However, identifying patients with intracranial aneurysms before they rupture still represents a diagnostic challenge. Gull [71], commenting on the rarity of the clinical diagnosis of SAH in 1859, considered that it was probably due to careless enquiry about the nature of headache by examining physicians and wrote: "the eye can see only that it brings with it the aptitude to see."

2.2.2 Incidence

Estimates of the incidence of SAH are derived from epidemiological studies performed in defined geographical areas. They are generally considered to be underestimates because of incomplete ascertainment caused by failures to recognise SAH as the cause of atypical headache or non-traumatic sudden death. Several authors have noted that patients presenting with ruptured intracranial aneurysm have experienced previous atypical headaches, so-called warning leaks, prior to the event leading to diagnosis [110, 183]. It is therefore probable that some patients never experience haemorrhage severe enough for SAH to be diagnosed and their aneurysm is not identified. Gudmunnson found an annual incidence of 10 per 100000 in the urban and 6 per 100000 in the rural populations of Iceland. This difference he attributed to the greater availability of medical services to the urban patient, in whom correct diagnosis was more likely to be made. At the other extreme of the symptomatic spectrum, major haemorrhage may be rapidly fatal. Up to a third of patients die within hours of SAH, and some never reach hospital medical care. The cause of death may then be incorrectly attributed to a cardiac or other cerebrovascular catastrophe, particularly in older patients. In Kiyohara et al.'s [105] study, for example, 35% of patients died within 8 h of the onset of symptoms and none of these deaths were attributed to SAH prior to autopsy. In a larger Finnish prospective population study of stroke the age-adjusted annual mean incidences were 4.0 per 1000 for men and 3.3 per 1000 for women. The cause of these events were SAH in 12%, cerebral haemorrhage in 10% and cerebral infarction in 30%, but in 49% of cases the type of stroke could not be defined [157].

All the reported incidences of SAH are to a greater or lesser extent subject to these ascertainment difficulties. They generally show an annual incidence of 10–16 per 100000 population (Table 2.1), with some regional variations. Variations may be due to differences in the size of study populations as well as ascertainment levels, but racial differences also account for some variation, e.g. higher incidences being reported from Japan. However, two Japanese studies performed between 1976 and 1984 reported incidences of 20–21 per 100000 [89, 189], whilst a third [105] an incidence of 96.1 per 100000. The higher incidence was thought by the authors to be due to improved ascertainment, particularly amongst the older population; a finding which emphasises the importance of methodology. A relatively low incidence has been reported amongst Danes [94, 104] and a racial difference was demonstrated by Kristensen [104]. In a study performed in Greenland, the risk of SAH amongst Eskimos was shown to be 4.4 times higher than amongst Danish Greenlanders. This report remains an exception to the general finding that racial variations are small and that much of the reported variation can be ascribed to the methodological difficulties of this type of research.

Table 2.1. Published annual incidence of subarachnoid haemorrhage (SAH)

Reference	Country	Incidence[a]
Brewis et al. [18]	United Kingdom	10.9
Pakarinen [144]	Finland	12.0
Gudmunsson [70]	Iceland	8.0
Kristensen [104]	Greenland	6.0
Bonita et al. [14]	New Zealand	14.3
Fogelholm [57]	Finland	19.4
Philips et al. [148]	United States	11.6
Joensen [94]	Denmark (Faroe Islands)	7.0
Tanaka [189]	Japan	20.0
Inagawara [89]	Japan	21.0
Kiyohara et al. [105]	Japan	96.1

[a]Per 100000.

Table 2.2. Relationship of age to annual incidence of subarachnoid haemorrhage (SAH)

Reference	Decade						
	3rd	4th	5th	6th	7th	8th	>9th
Brewis et al. [18]	3.4	12.7	22.1	23.1	13.7	11.4	12.5
Pakarinen [144]	6.1	13.4	26.9	38.6	30.6	26.6	–
Fogelholm [57]	8.0	16.0	38.0	35.0	41.0	49.0	–
Bonita et al. [14]	7.0	18.9	23.8	24.4	29.9	14.9	–
Kiyohara et al. [105]	–	–	34.9	38.4	97.4	148.9	281.7

The incidence of SAH increases with the patients' age and is generally higher in women. The majority of reports demonstrate a maximum incidence in middle and late middle age (Table 2.2), but two recent studies [57, 105] found maximum incidences in the oldest patients with a linear increase in incidence from 1.6 per 100000 per year in patients aged 10–19 years to 49.6 per 100000 per year in patients over 70 years [57]. In older patients female rates of SAH are generally 1.5–2.5 higher than for men [14, 18, 105, 144], and the median age of onset later for women [14]. As with the incidence of intracranial aneurysm, SAH is rare in children and young adults. Gender differences are less apparent amongst younger patients; Bonita et al. [14] found male rates to be greater than female up to the end of the third decade.

Survival rates at 30 days after SAH range from 39% to 60% [43, 57, 94, 105]. Most deaths occur in the first few days after haemorrhage; 15% before reaching hospital and 20% within 48 h in Bonita et al.'s study [14]. Kiyohara et al. [105] reported 35% of deaths occurring within 8 h of SAH and only 39% of their study population survived 30 days. They concluded that initial bleeding, rebleeding and delayed ischaemia were associated with the cause of death in 95% of fatalities. Survival rates after spontaneous SAH depends on the presence of a putative vascular lesion. Amongst patients with spontaneous SAH of unknown cause, the mortality rate was only a third of that in patients with intracranial aneurysms or arteriovenous malformation (AVM) [14], presumably because they are not at risk of rebleeding.

2.2.3
Clinical Consequences of Intracranial Aneurysm Rupture

The clinical consequence of intracranial aneurysm rupture is a syndrome of symptoms and signs which range from transient headache with minimal systemic disturbance to sudden death. In order to describe this spectrum the effects of aneurysm rupture will be divided into three groups: massive, major and minor haemorrhage.

2.2.3.1
Massive Haemorrhage

The loss of large volumes of blood into the subarachnoid, intraventricular or intracerebral compartments results in rapid loss of consciousness and an immediate rise in intracranial pressure. It occurs in up to a third of patients after aneurysm rupture [105, 144] and autopsy examinations demonstrate intracerebral and intraventricular haemorrhage (Fig. 2.2) in the majority of victims [29]. Patients present in coma and usually die within hours of ictus without regaining consciousness. The neurological signs on examination are initially a flaccid paralysis which progresses to decerebrate limb movements. Hypertension and bradycardia may develop in response to raised intracranial pressure, followed by unstable cardiovascular signs, pupillary irregularity and pyrexia due to loss of brain stem function, usually immediately prior to death.

Ictus and loss of consciousness may be associated with convulsions [74]. SAH should be considered in the differential diagnosis of the comatosed patients, including those with signs of head injury since sudden loss of consciousness may cause a fall. The resulting signs of trauma, in such cases, are usually minor compared with the severity of the neurological impairment.

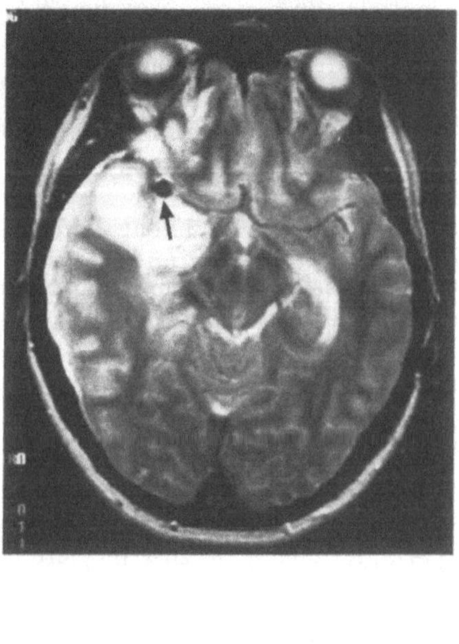

Fig. 2.2.
Axial T2-weighted magnetic resonance imaging at the level of the circle of Willis showing a saccular aneurysm in the region of the right middle cerebral artery bifurcation (*arrow*) and fresh intraparenchymal and extracerebral haemorrhage in the temporal lobe and middle cranial fossa

2.2.3.2
Major Haemorrhage

This type of presentation is the commonest amongst patients admitted to specialist neurosurgical hospitals. The syndrome is characterised by headache, loss of consciousness, vomiting, seizure, confusion and focal neurological deficits. Headache is the commonest feature, present in 70%–80% of cases [184], and is of sudden onset and typically of an unusual type for a particular patient. Loss of consciousness occurs in 30%–40% of patients [1, 98] and vomiting is a common feature. Vomiting is a non-specific feature of spontaneous intracranial haemorrhage which, if accompanied by diarrhoea, suggests bleeding in the posterior fossa. Seizures occur in less than 10% of patients, even with catastrophic haemorrhage [184]. The occurrence of convulsions at the time of rupture is not associated with an increased incidence of epilepsy developing later in the illness [74, 159]. Other symptoms include photophobia, blurring of vision, meningism and confusion. Focal neurological disturbances may be related to intracerebral extension of haemorrhage or direct involvement of a cranial nerve.

Activity, or the lack of it, at the time of SAH has been the source of some interest and controversy; in particular the relationship of aneurysm rupture to physical exertion. Locksley [117] found that SAH from all causes amongst the 6368 cooperative study patients occurred during sleep in 27% and during coitus in only 3% of patients. Fisher [55] considered that in 55% of his patients it was related to exertion; that in only 8% did it occur during sleep and then usually after coitus [9]. In 73% of the patients reported by Sengupta and McAlister [167] SAH occured when patients were awake and not involved in strenuous exertion. It can therefore be concluded that though episodes of hypertension and increased cerebral blood flow may theoretically increase the risk of aneurysm rupture, a link with physical exertion has not been proved.

2.2.3.3
Minor Haemorrhage

Rapid cessation of bleeding following aneurysm rupture will limit the volume of SAH and the severity of the clinical syndrome. Hemostasis results from the combined effects of reduced cerebral blood flow, probably the direct result of raised intracranial pressure [69, 138] and local clot formation. The latter depend on several factors, i.e. blood coaguability, size of the rupture point, aneurysm location and the tamponarde effect of fibrous membranes within the subarachnoid space. Leaks of small volumes of blood into the subarachnoid space are considered responsible for this syndrome in which headache may be mild, consciousness is not lost and signs of meningism are minimal and transient. Higher mental functions are preserved and abnormal physical signs, including disturbances of autonomic functions, are absent.

Patients with mild transient symptoms due to aneurysm rupture represent a diagnostic challenge with undoubtedly some undiagnosed, as discussed above. It is well recognised that patients not uncommonly give a history of transient unusual headache in the weeks prior to presentation with SAH.

Leblanc found retrospective evidence of minor leaks predating presentation by up to 4 weeks in 34 of 87 patients with proven SAH. Half of these patients had consulted physicians with symptoms such as hemicranial or periorbital pain and generalised headaches, but none were diagnosed as harbouring intracranial aneurysms [111]. Warnings of impending SAH or so-called sentinel headaches, have been described in 30%–50% of patients [44, 111, 140, 201], and are usually attributed to minor leaks in which bleeding due to aneurysm rupture rapidly ceases. An alternative explanation is that such headaches are caused by aneurysm enlargement or by haemorrhage into the wall and, as was discussed in Chap. 1, periods of aneurysm growth precede and might predispose to rupture. It is well recognised that sudden onset headaches typical of SAH may occur in patients without evidence of aneurysm rupture on computed tomography (CT) scan or CSF sampling, particularly patients with aneurysms in the region of the posterior communicating artery [32, 140].

2.2.4 Acute Signs of Intracranial Aneurysm Rupture

2.2.4.1 Non-localising Signs

The severity of presenting symptoms and signs are indicative of outcome and the likelihood of complications, apart from aneurysm rerupture. Neck stiffness and rigidity due to meningeal irritation is the commonest abnormal finding after SAH [55]. It is attributed to the stimulation of cervical sensory nerve roots by subarachnoid blood. In extreme cases neck retraction or opisthotonus is present. Spinal extension of haemorrhage is responsible for backache and the finding of a positive Kernig's sign. Back pain alone, and even sciatica, may dominate the clinical picture. Meningeal irritation is associated with photophobia, irritability, confusion and pyrexia. Absent or reduced tendon and abdominal reflexes with extensor plantar responses may be found in the absence of gross muscle weakness.

Retinal, subhyaloid or vitreous haemorrhages may cause unilateral or bilateral visual loss (Terson's syndrome) [192]. Intraocular bleeding probably results from transmission of raised intracranial pressure to the orbital optic nerve causing engorgement and rupture of retinal veins. This mechanism is considered more likely than the direct migration of SAH along the peri-optic subarachnoid space because at autopsy most of the blood is found in the subdural space [132]. Subhyaloid haemorrhages are found more often after aneurysmal SAH than other types of spontaneous intracranial bleeding. The finding is associated with a poor prognosis and an increased proportion of fatal outcomes [120, 147, 171]. It is commonest after anterior communicating artery aneurysm rupture [192]. On fundoscopic examination retinal haemorrhages are scattered and flame-shaped while subhyaloid collections are larger and typically flat-topped due to layering of blood. Extension of blood into the vitreous causes diffuse visual loss. In most patients haemorrhage clears and normal vision is restored within 3–12 months without surgical intervention [171], although recovery was quicker after vitrectomy in the series of Schultz et al. [165].

In addition, SAH may cause systemic abnormalities with disturbances of cardiac, respiratory and autonomic systems. The heart rate tends to fluctuate with moderate tachycardia. Progressive bradycardia occurs in response to rising intracranial pressure and combined with a deteriorating level of consciousness, is an ominous sign requiring urgent measures to prevent coning. Systemic hypertension may also occur in response to raised intracranial pressure. It is a frequent acute response to aneurysm rupture and systemic blood pressure may fluctuate over the first few post-ictal days. Pre-existing hypertension may be difficult to exclude and secondary features such as left ventricular enlargement, retinal artery changes and evidence of renal disease should be sought. Similarly, pre-existing respiratory disease may make recognition of changes in respiratory function difficult. Pulmonary oedema may occur as a response to SAH usually when intracranial pressure is elevated [209]. It develops acutely after massive haemorrhage and carries a poor prognosis. Impaired respiratory function causing tachyapnea and hypoxaemia is relatively common and may require treatment with oxygen supplement or assisted ventilation.

2.2.4.2 Localising Signs

The neurological status of patients recovering from aneurysm rupture frequently fluctuates in the first 24–48 h (Fig. 2.3). Intracerebral haematoma may cause fixed neurological deficits, but focal deficits are otherwise rela-

a

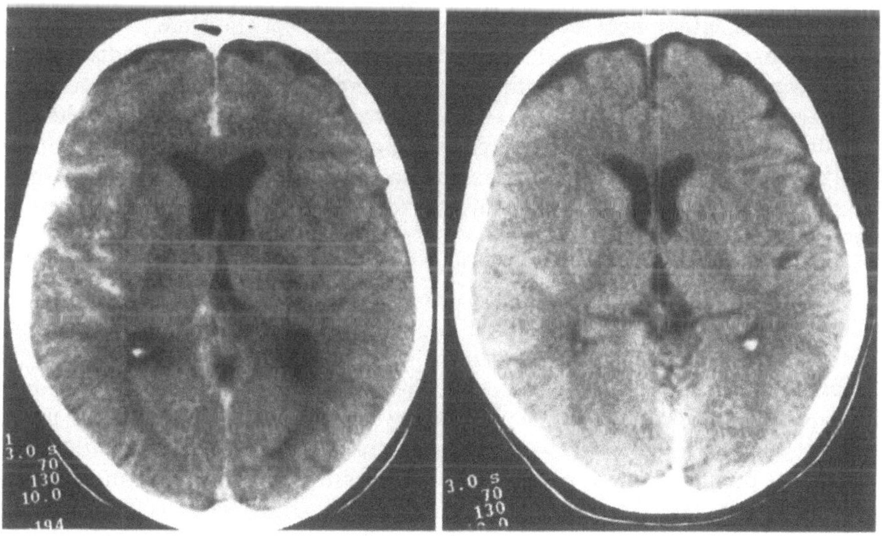

b

Fig. 2.3 a,b. Axial unenhanced computed tomography scans **a** 4 h and **b** 3 days after aneurysmal subarachnoid haemorrhage (SAH). The early scan shows high-density SAH with a moderate degree of ventricular enlargement; both have largely resolved by the fourth post-ictal day

tively uncommon and often transient with fluctuating abnormal signs. In the international cooperative study series of 3521 patients, severe focal motor deficits or homonymous hemianopsia were found at presentation to neurosurgical units in 7.1% of patients examined on the day of ictus, but in only 2.2% of patients admitted on the third day [100]. All the patients were assessed within 3 calendar days of ictus and 75.8% had normal motor responses, 12% mild focal deficits and 5.6% severe focal deficits. Dysphasic speech was also a transient finding, reported in 9.7% of patients admitted to hospital on day 0 and 4.7% of those admitted on day 3. Cranial nerve deficits were present in 12.2% of all patients, but the frequency of this sign did not fall in the first 48 h and the occulomotor nerve was by far the most commonly affected. Of 428 patients with cranial nerve deficits at presentation, 277 (64.7%) involved the third cranial nerve.

Acute hemispheric dysfunction causing fixed deficits such as hemiparesis, hemanopsia or dysphasia are uncommon after uncomplicated aneurysmal SAH. Paraparesis is classically associated with anterior communicating artery (ACoA) aneurysm rupture [67] and hemiparesis with middle cerebral artery (MCA) aneurysm rupture acutely or following the development of delayed vasospasm [158]. Dominant hemisphere MCA aneurysm rupture may cause dysphasia with or without intracerebral hematoma. Memory disturbance may occur, but in the acute period coincidental drowsiness and stupor often make assessment of higher mental functions difficult. Korsakoff's syndrome has been described due to ischaemia and/or infarction in the mammillary bodies, fornices and thalami in both operated and unoperated patients [73, 113]. Dementia and emotional liability occur after bifrontal damage, usually due to rupture of an ACoA aneurysm [168].

Cranial nerve palsies following aneurysm rupture may be due to direct compression, either because the aneurysm enlarges at the time of rupture or focal hematoma. Compression may anticede rupture so that patients present following aneurysmal SAH with long-standing signs of cranial nerve compression. Such localising signs and symptoms will be considered below in the discussion of symptomatic unruptured aneurysms. Mass effect due to focal hematoma or hydrocephalus may cause cranial nerve dysfunction indirectly by compressing the brain stem or distorting cranial nerves around the tentorial hiatus.

The oculomotor nerve is the cranial nerve most commonly affected after SAH. Dysfunction may result from both direct and indirect compression. The nerve lies immediately lateral to the posterior communicating artery (PCoA) in the interpeduncular cistern, where it is liable to compression by aneurysms arising at the PCoA origin, the distal basilar artery (BA), or more anteriorly from the intracavernous internal carotid artery (ICA). Third nerve paresis due to PCoA aneurysm rupture causes ophthalmoplegia with some degree of pupillary dilation due to direct pressure or extravasation of blood into the nerve fascicles [88]. Aneurysm was the single most common cause of third nerve palsy in the series of Green et al. [68] and the nerve is affected in the majority of patients presenting following PCoA aneurysm rupture [109, 153]. Pupillary sparing third nerve paresis, though rare, has been reported following PCoA aneurysm rupture [103]. The pupil is involved be-

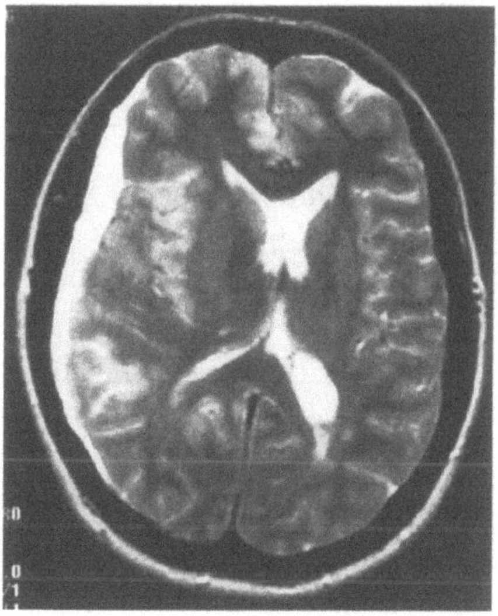

Fig. 2.4.
Axial T2-weighted magnetic resonance imaging following aneurysmal subarachnoid haemorrhage (SAH). There is a subdural haematoma on the right side causing displacement of the right hemisphere and mid-line structures. SAH is present in the right sylvian fissure. This subdural haematoma was caused by rupture of a middle cerebral artery aneurysm

cause the preganglionic parasympathetic fibres to the ciliary ganglion are carried in the superficial part of the nerve and are vulnerable to local pressure. Their interruption causes a dilated pupil which fails to constrict to light or in attempts at the near reflex.

In addition to direct pressure the third nerve may be compressed at the tentorial hiatus in the presence of hemispheric shifts with uncal herniation, brain stem haemorrhage or distortions caused by intracerebral, intraventricular or subdural haemorrhage (Fig. 2.4) [88]. Involvement of other cranial nerves is unusual after SAH. The fifth nerve, because of its vertical course in the subarachnoid space, is liable to distortion by downward pressure on the brain stem and sixth nerve palsy has been described after brain stem infarction [28]. Facial muscle weakness or palsies are usually due to hemispheric ischaemia or infarction and therefore upper motor neuron lesions.

2.2.5 Grading of Patients After Subarachnoid Haemorrhage

Several authors have employed grading scales to describe the neurological status of patients after SAH. They have been generally adopted since they provide physicians with a relatively simple method of describing a particular patient's condition to colleagues, recording fluctuations, comparing different treatments and estimating prognosis. The severity of the illness caused by aneurysm rupture and the likelihood of complications are to a large extent determined at the time of ictus. Early clinical grading is therefore relevant to final outcome and allows comparisons of different treatments to be made across the spectrum of symptomatology caused by SAH.

The most commonly adopted systems employ a five-point scale modelled on that described by Botterell et al. [15]. They graded their 23 patients according to operative risk using five grades as follows:

- *Grade 1.* A conscious patient with or without signs of blood in the subarachnoid space
- *Grade 2.* A drowsy patient without significant neurological deficit
- *Grade 3.* The drowsy patient with a neurological deficit and probably an intracerebral clot
- *Grade 4.* Patients with a major neurological deficit and deteriorating because of large intracerebral clots or older patients with less severe neurological deficit but pre-existing degenerative cerebrovascular disease
- *Grade 5.* A moribund or near moribund patient with failing vital centres and extensor rigidity

Subsequent modifications have been proposed by several authors (Nishioka [137], Hunt and Hess [86], Hunt and Kosnik [87], Nibbelink et al. [136]) in order to improve the objectivity of scoring and reduce inter-rater variations. The plethora of scoring systems that emerged has made comparison of reporting difficult and highlighted the need for a universally acceptable scale. The issue was considered by a committee of the World Federation of Neurological Surgeons set up in 1981 [41]. They concluded, from an analysis of data from the international cooperative aneurysm study [100], that the most important factors affecting outcome were the patient's level of consciousness, which predicted death and disability, and the presence or absence of hemiparesis and/or aphasia, which predicted disability but not mortality. They also considered that the presence of headache and neck stiffness in conscious patients had no significance on outcome and therefore that Hunt and Hess [137] grades I and II were identical for outcome. The resulting proposals were that: (a) a five-grade system be retained and unruptured aneurysm could be classed as grade 0, (b) the Glasgow Coma Scale [191] be used for evaluation of level of consciousness and (c) that the presence of major focal deficit (aphasia and/or hemiparesis or hemiplegia) be used to differentiate grades II and III (Table 2.3).

Not withstanding this applaudable attempt to achieve a consensus, a new scale for assessing neurological status after SAH was proposed the following year [91] and in 1994 a review of the neurological literature found that the Hunt and Hess (or Hunt and Kosnik) scales continue to be used for recording the clinical condition of patients in 71% of papers published since 1985

Table 2.3. World Federation of Neurological Surgeons (WFNS) grades and Glasgow Coma Scale (GCS)

WFNS grade	GCS score	Motor deficit
I	15	Absent
II	14–13	Absent
III	14–13	Present
IV	12–7	Present or absent
V	6–3	Present or absent

Table 2.4. Glasgow Outcome Scale (GOS)

GOS grade	Neurological status
1	Good recovery; patient can lead a full and independent life with or without minimal neurological deficit
2	Moderately disabled; patient has neurological or intellectual impairment but is independent
3	Severely disabled; patients are conscious but totally dependent on others to get through daily activities
4	Vegetative survival
5	Dead

[196]. This is despite two studies showing frequent inter-observer errors in grading the severity of headache and levels of consciousness due to the inherent vagueness in some of the definitions enshrined in the Hunt and Hess scale [114, 115].

However, the Glasgow Outcome Scale [93] has been generally adopted for recording outcome after aneurysmal SAH. This system, developed to evaluate the overall social outcome for survivors of brain damage, relies on assessment of a patient's ability to live independently. It is a five-point scale defined as: dead, vegetative state, severely disabled, moderately disabled and good recovery. In a "vegetative state", the patient is breathing spontaneously but remains unresponsive and speechless with no psychologically meaningful response. Severe disability is usually due to a combination of mental and physical disabilities which result in dependence on others for daily activities. It includes patients with devastating dementia without physical handicaps due to focal deficits. "Moderately disabled" covers a range of handicaps but the patient is able to cope independently in daily activities. The definition includes patients able to undertake work at a reduced level compared to their previous capabilities. The definition of "good recovery" does not imply complete recovery but indicates that the patient has regained the capacity to undertake work and leisure activites similar to those previously possible. These definitions are now scaled 1–5, with the higher levels indicating greater disability (Table 2.4). Its main competitor in rehabilitation assessments is the modified Rankin scale or Oxford Handicap Scale [16]. These are simular six-point scales which have both been shown to be reliable in inter-observer studies [4, 197].

2.3 Complications of Subarachnoid Haemorrhage

2.3.1 Medical Complications

Following aneurysmal SAH patients may develop non-neurological complications due to dysfunctions in the pulmonary, cardiac, endocrine, renal, hepatic or autonomic systems. In addition, pre-existing medical conditions may be exacerbated, complicating management and impeding recovery. SAH is also associated with the delayed development of epilepsy either post-craniotomy or following conservative management. Solenski et al. [176], in an analysis of 457 SAH patients forming the placebo group of a multicentre trial, showed that medical complications were a major cause of mortality. They found that, at 3 months, 19% of the patients had died; and that these deaths were due to the direct effect of SAH in 19%, rebleeding in 22%, vasospasm in 23% and medical complications in 23%.

Pulmonary complications were responsible for 50% of the deaths due to medical complications reported by Solenski et al. [176]. These were diagnosed pneumonia, neurogenic pulmonary oedema, pulmonary embolus and aspiration. Neurogenic pulmonary oedema may occur after any cerebral insult associated with raised intracranial pressure and is a well recognised complication of aneurysmal SAH [209]. It usually occurs in the first few days after SAH [176] and is caused by capillary leakage of protein-rich fluid in the absence of left-sided cardiac failure [193]. The mechanism is unclear, but it is thought to be the result of a massive adrenergic discharge which decreases left ventricular compliance or acts directly on pulmonary adrenergic receptors to increase capillary permeability [173, 180]. Amongst Solenski et al.'s patients, it was evident in 23% and severe in 6%. Patients in poor clinical grades are more likely to be affected [176] and they are also more liable to develop other pulmonary complications such as pneumonia or pulmonary embolism [209].

The most frequent cardiovascular complications after SAH are systemic hypertension and cardiac arrhythmia. The difficulty in distinguishing pre-existing systemic hypertension from reactive hypertension in patients after aneurysm rupture has been discussed. It has been reported in 16%–36% of patients and may be a non-specific sympathetic response to stress or the Cushing's response to raised intracranial pressure and brain stem ischaemia [100, 176]. Cardiac dysrhythmia and electrocardiac abnormalities may be found in 35%–50% of patients [121, 176]. The described changes on electrocardiograms are prolongation of the Q–T interval, T wave abnormalities including inversion, ST segment changes and prominent U waves. A variety of arrhythmias have been described; these are usually not life threatening [199, 206]. Cardiac arrhythmia are commonest in the first few days after SAH and immediately after acute aneurysm surgery [199]. They are also thought to result from excessive sympathetic activity and treatment with adrenergic blocking drugs has been shown to be of benefit [202].

A variety of electrolyte disturbances have been found after SAH including hyponatraemia and diabetes insipidus. The latter is relatively rare in uncomplicated SAH except in poor grade patients after severe and prolonged episodes of raised intracranial pressure. Hyponatraemia, however, which may be defined as plasma sodium levels below 135 mEq/l for 2 consecutive days, occurs in 27%–35% of patients [34, 212]. Initially considered to be due to the syndrome of inappropriate secretion of antidiuretic hormone [35, 95] it is now thought to be due to salt wasting, i.e. primary natriuresis associated with cerebral injury [134, 211]. Since in animal studies of SAH, hyponatraemia did not correlate with raised serum antidiuretic hormone [135] and, though transiently elevated in patients, raised levels have been shown to be unrelated to the subsequent development of hyponatraemia [212, 214]. Wijdicks et al. [212] found the severity of hyponatraemia to be proportional to the severity of SAH and, importantly, that its treatment by fluid restriction may increase the risks of cerebral infarction.

The pathophysiological mechanisms for electrolyte and autonomic disturbances after SAH remain uncertain. It is well recognised that hypothalamic lesions occur after fatal SAH more frequently than after other causes of death associated with raised intracranial pressure [30, 38], and it has been postulated that this is due to the effects of local haemorrhage. The occurrence of hyponatraemia has been linked with the presence of haemorrhage in the chiasmatic cistern and third ventricle, usually due to rupture of an anterior communicating artery aneurysm [30, 187, 213]. Hypothalamic injury presumably results from ischaemia or infarction due to vasospasm of perforating arteries or secondary to pressure from enlargement of the third ventricle [213]. Elevated levels of atrial natriuretic factor (ANF) or peptide in blood [160, 207] and CSF [160] have been observed after SAH, both alone and in association with hyponatremia [214]. ANF is a diuretic natriuretic hormone produced in the heart and brain. However, Diringer et al. [34] did not show a correlation between blood levels and hyponatraemia. They did however show that the presence of suprasellar and intraventricular haemorrhage correlated with raised plasma ANF levels. The current evidence therefore suggests that ANF does play a role in urinary salt loss after SAH, particularly as both hypothalamic and myocardial lesions have been demonstrated at autopsy [38]. But other factors contribute to the electrolyte balance of SAH patients and hypokalaemia, as well as hypernatramia and hyperkalaemia may develop, particularly during diuretic and hypervolaemic treatments [34, 176].

In addition to these electrolyte disturbances, other metabolic abnormalities may less commonly occur as a consequence of hepatic or renal dysfunction. In the majority of Solenski et al.'s patients, these were not severe, unless they occurred in association with another complication such as sepsis or pulmonary oedema [176].

Epilepsy after aneurysmal SAH has been reported in 9%–15% of patients [74, 75, 139, 159, 181]. The onset of siezures is usually in the first 4 weeks but may be delayed. Ictal seizures, i.e. siezures at the time of aneurysm rupture, occurred in 3% of 381 patients reported by Hasan et al. [74], but none of these patients had further fits. The clinical factors most often found in association with seizures in four studies reviewed by Hasan et al. were aneurysm rebleeding [74, 75, 159], MCA aneurysm rupture [75, 159], age less than 50 years [159], loss of consciousness for 1–8 h [139], systemic hypertension [139] and large volumes of cisternal blood on CT scan [74]. Therefore, apart from rebleeding and MCA aneurysm rupture, no clear consensus has emerged about the factors predisposing to, nor the mechanism that causes, delayed epilepsy after SAH on its own. Craniotomy and aneurysm clipping undoubtably contributes to the incidence since Cabal et al. [23] found that the overall post-operative incidence was 22%; the highest being 35% after clipping of MCA aneurysms and lowest 5% in patients undergoing carotid artery ligation only.

2.3.2
Aneurysm Rebleeding

Aneurysm rerupture is currently the single largest preventable cause of morbidity due to aneurysmal SAH, and therefore its prevention represents the greatest therapeutic challenge facing physicians caring for victims of aneurysmal SAH. The incidence of rebleeding has been calculated by various authors. These estimates depend on: (a) accurate diagnosis and differentiation of rebleeding from other causes of sudden deterioration in patients recovering from aneurysm rupture, (b) calculations based on an accurate estimate of the size of the population at risk and (c) allowances for the effects of medical management such as the use of antifibrinolytics as prophylaxis against aneurysm rerupture.

The availability of CT scanning or magnetic resonance imaging (MRI) for confirmation of the diagnosis of rerupture is therefore critical. In calculating the risk of fatal rebleeding amongst the 1232 patients managed conservatively in the pre-CT cooperative study, Nishioka [137] excluded other causes of death and then distinguished those patients in whom rebleeding was proven from a larger group which included those patients in whom it had been suspected but not proven. The risks calculated from the day of haemorrhage in the two groups were 25% and 33%, respectively. The lower incidence of fatal rebleeding is similar to that of later studies in which planar scanning was used to confirm rebleeding [176, 81].

The time interval to rebleeding determines the period when preventative treatments should be performed. The risk of rebleeding appears to fall exponentially from the day of ictus. Although it had been suggested that a peak incidence occurs towards the end of the first week [117], more recent reports found incidences of 4%–10% in the first 24 h falling thereafter [82, 97]. Inagawa et al. [90] reported a rate of 15.3% in the first 6 h – such statistics obviously depending on rapid admission to hospital. Kassel and Torner [97] estimated the rebleeding risk at 1%–5% per day after 48 h with a cumulative risk of 26.5% by 14 days. A flat incidence of rebleeding was also reported by Maurice-Williams et al. [123]. It is generally agreed that by 3–6 months the risk has fallen to the annual rebleeding rate of 3%–4% [137, 217].

These data are consistent with the concept that aneurysmal bleeding ceases with the formation of a sealing clot, the subsequent organisation of which takes up to 3 months or more. The potential effects of investigations and treatment during the acute period have to be considered. Inagawa [90] estimated that early angiography (within 6 h of rupture) doubled the risk of rerupture. Alternatively, early surgical clipping halved the mortality due to rebleeding in the international cooperative study on the timing of aneurysm surgery (rebleeding occurred in 5.7% of patients operated on days 0–3 and in 13.9% of patients operated on days 11–14); a benefit offset by an increase in the morbidity of early surgery [100]. Early surgical clipping to secure the aneurysm and removing the spectra of rebleeding, is now generally practised. Furthermore, it allows more aggressive medical treatment of vasospasm, should it occur [116]. The mortality associated with rebleeding has been consistently reported as higher than that following the initial haemorrhage with estimates ranging from 50% to 90% [123, 137, 176], which emphasise the need for its prevention by early intervention.

2.3.3 Delayed Cerebral Vasospasm

Subarachnoid haemorrhage may cause acute or delayed cerebral vasospasm. Acute transient constriction of basal cerebral arteries is evident on angiography soon after aneurysm rupture and contributes to the presenting illness. Its cause is probably a combination of the sudden rise in intracranial pressure, mechanical disruption of the basal arteries and the release of short-acting vasoconstrictors such as adrenaline, thrombin and 5-hydroxytryptamine from platelets. Delayed cerebral vasospasm, on the other hand, is seen in patients recovering from the acute effects of aneurysmal SAH and is associated with delayed neurologic deterioration. This complication is a potentially preventable cause of additional morbidity and its elucidation has generated an enormous literature with five international symposia held on the subject since 1975 [54, 163, 174, 215, 216]. It is caused by the adventitial exposure of cerebral arteries to the breakdown products of blood and subsequent changes in vascular smooth muscle function. The mechanism or mechanisms (several factors are almost certainly involved) have yet to be understood and there is currently no universally effective therapy.

The clinical syndrome of symptomatic vasospasm or delayed ischaemic deficit due to cerebral ischaemia is an inconsistent consequence of angiographic vasospasm. It was first described by Robertson [158] in 1949 and is characterised by the insidious onset of confusion, decreased conscious level and focal neurological deficits. Occasionally, the onset is sudden and may be mistaken for rebleeding [123]. Angiographic vasospasm of cerebral arteries after SAH was first described by Ecker and Riemenschneider in 1951 [47]. They reported finding focal narrowing of basal cerebral arteries in patients with ruptured berry aneurysms. They defined vasospasm as transient narrowing of at least 0.5 mm in the larger basal cerebral arteries, which was visible in two angiographic projections. This phenomenon was observed only in patients examined within 23 days of haemorrhage and usually involved arteries adjacent to an aneurysm. They felt it was provoked by arterial disruption at the time of the ictus and that its role was protective, i.e. to limit the amount of haemorrhage. The time course of symptomatic vasospasm parallels that of angiographic vasospasm (Fig. 2.5), the onset being rare before the third post-ictal day, with a peak incidence at about the seventh day [208]. It rarely persists for longer than 3 weeks after SAH [42].

In an extensive survey of the literature Dorsch and King [36, 37] found the average incidence of angiographic vasospasm to be 43.3% (range, 19%–97% in 222 studies), whilst the average incidence of symptomatic vasospasm

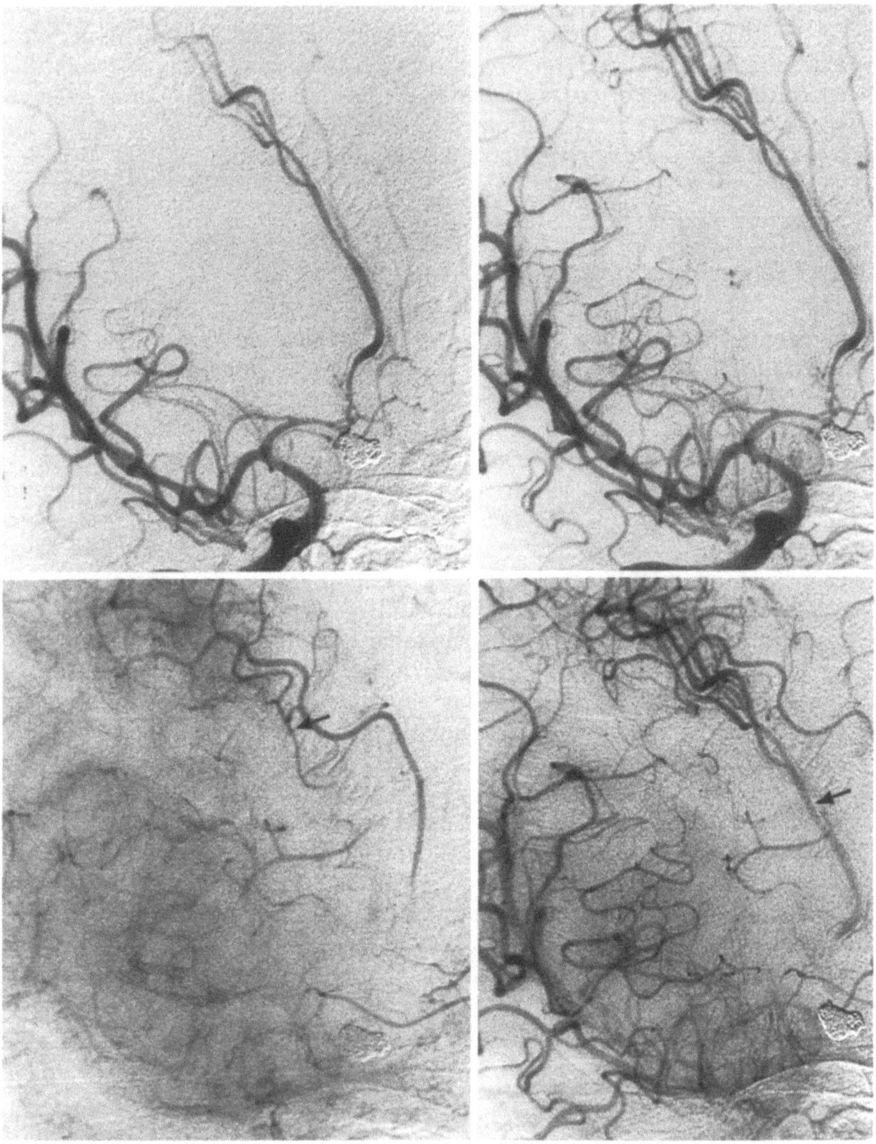

a c b d

Fig. 2.5 a–d. Delayed vasospasm. A series of images from an oblique frontal intra-arterial digital subtraction angiography of the right carotid artery. A ruptured aneurysm of the anterior communicating artery was treated acutely by coil embolisation without complication. Four days after treatment and 6 days after subarachnoid haemorrhage, the patients developed increasing drowsiness and weakness of both legs. The angiograms show vasospasm of the anterior cerebral arteries. This is most marked in the left anterior cerebral artery (**a** and **b**). The delayed images show retrograde flow (*arrows* in **c** and **d**) providing collateral flow to the left frontal lobe

was 32.4% (range, 5%–90% in 296 studies). The incidence of angiographic vasospasm increased to 67.3% (range 40–97% in 38 studies) when they restricted the survey to reports of diagnosis between 4 and 11 days after SAH. A similar exercise, analysing only studies with strict criteria for the diagnosis of symptomatic vasospasm and the exclusion of other causes of delayed neurological deterioration, did not change the average incidence of symptomatic vasospasm significantly (32.6%), but narrowed the range of incidences (range, 12%–57% in 132 studies). Thus only about half the number of patients with evidence of angiographic vasospasm will develop neurological symptoms [106]. Asymptomatic patients may have evidence of vasospasm on serial transcranial doppler velocity studies performed over several days [166]. Whether individual patients experience symptoms of cerebral ischaemia or not depends on the degree of arterial narrowing, its location and the adequacy of collateral blood flow [43], as well as other factors such as increased intracranial pressure or the presence of cerebral oedema [200]. Specific neurological deficits are determined by the arterial territory(ies) involved; for example, vasospasm of the anterior cerebral artery (ACA) causes a characteristic syndrome of paraparesis, cognitive and affective impairment [67].

The cause of cerebral vasospasm remains uncertain despite considerable research efforts over the last 30 years. The single term cerebral vasospasm has been generally adopted and defined as angiographic narrowing of the cerebral vessels, which may be symptomatic or asymptomatic [215]. Early workers noted that vasospasm did not occur without a significant amount of blood around the basal cerebral arteries [46, 151]. Since the introduction of CT, it has been demonstrated that the locations of peri-arterial blood clots correlate with sites of arterial narrowing [56, 127, 188]. The presence of sub arachnoid blood thus appears to initiate and/or sustain the phenomenon, but conclusive evidence as to the causative factor(s) is still lacking. Controversy still remains as to whether cerebral vasospasm is an abnormal contraction, a failure of relaxation of arterial smooth muscle or whether it represents pathological thickening of the arterial wall.

Various components of whole blood have been suspected as potential spasmogen; most recently haemoglobin and its breakdown products, in particular oxyhaemoglobin, have been incriminated. The delay of 3–4 days in onset of delayed cerebral vasospasm is characteristic and coincides with maximum concentrations of oxyhaemoglobin in subarachnoid clots [25, 141, 143]. Oxyhaemoglobin has a vasoconstricting action which has been attributed to its multiple effects on vascular physiology. The possible mechanisms are: that it acts as a generator of superoxides [190], inhibits endogenous dilators such as nitric oxide either directly [77, 122] or indirectly by affecting smooth muscle cyclic guanosine monophosphate [48, 50], or by stimulation of vasoconstrictors such as the endothelins produced by endothelial cells [101].

There is no doubt that cerebral vasospasm complicating SAH affects outcome. Mortality rates amongst patients with symptomatic vasospasm are at least twice those for patients without this complication and Dorsch [36] calculated that the odds of a fatal outcome were three times greater for patients with vasospasm. The likelihood of a good outcome (i.e. Glasgow Outcome

Score of 1) was two to three times better if symptomatic vasospasm did not develop. Analysis of 101 references with complete data on 3193 patients who developed delayed ischaemic deficits, revealed a fatal outcome in 31.0%, permanent neurological deficit in 34.7% and more or less complete recovery (sic) in 34.3% [36]. Its prevention, therefore, represents a continuing therapeutic challenge.

2.3.4 Hydrocephalus

Obstruction to the circulation of CSF may occur after SAH. The resulting hydrocephalus, like delayed cerebral vasospasm, may or may not be associated with symptoms. Furthermore, hydrocephalus may develop immediately following aneurysm rupture, i.e. acutely or its onset may be delayed for days or weeks (Figs. 2.3, 2.6). Ventriculomegaly, evident on CT scan or MRI, implies an impediment to normal CSF flow but its clinical consequences are variable and dictate the need for surgical intervention to re-establish CSF drainage. Since spontaneous resumption of normal CSF flow can be anticipated within 24 h in approximately 50% of patients presenting with acute hydrocephalus, primary treatment is usually provided by a temporary ventricular or lumbar drain [76].

The incidence of acute hydrocephalus following spontaneous SAH is 15%–20% [66, 76, 198]. Yasagil et al. [221] reported, in a study of patients treated prior to CT scanning, incidences of 9% in operated and 15% in unoperated patients. Subsequently, Vassilouthis and Richardson [198] described incidences of 15.5% in the first 2 weeks and 10.5% after 2 or more weeks after

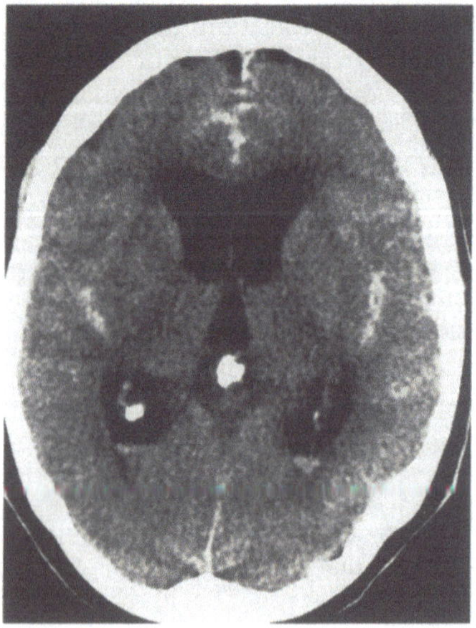

Fig. 2.6. Axial computed tomography scan 5 days after aneurysmal subarachnoid haemorrhage showing hydrocephalus of the lateral and third ventricles with dependent high-density intraventricular haemorrhage

SAH diagnosed by CT. Despite the CT finding of ventriculomegaly, clinically significant hydrocephalus occurred in only 7% of the total 167 patients. Graff-Radford et al. [66] distinguished hydrocephalus diagnosed by CT on admission within 3 days of SAH (which affected 15% of patients) from symptomatic hydrocephalus diagnosed at any time (which affected 13.2% of patients). In all, 22.3% of 3521 patients in the international cooperative study were affected since overlap between the two groups occurred in 5.9% of patients [66].

Acute ventriculomegaly is caused by blood cells and cellular debris obstructing CSF flow in the ventricles, basal cisterns, or around the exit foramina of the fourth ventricle. Alternatively, ventricular enlargement also occurs due to haematomas, particularly in the posterior fossa compressing CSF pathways. Chronic hydrocephalus is due to the development of fibrosis and adhesions within the leptomeninges which impede CSF flow and/or its absorption by arachnoid granulations.

The amount and distribution of SAH is a factor in the pathogenesis of both acute and chronic hydrocephalus. The presence of intraventricular haemorrhage is obviously more likely to cause acute hydrocephalus. Mohr [128] found that acute ventricular dilation was evident in 85% of 91 patients with intraventricular haemorrhage. These findings were confirmed by Graff-Radford et al. in a detailed analysis of factors associated with hydrocephalus [66]. In this study, acute hydrocephalus was associated with intraventricular haemorrhage, the diffuse spread of subarachnoid haemorrhage and rupture of posterior circulation aneurysms. Multiple factors were found to be related to the development of clinical hydrocephalus at any stage; these included: CT demonstrated hydrocephalus, intraventricular haemorrhage, the patient's level of consciousness on admission to hospital, pre-existing systemic hypertension, increasing age, subarachnoid blood on CT, posterior circulation aneurysm rupture and hypertension postoperatively. They also confirmed a previously described observation that use of antifibrinolytic drugs increased the risk of chronic hydrocephalus [146], but not the finding of Shulman et al. [172] that the ACoA was the most likely aneurysm location to be associated with hydrocephalus after rupture.

The clinical consequences of acute hydrocephalus vary from sudden death to mild reduction in the level of consciousness. In Hasan et al.'s [76] series, 91 patients had hydrocephalus on their initial CT; their levels of consciousness were normal in 28%, slightly impaired in 14% and moderately or severely impaired in 58%. Impairment of consciousness may improve dramatically once ventricular drainage has been established [7]. Patients who develop subacute and chronic hydrocephalus complain of headaches, drowsiness with fluctuating levels of consciousness, ataxia, dementia and incontinence. The onset of symptoms are typically insidious but may be rapid and simulate rebleeding [76]. Acute relief of intracranial hypertension by ventricular drainage is considered by some to increase the risk of rebleeding. Reported rebleeding rates after ventricular drainage vary from 14% to 43% [76, 154]. A cautious reduction in intraventricular pressure is generally advocated when drainage is performed prior to surgical clipping. In this situation, the less invasive endovascular route has the potential of securing the aneurysm without changing intracranial pressure and, therefore, is theoretically of benefit prior to CSF shunting. A definitive CSF drainage procedure either by ventricular-peritoneal or lumbar-peritoneal shunt is necessary in only 5%–8% of SAH patients [66, 198], and often symptoms can be relieved during the subacute period by lumbar puncture(s). In the patients of the international cooperative study, 8.7% morbidity and 1% mortality overall was attributed to hydrocephalus [99, 100].

2.4 Symptomatology of Unruptured Intracranial Aneurysms

Unruptured aneurysms are diagnosed as the result of symptoms referable to the lesion or incidentally during investigations for other reasons. Asymptomatic aneurysms are most commonly discovered coincidental to SAH in patients with multiple intracranial aneurysms or AVM. Multiple aneurysms are found in approximately 19%–25% of patients presenting after aneurysmal SAH [99, 102, 117, 167]. The unruptured aneurysms of patients with multiple aneurysms presenting following SAH have been the subjects for most studies of the natural history of unruptured aneurysms. Data on other incidentally discovered aneurysms and symptomatic unruptured aneurysms have come from surgical series and therefore tend to be biased towards treatable lesions.

2.4.1 Natural History

The risk of SAH due to rupture of an incidental aneurysm has been estimated by Winn et al. [218] at 1% per annum. This estimate was made in a follow-up study of 182 SAH patients with multiple aneurysms of whom over two thirds (132 patients) were treated conservatively. Over the study period (mean, 8 years) the rebleed rate was 3% per annum amongst those treated conservatively (all of whom rebled due to aneurysm rerupture), but only 1% per annum amongst patients who had the originally ruptured aneurysm successfully clipped. The rerupture rate (3% per annum) in patients with multiple aneurysms is therefore similar to that of patients with single aneurysms [137, 217].

The risk of haemorrhage posed by the discovery of an unruptured intracranial aneurysm was estimated according to age at diagnosis by Dell [33] as follows: 16.6% at 20 years, 16.1% at 30 years, 14.4% at 40 years, 10.3% at 50 years and 4.7% at 60 years. It is currently the subject of a large multicentre evaluation study [58].

However, the natural history of symptomatic aneurysms, as regards the risk of SAH, is likely to be different from that of incidental aneurysms [150]; the risk of rupture in the former appears to be greater. Graf [65] followed 35 patients with untreated symptomatic aneurysms for 2–12 years; 26% died following SAH. Over the same period only two of 52 patients with untreated coincidental aneurysms died. This difference in subsequent rupture rates may be because symptomatic aneurysms tend to be larger than incidental aneurysms when they are discovered. This deduction is supported by Weibers et al. [205] who found that rupture in a mixed cohort of symptomatic and incidental unruptured aneurysms (followed for a mean of 8.3 years) only occurred in those over 9 mm in size and that all aneurysms causing symptoms due to mass effect were over 10 mm in size. Furthermore, size has been shown to be the only significant predictor of rupture of previously unruptured aneurysms [96, 205] and is therefore more likely to occur in patients with larger symptomatic aneurysms.

2.4.2 Modes of Presentation

The relative frequency of symptomatic and incidental unruptured aneurysms is difficult to estimate. In 130 patients with unruptured aneurysms diagnosed at the Mayo Clinic between 1955 and 1980 [205], angiography was performed for the following reasons: ischaemic cerebrovascular symptoms (32%), headache (15%), cranial nerve palsies (10%), seizures (8%), mass effects (5%) and other symptoms unrelated to intracranial aneurysms (30%) (see Fig. 2.11). Symptoms due to the discovered aneurysms were present in 31 of 130 patients (24%) and half were attributable to cranial nerve compression. It is therefore not surprising that symptomatic unruptured aneurysms are usually larger than incidental aneurysms and are often discovered on arteries below the circle of Willis, where they are more likely to affect cranial nerves.

In two recent surgical series of unruptured aneurysms [102, 155], 17%–18% presented due to symptoms of mass effect, 5% due to seizures, 5% in association with AVM, 14%–17% were incidental and 10%–30% of the rest were discovered in patients with non-specific symptoms of cerebral ischaemia. There was a female preponderance of 3:1, largely due to a ten times greater female incidence of cavernous carotid aneurysms [177]. The majority of operated aneurysms in the reports of Solomon et al. [177] and Khanna et al. [102] were giant or large: 61.8% and 63.9%, respectively. In Khanna et al.'s [102] series aneurysms involved the anterior cerebral circulation in 87.2% and posterior cerebral circulation in 12.8%. The commonest location for unruptured aneurysms in most series was the ICA (Table 2.5).

Symptoms attributable to unruptured aneurysms are pain, neural dysfunctions due to compression, i.e. cranial nerve palsies, visual disturbances, motor weakness, sensory loss, dysaesthesia and seizures; or symptoms due to cerebral ischaemia or infarction, i.e. transient ischaemic attacks (TIA), hemiparesis, dysphasia and hemianopsia. Except for symptoms due to thromboemboli, their nature depends largely on the aneurysm's location. Presentation with symptoms of cerebral ischaemia or TIA is not directly related to aneurysm site [102]. Intra-aneurysmal thromboemboli are typically associated with large and giant aneurysms, but it is noteworthy that one of Weibers et al.'s patients presented with symptoms of thromboembolism arising from an angiographically small aneurysm [205]. Unstable intraluminal

Table 2.5. Incidence of unruptured aneurysms according to site

Reference	Aneurysms (n)	Aneurysm locations					
		ICA	PCoA[b]	MCA	ACA	BA/VA	PCA
Asari et al. [5][a]	72	26 (36%)	7 (10%)	14 (19%)	15 (20%)	14 (19%)	3 (5%)
Solomon et al. [177][a]	202	100 (50%)	–	38 (19%)	28 (14%)	29 (16%)	–
Juvela et al. [96]	181	79 (44%)		81 (45%)	16 (9%)	5 (3%)	–
Weibers et al. [205]	161	98 (61%)	26 (16%)	30 (19%)	14 (9%)	14 (9%)	5 (3%)
Eskesen et al.[a] [49]	53	30 (56%)		10 (14%)	7 (13%)	6 (11%)	–

ICA, internal carotid artery; PCoA, posterior communicating artery; MCA, middle cerebral artery; ACA, anterior cerebral artery; BA, basilar artery; VA, vertebral artery; PCA, posterior cerebral artery.
[a] Surgical series.
[b] Aneurysms in this column are also included in the overall ICA figures.

thrombus increases the risk of morbidity due to surgical and endovascular treatments [205, 219]. The rest of this chapter will be devoted to the symptoms caused by unruptured aneurysms at specific locations.

2.5 Anterior Cerebral Circulation Aneurysms

2.5.1 Intrapetrous Carotid Aneurysms

Aneurysms of the intrapetrous portion of the ICA are rare. Only 54 cases have been reported [63, 118, 145]. The intrapetrous section of the ICA extends from the skull base to the cavernous sinus. The artery initially ascends vertically in the bony carotid canal, turns anteromedially to run horizontally above the fibrocartilage which fills the foramen laceram in life and then turns upwards at the petrous apex to run forwards into the cavernous sinus. Aneurysms are usually fusiform, though pseudo-aneurysms [145] and saccular aneurysms [72] of the intrapetrous carotid artery have been described (Fig. 2.7). This section of the ICA is rarely affected by atherosclerosis and aneurysms commonly occur in young patients [63, 72]; the mean age of patients at the time of treatment was 30 years in the small series reported by Halbach et al. [72]. No specific cause can be defined in most patients, but in approximately 10% of patients aneurysms are due to trauma (either accidental or surgical) and in a further 10% occur in association with middle ear sepsis [72, 156]. Males and females are equally likely to be affected [156].

The majority of patients present with symptoms caused by the pressure effects of aneurysms on local structures. The commonest presenting symptoms are headache and hearing loss due to dysfunction of the eighth cranial nerve

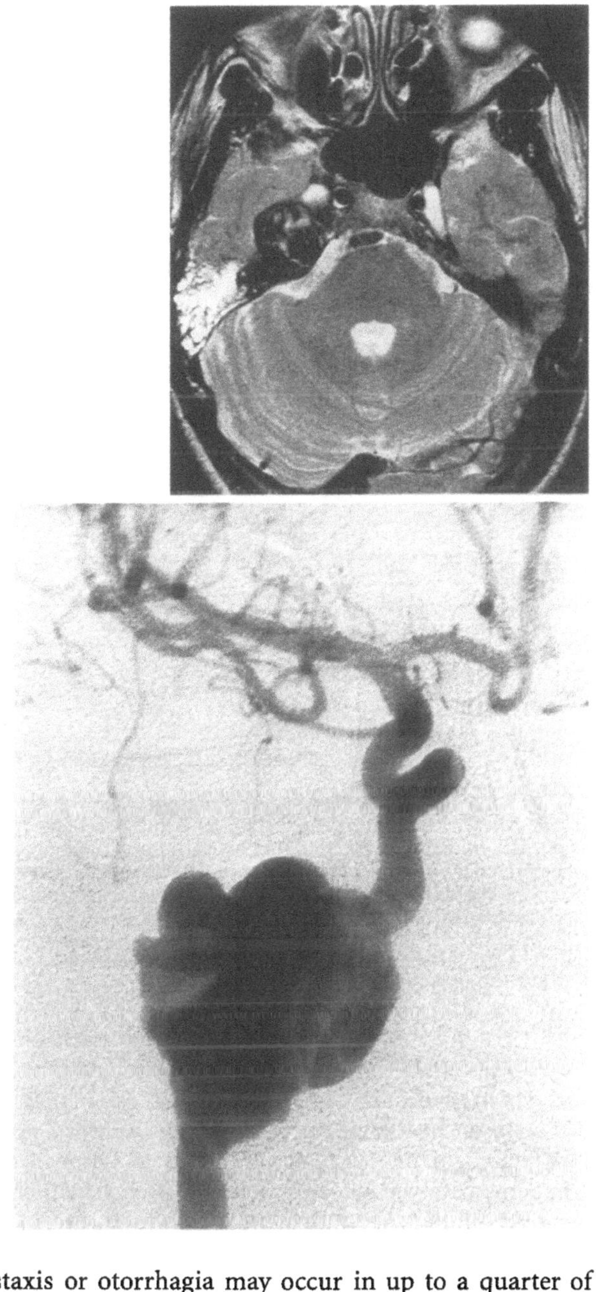

a

b

Fig. 2.7.
a Axial T2-weighted magnetic resonance imaging and b oblique frontal intra-arterial digital subtraction angiography showing a giant aneurysm of the intrapetrous right carotid artery. This patient presented complaining of deafness and was treated by balloon occlusion of the carotid artery. (Case previously reported by Goodman et al. [63])

[3]. Rupture causing epistaxis or otorrhagia may occur in up to a quarter of patients [3, 27] and neurological deficits due to migration of thromboemboli formed within the aneurysm sac have been described [72]. Expansion of the aneurysm causes bone erosion and may lead to the sac extending into the nasopharynx, middle ear or posterior fossa [118]. Aneurysms are usually large or giant at the time of presentation.

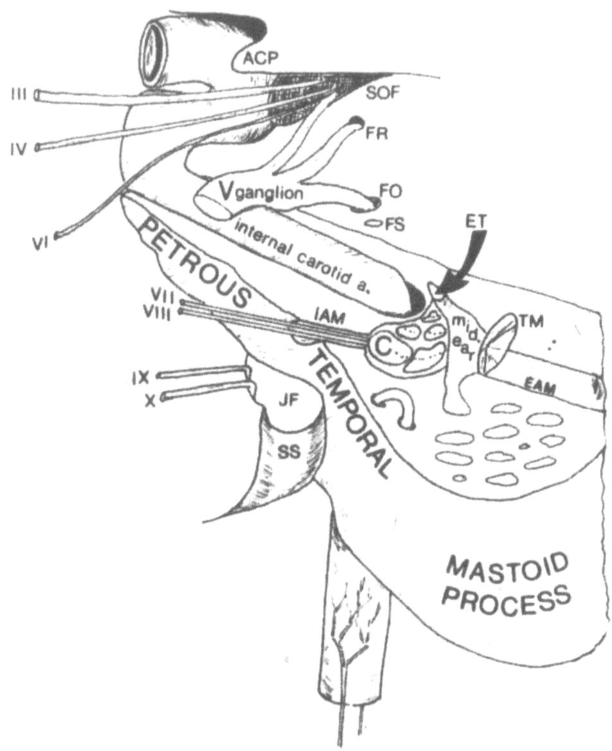

Fig. 2.8. Relationship of the intrapetrous internal carotid artery to adjacent structures. The artery lies (from proximal to distal) close to cranial nerves IX and X in the jugular fossa (*JF*), the middle ear and internal acoustic canal containing the VII and VIII cranial nerves before coursing under the trigeminal ganglion to reach the cavernous sinus and the VI, IV and III cranial nerves. *ACP*, anterior clinoid process; *C*, cochlear; *EAM*, external auditory meatus; *ET*, eustachian tube; *FO*, foramen ovale; *FR*, foramen rotundum; *FS*, foramen spinosum; *IAM*, internal auditory meatus; *JF*, jugular foramen; *SOF*, superior orbital fissure; *SS*, sigmoid sinus; *TM*, tympanic membrane. (From Rawlinson and Colquhoun [156])

The clinical effects of aneurysm enlargement vary according to the direction in which it occurs, thus: medial extension may cause diplopia due to third, fourth and sixth nerve compression; upward extension facial pain due to involvement of the fifth nerve and its ganglion; lateral extension hearing loss, hyperacusis, vertigo and pulsitile tinnitus; inferior extension, involvement of the ninth and tenth cranial nerves in the jugular canal or the seventh nerve in the hypoglossal canal (Fig. 2.8). Posterior extension into the cerebellar-pontine angle has been described [118] but, like postero-inferior growth, is relatively uncommon [156]. Patients may develop Horner's syndrome with a constricted pupil and ptosis due to involvement of the sympathetic nerve fibres to the orbit carried in the ICA sheath [156]. There is general consensus amongst the reports that hearing loss due to direct involvement of middle ear structures or Eustachian tube compression, together with headache, are the most common symptoms, affecting 40%–50% of patients [72, 145]. Erosion into the middle ear cleft may simulate a glomus tumour on inspection of the tympanic membrane and fatal biopsies have been described [21].

2.5.2 Cavernous Carotid Aneurysms

Aneurysms of the cavernous carotid artery represent approximately 5%–10% of all intracranial aneurysms [52, 175]. Most are attributed to atherosclerotic degeneration of the artery wall, but the cavernous portion of ICA is a relatively common site for traumatic or false aneurysms. They are extradural and their rupture usually causes cavernous carotid fistulas, though rarely aneurysms may extend intradurally and cause subarachnoid or subdural haemorrhage [175]. They are commoner in women [177] and present in late middle or old age – the increased frequency amongst women at this site accounting for much of the overall female preponderance in surgical series of intracranial aneurysms. This factor probably explains the near equal frequency of male and female patients in a series treated by coil embolisation [22], since cavernous carotid aneurysms are rarely suitable for endosaccular packing because of their wide necks.

Small aneurysms are often asymptomatic [49]. Patients with large or giant aneurysms present with pain, progressive cranial nerve palsies and thromboemboli. Pain is the commonest symptom and is rarely absent at some stage in the illness [108]. It is usually chronic and may be intractable and at times explosive. It is orbital, periorbital or facial, usually involving the orbital and/or maxillary divisions of the trigeminal nerve. Involvement of the intracavernous third to sixth cranial nerves causes diplopia, ptosis, blurring of vision due to accommodation paresis and facial pain or numbness. The onset of ophthalmoplegia is insidious and progressive but may be rapid and very occasionally sudden (presumably due to acute interruption of cranial nerve blood supply). Combined third, fourth and sixth nerve paresis occurs with larger aneurysms but isolated third or sixth nerve paresis may occur; an isolated fourth nerve paresis is extremely rare. Variations in symptoms and signs can be explained by the positions of the cranial nerves in the cavernous sinus. An isolated sixth nerve palsy occurs because the nerve lies closer to the intracavernous ICA than the third nerve; it is particularly liable to compression by aneurysms in the posterior part of the cavernous sinus because the sixth nerve enters the back of the sinus inferior to the third nerve (Fig. 2.9). In a truly illuminating paper, Jefferson described three syndromes determined by the position of aneurysms in the cavernous carotid; group A comprised patients with posteriorly situated aneurysms and symptoms in all divisions of the fifth nerve, together with sixth nerve palsy; group B were patients with aneurysms in the mid-portion of the sinus which affected the first and second divisions of the fifth nerve and to a varying degree the third, fourth and sixth nerves causing ophthalmoplegia; and group C consisted of aneurysms in the anterior part of the sinus where only the ophthal-

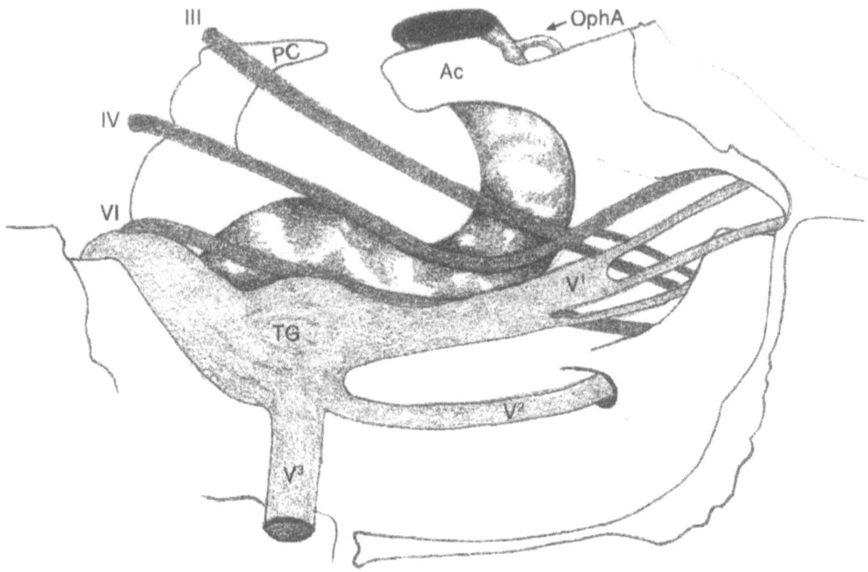

Fig. 2.9. The cavernous carotid artery and adjacent cranial nerves. Lateral view: the sixth and fifth cranial nerves are in close proximity to the proximal portion of the intracavernous internal carotid artery, whilst the third and fourth cranial nerves lie lateral to the distal portion. The third cranial nerve is shown dividing into superior and inferior branches and the ophthalmic division of the fifth cranial nerve V^1 into the frontal, lacrimal and nasociliary nerves as they run forward into the orbit via the superior orbital fissure. Posteriorly sited aneurysms are therefore more likely to cause pain due to compression of the trigeminal nerve, whilst anterior aneurysms cause ophthalmoplegia due to compression of the occulomotor nerves. *Ac*, anterior clinoid process; *PC*, posterior clinoid process; *OphA*, ophthalmic artery; *TG*, trigeminal ganglion; V^1 ophthalmic division; V^2, maxillary division; V^3, mandibular division

mic division of the fifth nerve was involved but all the oculomotor nerves were affected [92].

The larger the aneurysm the more complete the degree of resulting ophthalmoplegia due to compression of the oculomotor nerves [125]. Unlike third nerve compression due to PCoA aneurysms, involvement of the pupil may be relatively late because the pupillary parasympathetic fibres are carried in the inferior division. However, afferent fibres to levator superioris and superior rectus muscle are carried in the upper division of the third nerve and are commonly affected early. Likewise, sympathetic dysfunction (Horner's pupil and slight ptosis) may occur with sixth nerve compression because the sympathetic fibres are carried in the sixth nerve sheath for a short distance during its intracavernous course. Loss of facial or corneal sensation is a relatively late finding suggesting chronic compression.

Other features, which include visual loss due to compression of the optic nerve, and/or proptosis are due to forward expansion of larger aneurysms. Medial extension and erosion of the sphenoid bone may cause epistaxis if the aneurysm ruptures, while posterior expansion into the posterior fossa can cause compression of the seventh or eight cranial nerves and facial weakness or deafness. In Kupersmith et al.'s series the third nerve was affected in 82%, the sixth nerve in 71% and the fourth nerve in 47% of patients. Pain was the most common presenting feature and only a third of patients initially complained of diplopia [108].

2.5.3 Carotid-Ophthalmic Aneurysms

Intradural aneurysm arising from the ICA at or just above the ophthalmic artery origin are generally termed carotid-ophthalmic aneurysms (COA), though if large their point of origin may be difficult to define (see Chap. 6). They most commonly present with SAH but because of their proximity to the intracranial optic nerve, patients presenting with both ruptured or unruptured aneurysm commonly have signs of visual disturbance [220]. Carotid ophthalmic aneurysms represent 1.5%–8% of all intracranial aneurysms [169, 220], but a higher proportion of symptomatic unruptured aneurysms; 13% in the cooperative study [117]. They were bilateral in 20% of Drakes series [40] and are more common in women; the female preponderance being higher at this site than all others, except the cavernous carotid artery [117].

Aneurysm enlargement causes compression of the ipsilateral optic nerve, usually initially from its infero-lateral aspect (Fig. 2.10). Symptoms and signs are therefore more likely with larger aneurysms; 45% of aneurysms in Ferguson and Drake's series were over 12 mm in size at presentation [53]. Patients sometimes tolerate unilateral visual loss, only becoming aware of blindness and seeking medical advice when the other eye is affected. Symptoms include: pain (either orbital or more generalised headache); visual disturbances due to visual field loss or deterioration in visual acuity; pituitary

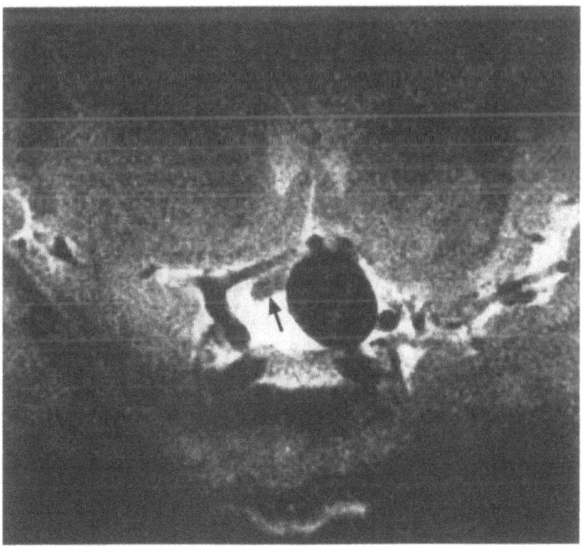

Fig. 2.10. Coronal T2-weighted magnetic resonance imaging through the chiasmatic cistern. The optic chiasm is displaced to the left (*arrow*) and the anterior cerebral arteries elevated by a large right carotid-ophthalmic aneurysm. This patient presented with visual disturbance and examination revealed an ipsilateral temporal quadrantanopia

dysfunction and non-specific symptoms due to thromboembolism. Optic nerve or chiasm compression causes unilateral or bilateral visual loss with an asymmetric pattern. An ipsilateral central scotoma is common with nasal or temporal quadrantanopia or hemianopia. If the aneurysm extends medially to involve the optic chiasm and compresses crossing fibres then a contralateral temporal field defect is present [53]. In Ferguson and Drake's series [53], ipsilateral scotoma was present in 78% of patients and in 44% of patients a field defect was present in the contralateral eye. Involvement of the chiasm and pituitary dysfunction may simulate a pituitary tumour, but investigation by MRI will differentiate blood flow in an aneurysm from pituitary macroadenoma. Hormonal disturbances associated with COA are variable, not well documented and usual resolve after treatment.

Impairment of visual acuity is associated with prolonged compression of the optic pathway. Visual loss is usually insidious and progressive but may be percipitous in the absence of SAH. The optic disc is pale and some degree of optic atrophy is common, even in patients presenting with SAH. In fact, evidence of chronic compression i.e., optic nerve atrophy, is rarely absent at presentation [108].

2.5.4 Distal Internal Carotid Artery Aneurysms

Aneurysms of the ICA distal to the ophthalmic artery are described by the nearest branch artery. Thus, aneurysms occur at: the origins of the superior hypophyseal, posterior communicating, anterior choroidal arteries and the ICA termination. Pressure effects caused by superior hypophyseal artery aneurysms may be difficult to distinguish from COA; both cause symptoms due to optic pathway compression. PCoA aneurysms arise at the level of the branch artery and only rarely from PCoA itself (so-called true PCoA aneurysms). Anterior choroidal artery (AChA) aneurysms are uncommon, representing only 1%–2% of all intracranial aneurysms in the cooperative study [161]. They rarely cause symptoms and signs unless large or giant and then these are similar to either PCoA or ICA termination aneurysms. ICA termination aneurysms represent approximately 4%–5% of intracranial aneurysms [161], though this is a relatively more frequent site for aneurysms in younger patients presenting with SAH [79].

The PCoA aneurysm is the commonest site for aneurysms of the supraclinoid ICA and comprised approximately 30% of a series of ruptured aneurysms [161] and 7%–16% of patients presenting with symptomatic unruptured aneurysms [5, 205]. Symptoms and signs are due to third cranial nerve compression causing oculomotor paresis as described above. In Raga's series of 42 patients with third nerve palsy due to intracranial aneurysms, 37 were due to PCoA aneurysms and 22 presented with evidence of rupture [153]. Symptomatic PCoA aneurysms are also commonly associated with pain in the first division of the fifth cranial nerve, which may precede the onset of ophthalmoplegia or SAH. Patients therefore complain of pain involving the forehead or orbit, diplopia, blurring of vision and ptosis. The oculomotor

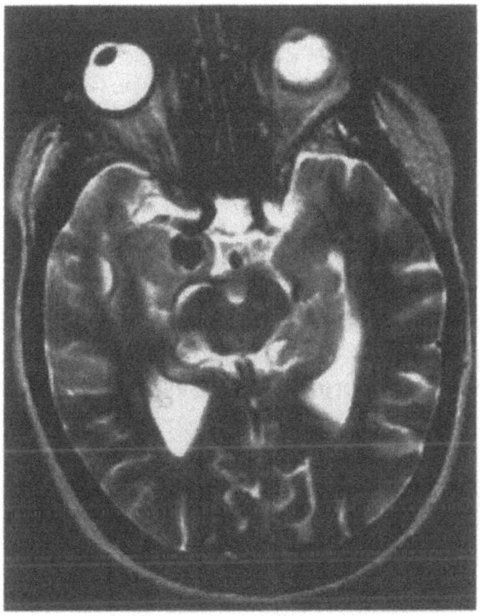

Fig. 2.11.
Axial T2-weighted magnetic resonance imaging at the level of the circle of Willis. There is an aneurysm of the terminal right internal carotid artery which projects posteriorly into the medial temporal lobe. This patient presented with complex partial seizures of recent onset

paresis characteristically involves the pupil, which is enlarged and poorly reactive to light. Early treatment improves the chances of third nerve recovery. Failure of complete resolution results in a characteristic misdirection syndrome, described by Gowers [64], due to aberrant regeneration of the nerve. Also called oculomotor synkinesis, this syndrome is associated, for instance, with a normal position of the upper eyelid in the neutral position and paradoxical elevation of the lid on adduction of the eye due to overaction of the levator when medial rectus is activated. Levator palprabrae superioris is usually the first muscle to recover from third nerve compression, followed in sequence by medial and lateral rectus, with superior rectus typically the last to recover. Full recovery rarely occurs if symptoms are present for more than 10 days [178].

Giant or large aneurysms of the distal ICA, i.e. at or close to the bifurcation, may cause headache, hemiparesis, visual disturbance, pituitary dysfunction or epilepsy. As with compression of the optic pathway by carotid-ophthalmic aneurysms, the resulting visual disturbance depends on the direction in which the aneurysm grows. The intracranial optic nerve, lateral chiasm or optic tract, together or individually, may be compressed. There is, therefore, a range of possible visual field deficits from ipsilateral scotoma and quadrantanopia if the optic nerve is involved, contralateral temporal quadrantanopia if the chiasm is affected and incongruous homonomous hemianopia if the optic tract is compressed. Compression of the pituitary stalk or hypothalamus may cause endocrine abnormalities, typically hypopituitarism [170] and pressure on the ipsilateral temporal lobe may cause partial complex seizures (Fig. 2.11). However, epilepsy due to local pressure effects is uncommon; amongst 380 patients with both ruptured and unruptured aneurysms referred to the Radcliffe Infirmary in Oxford for endovascular treatment between 1992 and 1996, only six presented with epilepsy. The aneurysms in these patients were large or giant in size and four were located at the ICA bifurcation. Other modes of presentation are with signs of ipsilateral hemispheric dysfunction due to thromboembolism causing stroke or non-specific progressive signs of an expanding cerebral tumour.

2.5.5 Anterior Cerebral Artery Aneurysms

Symptoms due to unruptured aneurysms occurring above the level of the circle of Willis are rare unless the aneurysm is of very large or giant proportions. Unruptured aneurysms of the ACA usually occur at or close to the anterior communicating artery and are found as commonly at this location as those at the MCA bifurcation (see Table 2.5). Rarely, giant aneurysms arising from the ACA proximal to the ACoA or from the pericallosal artery have been reported [61, 119]. Presenting symptoms include headache, visual disturbance, dementia and epilepsy. Visual disturbance is caused by compression of the anterior optic pathway and occurs in 28% of large or giant ACA aneurysms. It may be unilateral or bilateral [80]. If symptoms are bilateral visual loss is often asymmetric and occurs due to compression of the optic nerve or chiasm [45, 83]. Typically, compression of the chiasm causes bitemporal hemianopia. The contralateral eye is affected if the aneurysm expands across the midline away from its side of origin [31, 83]. Very large lesions which extend posteriorly may cause compression of the optic tract, pituitary stalk and hypothalamus. Symptoms of dementia result from frontal lobe compression and distortion of the anterior portion of the third or lateral ventricles may cause hydrocephalus.

2.5.6 Middle Cerebral Artery Aneurysms

The incidence of unruptured aneurysms of the MCA is approximately 20% (Table 2.5), though they represented 45% of Juvella et al.'s non-surgical series [96]. The MCA is a common site for incidental aneurysms and was found by Nehls et al. to be the least likely site of rupture in patients with multiple aneurysms [133]. In this study, 205 patients presenting with SAH were reviewed; 69 (33.5%) were found to have multiple aneurysms and, although the PCoA and MCA were the most common aneurysm locations, the presenting haemorrhage was more commonly due to rupture of ACA, the posterior inferior cerebellar artery (PICA) or BA termination aneurysms. The "probability of rupture" (calculated by dividing the number of ruptured aneurysms by the total number at individual sites) was 62% for ACA, compared with 27% for MCA aneurysms. Small aneurysms are rarely symptomatic and most unruptured aneurysms present when large or giant. Giant aneurysms most commonly occur on the ICA, but their relative frequency elsewhere in the anterior circulation is controversial. Hosobuchi [84], in a series of 84 giant aneurysms, reported that nine (11%) arose from ACA and only four (5%)

from the MCA, but others have found the MCA to be a more common site than the ACA [6].

Symptoms due to MCA aneurysms are typically headache, hemiparesis and epilepsy. Large lesions may present with progressive hemisphere dysfunction simulating a neoplasm such as speech or visual disturbances, motor weakness and non-specific mental disturbances. Hemiparesis may be caused by ischaemia secondary to local compression of middle cerebral branch arteries, as well as neural compression.

2.6 Posterior Cerebral Circulation Aneurysms

About 15% of unruptured aneurysms are found in the posterior circulation [102, 162, 205] (Table 2.5). They are more frequently reported in series of giant aneurysms, in which they account for 20%–30% of aneurysms [6, 84, 149, 182]. It has been suggested that because they present only after massive enlargement they are less likely to rupture [59]. Aneurysms of the posterior circulation are in close proximity to cranial nerves and the brain stem, so their enlargement is likely to cause symptomatic neural compression.

2.6.1 Distal Basilar Artery Aneurysms

Presenting symptoms and signs due to unruptured posterior circulation aneurysms are highly variable. Aneurysms of the terminal basilar artery cause signs due to progressive or intermittent compression of the mesencephalon, pons, oculomotor or abducens nerves (Fig. 2.12). Larger lesions may compress the thalamus, medial temporal lobes and optic tracts, thus simulating a brain stem mass lesion. The large number of eloquent areas that may be affected by distal basilar aneurysms account for the wide variability in clinical presentations.

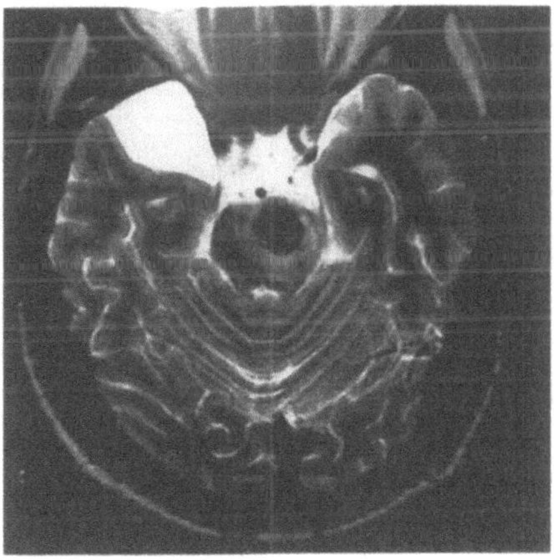

Fig. 2.12. Axial T2-weighted magnetic resonance imaging at the level of the mesencephalon. A large aneurysm of the basilar artery termination is compressing the brain stem. On this image, the aneurysm appears embedded in the left side of the mesencephalon. It was the cause of right hemiplegia. An arachnoid cyst is present in the right middle cranial fossa

The BA termination is the commonest site for all aneurysms in the posterior fossa. Small aneurysms arising at the termination of the distal BA between the posterior cerebral (PCA) and superior cerebellar artery (SCA) may cause unilateral third nerve paresis and an isolated fourth nerve palsy has been described [2]. Bilateral third nerve palsies may occur due to direct compression or disruption of small arteries supplying the nerve or its nuclei. Concurrent compression of the adjacent cerebral peduncle causes ipsilateral oculomotor palsy and contralateral hemiparesis (Weber's syndrome) [204].

Anterior aneurysm growth may affect the optic chiasm and floor of the third ventricle to simulate growth of a pituitary tumour by causing bitemporal hemianopia. Patients present with signs of hydrocephalus, dementia, gait disturbances and memory deficits or complex partial seizures [112, 194].

Ocular findings are common; they affected 50% of patients with posterior fossa aneurysms reported by McKinna [124]. Upward and backward extension will cause midbrain compression and gaze disturbances such as skew deviation, internuclear ophthalmoplegia, paresis of upward gaze (Parinaud's syndrome) or horizontal gaze paresis [107, 179, 194]. Visual field defects may result from distal thromboemboli to the PCA causing homonymous hemianopia. Nystagmus can be due to midbrain or pontine compression. Horizontal, rotatory or upbeat nystagmus may occur in primary gaze, upbeat nystagmus on upward gaze and horizontal or rotatory nystagmus on lateral gaze [124]. Symptoms due to compression of the mesencephalon, posterior thalamus and medial temporal lobes may simulate the "top of the basilar syndrome" described in thromboembolic disease [24, 126].

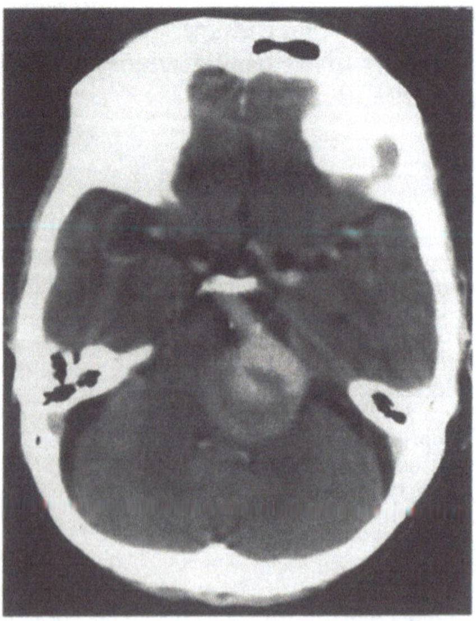

a

Fig. 2.13.
a Axial enhanced computed tomograph at the level of the pons. The brain stem is deformed and the fourth ventricle compressed by a large basilar artery aneurysm

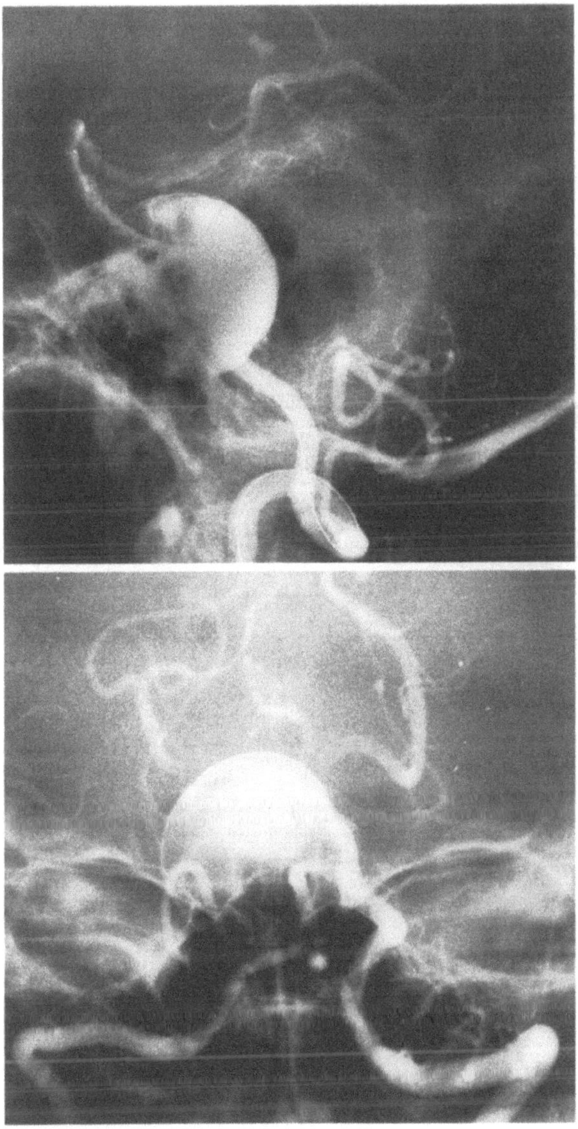

b

c

Fig. 2.13.
b Lateral and **c** frontal angiograms showing an aneurysm of the basilar artery trunk. This patient presented with progressive symptoms and signs of brain stem compression. Contrast filling of the aneurysm appears incomplete due to slow blood flow and poor contrast mixing within the sac

2.6.2
Vertebral and Proximal Basilar Artery Aneurysms

Aneurysms of the more proximal BA and intracranial vertebral artery (VA) cause symptoms and signs due to dysfunction of the fifth to twelfth cranial nerves, the pons and medulla oblongata (Fig. 2.13). The mechanism is usually direct compression secondary to aneurysm growth and the chronic effects of systolic pulsation (Fig. 2.12). Patients suffer headache, facial pain, diplopia, vertigo, tinnitus, dysarthria and dysphasia. Mid basilar aneurysms cause symptoms and signs due to involvement of the fifth to eighth cranial nerves which simulate tumours in the cerebellar-pontine angle. Aneurysms at the vertebro-basilar junction or PICA origin cause progressive lower cranial nerve involvement with unilateral or bilateral palatal and lingual paralysis or a partial lateral medullary (Wallenberg's) syndrome. Limb ataxia and gait disturbances with crossed hemiparesis occur due to compression of corticospinal and cerebellar outflow pathways at both levels [162].

Distal aneurysms of the anterior inferior cerebellar artery (AICA), the PICA, SCA or PCA are rare and most commonly present following rupture. Rupture of posterior fossa aneurysms is more often associated with sudden death than supra-tentorial aneurysms presumably because of acute brain stem compression or hydrocephalus may result if rupture occurs directly into the fourth ventricle [164]. Despite the proximity of the PICA origin to the ninth to twelfth cranial nerves as they emerge from the lateral medulla oblongata (see Chapter 6, Fig. 6.20), unilateral palsies are uncommon and unruptured aneurysms may enlarge to cause compression of the fourth ventricle and hydrocephalus before they are diagnosed [10].

References

1. Adams HP, Jergenson DD, Kassell NF, Sahs AL (1980) Pitfalls in the recongition of SAH. JAMA 244:794–796
2. Agostinis C, Caverni L, Moschini L et al (1992) Paralysis of fourth cranial nerve due to superior-cerebellar artery aneurysm. Neurology 42:457–458
3. Anderson RD, Liebeskind A, Schechter M et al (1972) Aneurysms of the internal carotid artery in the carotid canal of the petrous temporal bone. Radiology 102:639–642
4. Anderson SI, Housley AM, Jones PA et al (1993) Glasgow Outcome Score an inter-rater reliability study. Brain Injury 7:309–317
5. Asari S, Takashi O (1993) Natural history and risk factors of unruptured cerebral aneurysms. Clin Neurol Neurosurg 95:205–214
6. Atkinson JLD, Piepgras DG (1994) Giant aneurysms Supratentorial. In: Carter LP, Spetzler RF (eds) Neurovascular surgery. McGraw-Hill, New York, pp 815–828
7. Bailes JE, Spetzler RF, Hadley MN, Baldwin HZ (1990) Management morbidity and mortality of poor-grade aneurysm patients. J Neurosurg 72:559–566
8. Bartholow R (1872) Aneurisms of the arteries at the base of the brain; their symptomatology, diagnosis and treatment. Am J Med Sci 64:373
9. Barton E, Tudor J (1982) Subdural haematomas in association with intracranial aneurysms. Neuroradiology 23:157–160
10. Batjer HH, Kopitnik A, Pardy PD, Samson DS (1994) Vertebral and PICA aneurysms. In: Carter LP, Spetzler RF (eds) Neurovascular surgery. McGraw-Hill, New York, pp 763–765
11. Biumi F (1778) Observationes anatomicae. Observatio V. In: Sandifort E (ed) Thesaurus dissertationum, vol 3. Milan, S&J Luchtmans (reprinted 1778), pp 373–379
12. Blackhall L (1813) Observations on the nature and cure of dropsies. Longman, London, p 126
13. Blane G (1880) History of cases of diseases in the brain. Transactions of a Society for the Improvement of Medical and Chiruriginal Knowledge, vol 2, p 192
14. Bonita R, Thompson S (1985) Subarachnoid hemorrhage: epidemiology, diagnosis, management and outcome. Stroke 4:591–594
15. Botterell EH, Lougheed WM, Scott JN, Vandewater SL (1956) Hypothermia, and interruption of carotid, or carotid and vertebral circulation, in the surgical management of intracranial aneurysms. J Neurosurg 13:1–42

16. Bramford JM, Sandercock PAG, Warlow CP, Slattery J (1989) Interobserver agreement for the assessment handicap in stroke patients (letter to editor). Stroke 20:828
17. Bramwell B (1886) Clinical and pathological memoranda illustrated. Edinb Med J 32:97–108
18. Brewis M, Poskanzer DC, Rolland C, Miller H (1966) Neurological disease in an English city. Acta Neurol Scand 42 [Suppl 24]:1–89
19. Brinton W (1850) Report on cases of cerebral aneurysms. Trans Pathol Soc Lond 3:47–49
20. Bull J (1962) A short history of intracranial aneurysms. Lond Clin Med J 3:47–61
21. Busby DR, Slemmons DH, Miller TF (1968) Fatal spistaxis via carotid aneurysm and eustachian tube. Arch Otolaryngol 87:293–296
22. Byrne JV, Adams CBT, Kerr RSC, Molyneux AJ (1995) Endosaccular treatment of inoperable intracranial aneurysms with platinum coils. Br J Neurosurg 9:585–592
23. Cabal RJ, King TT, Scott DF (1976) Epilepsy after two different neurosurgical approaches to the treatment of ruptured intracranial aneurysms. J Neurol Neurosurg Psychiatr 39:1052–1056
24. Caplan LR (1980) Top of the basilar syndrome selected clinical aspects. Neurology 30:72–79
25. Chokyu M (1975) An experimental study of cerebral vasospasm, especially on spasmogenic factors in red blood cells. J Osaka City Med Centre 24:211–221
26. Collier J, Spontaneous SAH (1922) In: Price FW (ed) A textbook of the practice of medicine. Oxford University Press, London, p 1351
27. Constantino PD, Russell E, Reisch Z et al (1991) Ruptured petrous carotid aneurysm presenting with otorrhagia and epistaxis. Am J Otol 12:378–383
28. Crevits L, De Reuck J, Eecken VH (1975) Paralytic pontine exotropia in subarachnoid haemorrhage. Clin Neurol Neurosurg 78:269–276
29. Crompton MR (1962) Intracerebral haematoma complicating ruptured berry aneurysms. J Neurol Neurosurg Psychiatry 25:378–386
30. Crompton MR (1963) Hypothalamic lesions following the rupture of cerebral berry aneurysms. Brain 86:301–304
31. Cullen JF, Haining WM, Crombie AL (1966) Cerebral aneurysms presenting with visual field defects. Br J Ophthalmol 50:251–256
32. Day JW, Raskin NH (1986) Thunderclap headache: symptom of unruptured cerebral aneurysm. Lancet 2:1247–1248
33. Dell S (1982) Asymptomatic cerebral aneurysm. Assessment of its risk of rupture. Neurosurgery 10:162–166
34. Diringer MN, Lim JS, Kirsch JR, Hanley DR (1991) Suprasellar and intraventricular blood predict elevated plasma atrial natriuretic factor in SAH. Stroke 22:577–581
35. Dòczi T, Bende J, Huszka E et al (1981) Syndrome of inappropriate secretion of antidiuretic hormone after subarachnoid hemorrhage. Neurosurgery 4:394–396
36. Dorsch NWC (1995) Cerebral arterial spasm – a clinical review. Br J Neurosurg 9:403–412
37. Dorsch NWC, King MT (1994) A review of cerebral vasopasm in aneurysmal subarachnoid haemorrhage. I. Incidence and effects. J Clin Neurol 1:19–26
38. Doshi R, Neil-Dwyer G (1980) A cinicopathological study of patients following a subarachnoid hemorrhage. J Neurosurg 52:295–301
39. Dott N (1933) Intracranial aneurysms. Cerebral arterioradiography: surgical treatment. Trans Med Chir Soc Edinb 40:219–236
40. Drake CG, Vanderlinden RG, Amacher AL (1968) Carotid-ophthalmic aneurysms. J Neurosurg 29:24–31
41. Drake CG, Hunt WE, Sano K et al (1988) Report of World Federation of Neurological Surgeons Committee on a universal subarachnoid hemorrhage grading scale. J Neurosurg 68:985–986
42. du Boulay GH (1963) Distribution of spasm in the intracranial arteries after subarachnoid haemorrhage. Acta Radiol (Diagn) 1:256–266
43. du Boulay GH, Marshall J, Merory J, Symon L (1980) The location of spasm and it's relationa to symptoms. In: Wilkins RH (ed) Cerebral arterial spasm. Williams and Wilkins, Baltimore, pp 394–396
44. Duffy G (1983) The "warning leak" in spontaneous subarachnoid haemorrhage. Med J Aust 1:514–516
45. Durston JHJ, Parsons-Smith BG (1970) Blindness due to aneurysms of anterior communicating artery. With recovery after carotid ligation. Br J Ophthalmol 54:170–176
46. Echlin FA (1965) Spasm of basilar and vertebral arteries caused by experimental subarachnoid haemorrhage. J Neurosurg 23:1–11

47. Ecker A, Riemenschneider PA (1951) Arteriographic demonstration of spasm of the intracranial arteries with special reference to saccular arterial aneurysms. J Neurosurg 8:660–667
48. Edwards DH, Byrne JV, Griffiths TM (1992) The effect of chronic subarachnoid hemorrhage on basal endothelium-derived relaxing factor activity in intrathecal cerebral arteries. J Neurosurg 76:830–837
49. Eskesen V, Rosenøren J, Schmidt K et al (1987) Clinical features and outcome in 48 patients with unruptured intracranial saccular aneurysms: a prospective consecutive study. Br J Neurosurg 1:47–52
50. Faraci FM, Brian JE (1994) Nitric oxide and the cerebral circulation. Stroke 25:692–703
51. Fearnsides EG (1916) Intracranial aneurysms. Brain 39:224–296
52. Fergurson GG (1989) Intracranial arterial aneurysms – a surgical perspective. In: Vinken PJ, Bruyn GW, Klawans HL (eds) Handbook of clinical neurology, vol II. ElsevierScience, New York, pp 41–87
53. Ferguson G, Drake CG (1981) Carotid-ophthalmic aneurysms visual abnormalities in 32 patients and the results of treatment. Surg Neurol 16:1–8
54. Findlay JM (ed) (1993) Cerebral vasospasm. Proceedings of the V International Conference on Cerebral Vasospasm, Edmonton. Elsevier, Amsterdam
55. Fisher CM (1975) Clinical syndrome in cerebral thrombosis, hypertive hemorrhage and ruptured saccular aneurysm. Clin Neurosurg 22:117–121
56. Fisher CM, Kistler JP, Davies JM (1980) Relation of cerebral vasospasm to subarachnoid haemorrhage, visualised by computerised tomographic scanning. J Neurosurg 6:1–9
57. Fogelholm R (1981) Subarachnoid hemorrhage in Middle-Finland: incidence, early diagnosis and indications for neurosurgical treatment. Stroke 3:296–301
58. Forbes G, Fox AI, Huston J et al (1996) Interobserver variability in angiographic measurement and morphologic characterization of intracranial aneurysms report from the international study of unruptured intracranial aneurysms. AJNR 17:1407–1415
59. Fox JL (1983) Intracranial aneurysms, vol 1. Springer, Berlin Heidelberg New York
60. Froin G (1904) Les hemorragies sous-arachnoidiennes et le mecanisme de l'hematolyse en general. Thèse de Paris, Steinher, Paris
61. Gerwitz RJ, Awad IA (1993) Giant aneurysms of the proximal anterior cerebral artery. Report of three cases. Neurosurgery 33:120–124
62. Gintrac E (1869) Traite theorique et pratique de l'appareil nerveux. Germer-Bailliere, Paris
63. Goodman TR, Renowden S, Byrne JV (1996) Petrous internal carotid artery aneurysm an unusual cause of Rustacian tube dysfunction. Clin Radiol 51:658–660
64. Gowers W (1879) The movements of the eyelids. Med Chir Trans 62:429–449
65. Graf C (1971) Prognosis for patients with non-surgically treated aneurysms. Analysis of the co-operative study of intracranial aneurysms and subarachnoid hemorrhage. J Neurosurg 35:438–443
66. Graff-Radford NR, Torner J, Adams HP, Kassell NF (1989) Factors associated with hydrocephalus after subarachnoid hemorrhage. Arch Neurol 46:744–752
67. Green KA, Marciano FF, Dickman CA et al (1995) Anterior communication artery aneurysm paraparesis syndrome clinical manifestations and pathologic correlates. Neurology 45:45–50
68. Green WR, Hackett ER, Schlezinger NS (1964) Neuro-ophthalmologic evaluation of oculomotor nerve paralysis. Arch Ophthalmol 72:154–167
69. Grote E, Hassler W (1988) The critical first minute after SAH. Neurosurgery 22:654–661
70. Gudmunsson G (1973) Primary subarachnoid hemorrhage in Iceland. Stroke 4:764–767
71. Gull W (1859) Cases of aneurysms of the cerebral vessels. Guy's Hosp Rep 3rd Ser 5:281–304
72. Halbach VV, Higashida RT, Hieshima GB et al (1990) Aneurysms of the petrous portion of the internal carotid artery results of treatment with endovascular or surgical occlusion. AJNR 11:253–257
73. Hall AJ (1929) Lecture on three cases of spontaneous subarachnoid haemorrhage with special reference to the occurrence of massive albuminuria and Korsakoff's syndrome. Br Med J 1:1025–1139
74. Hansan D, Schonck RSM, Arezaat CJJ et al (1993) Epileptic seizures after subarachnoid hemorrhage. Ann Neurol 33:286–291

75. Hart RG, Byer JA, Slaughter JR et al (1981) Occurrence and implications of seizures in subarachnoid hemorrhage due to ruptured intracranial aneurysms. Neurosurgery 8:417–421
76. Hasan D, Vermeulen M, Wijdicks EFM et al (1989) Management problems in acute hydrocephalus after subarachnoid hemorrhage. Stroke 20:747–753
77. Hatake K, Wakabayashi I, Kakishita E, Hishida S (1992) Impairment of endothelium-dependent relaxation in human basilar artery after subarachnoid hemorrhage. Stroke 23:1111–1117
78. Hayem G (1872) Les hemorragies intra-arachnoidiennes. Thèse de Paris, Delahave, Paris
79. Heiskanen O (1989) Ruptured intracranial arterial aneurysms of children and adolescents. Surgical and total management results. Childs Nerv Syst 5:66–70
80. Henderson JW (1955) Intracranial arterial aneurysms. A study of 119 cases, with special reference to the ocular findings. Trans Am Ophthalmol Soc 53:349–462
81. Hijdra A, Vermeulen M, van Gijn J, van Creval H (1987) Rerupture of intracranial aneurysms. A clinicoanatomic study. J Neurosurg 67:29–33
82. Hillman J, Von Essen C, Lesniewski W, Johansson I (1988) Significance of "ultra-early" rebleeding in subarachnoid hemorrhage. J Neurosurg 68:901–907
83. Hojer-Pederson E, Haase J (1981) Giant anterior communicating artery aneurysm with bitemporal hemianopia case report. Neurosurgery 8:703–706
84. Hosobuchi Y (1985) Giant intracranial aneurysms. In: Wilkins RH, Rengachary SS (eds) Neurosurgery. McGraw-Hill, New York, pp 1404–1414
85. Hounsfield GN (1973) Computerised transverse axial scanning (tomography). I. Description of system. BJR 46:1016–1022
86. Hunt WE, Hess RM (1968) Surgical risk as related to time of intervention in the repair of intracranial aneurysm. J Neurosurg 28:14–19
87. Hunt WE, Kosnik EJ (1974) Timing and pre-operative care in intracranial aneurysm surgery. Cong Neurol Surg 21:79–80
88. Hyland HH, Barnett HJM (1954) The pathogenesis of cranial nerve palsies associated with intracranial aneurysms. Proc R Soc Med 47:141–146
89. Inagawara T, Ishikawa S, Aoki H et al (1988) Aneurysmal subarachnoid hemorrhage in Izumo city and Shimane prefecture of Japan. Incidence. Stroke 19:170–175
90. Inawara T, Kamiya K, Ogasawara H, Yano T (1987) Rebleeding of ruptured intracranial aneurysms in the acute stage. Surg Neurol 28:93–99
91. Jagger J, Torner JC, Kassell NF (1989) Neurological assessment of subarachnoid hemorrhage in a large patients series. Surg Neurol 32:327–333
92. Jefferson G (1938) On the saccular aneurysms of the internal carotid artery in the cavernous sinus. Br J Surg 26:267–302
93. Jennett B, Bond M (1975) Assessment of outcome after severe brain damage: a practical scale. Lancet 1:480–484
94. Joensen P (1984) Subarachnoid hemorrhage in an isolated population. Incidence on the Faroes during the period 1962–1975. Stroke 15:438–440
95. Joynt RJ, Afifi A, Harrison J (1965) Hyponatremia in subarachnoid hemorrhage. Arch Neurol 13:633–638
96. Juvela S, Porras M, Heiskanen O (1993) Natural history of unruptured intracranial aneurysms: a long-term follow-up study. J Neurosurg 79:174–182
97. Kassel NF, Torner JC (1983) Aneurysmal rebleeding: a preliminary report from the Cooperative Aneurysm Study. Neurosurgery 13:479–481
98. Kassell NF, Kongable GL, Torner JC et al (1985) Delay in referral of patients with ruptured aneurysms to neurosurgical attention. Stroke 16:587–590
99. Kassel NF, Torner JC, Haley C, Jane JA et al (1990) The international cooperative study on the timing of aneurysm surgery. Part 1: overall management results. J Neurosurg 73:18–36
100. Kassel NF, Torner JC, Jane JA et al (1990) The international cooperative study on the timing of aneurysm surgery. Part 2: surgical results. J Neurosurg 73:37–47
101. Kasuya H, Weir B, White et al (1993) Mechanism of oxyhemoglobin induced release of endothelin-1 from cultured vascular endothelial cells and smooth muscle cells. J Neurosurg 79:892–898
102. Khanna RK, Malik GM, Qureshi N (1996) Predicting outcome following surgical treatment of unruptured intracranial aneurysms: a proposed grading system. J Neurosurg 84:49–54

103. Kissel JT, Burde RM, Klingele TG, Zeiger HE (1983) Pupil-sparing oculomotor palsies with internal carotid-posterior communicating artery aneurysms. Ann Neurol 13:149–154
104. Kristensen M (1983) Increased incidence of bleeding intracranial aneurysms in Greenlandic Eskimos. Acta Neurochir (Wien) 67:37–43
105. Kiyohara Y, Ueda K, Hasan Y et al (1989) Incidence and prognosis of subarachnoid hemorrhage in a Japanese rural community. Stroke 20:1150–1155
106. Kodamo N, Mizoi K, Sakurari J, Suzuki J (1980) Incidence and onset of vasopasm. In: Wilkins RH (ed) Cerebral arterial spasm. Williams and Wilkins, Baltimore, pp 361–365
107. Koga H, Mori K, Kawano T et al (1983) Parinaud's syndrome in hydrocephalus due to a basilar artery aneurysm. Surg Neurol 19:548–553
108. Kupersmith MJ, Berenstein A, Choi IS et al (1984) Percutaneous transvascular treatment of giant carotid aneurysms neuro-ophthalmologic findings. Neurology 34:328–335
109. Kupersmith MJ (1993) Aneurysms involving the motor and sensory visual pathway. In: Kupersmith MJ (ed) Neurovascular neuro-ophthalmology. Springer, Berlin Heidelberg New York, pp 239–299
110. Leblanc R (1987) The minor leak preceding subarachnoid haemorrhage. J Neurosurg 66:35–39
111. Leblanc R, Winfield JA (1984) The warning leak in subarachnoid haemorrhage and the importance of its early diagnosis. Can Med Assoc J 131:1235–1236
112. Leibrock LG, Bennett DR, Bloch S (1983) Complex partial seizures associated with unruptured thrombosed basilar apex aneurysm. Surg Neurol 19:17–20
113. Lindquist G, Norlen G (1996) Korsakoff's syndrome after operation on ruptured aneurysm of anterior communicating artery. Acta Psychiatr Scand 42:24–34
114. Lindsay KW, Teasdale G, Knill-Jones RP, Murray L (1982) Observer variablitity in grading patients with subarachnoid hemorrhage. J Neurosurg 56:628–633
115. Lindsay KW, Teasdale GM, Knill-Jones RP (1983) Observer variablitity in assessing the clinical features of subarachnoid hemorrhage. J Neurosurg 58:57–62
116. Ljunggren B, Sαveland H, Brandt L, Zygmunt S (1985) Early operation and overall outcome in aneurysmal subarachnoid hemorrhage. J Neurosurg 62:547–551
117. Locksley HB (1966) Report on the cooperative study of intracranial aneurysms and subarachnoid hemorrhage, section 5, part 1. Natural history of subarachnoid hemorrhage, intracranial aneurysms, and arteriovenous malformations. J Neurosurg 25:219–239
118. Love MHS, Bell KE (1996) Giant aneurysm of the intrapetrous carotid artery presenting as a cerebellopontine angle mass. Clin Radiol 51:587–588
119. Maiuri F, Corriero G, D'Amico L, Simonetti L (1990) Giant aneurysm of the pericallosal artery. Neurosurgery 26:703–706
120. Manschot WA (1944) The fundus oculi in subarachnoid haemorrhage. Acta Ophthamol 22:281–299
121. Marion DW, Segal R, Thompson ME (1986) SAH and the heart. Neurosurgery 18:101–106
122. Martin W, Villani GM, Jothianandan D, Furchgott RF (1985) Selective blockage of endothelium-dependent and glyceryl trinitrate-induced relaxation by hemoglobin and methylene blue in the rabbit aorta. J Pharmacol Exp Ther 232:708–716
123. Maurice-Williams RS (1982) Ruptured intracranial aneurysms has the incidence of early rebleeding been over-estimated. J Neurol Neurosurg Psychiatry 45:774–779
124. McKinna AJ (1983) Eye findings in 611 cases of posterior fossa aneurysms. Their diagnostic and prognostic value. Can J Ophthalmol 18:3–6
125. Meadows SP (1959) Intracavernous aneurysms of the internal carotid artery. Their clinical features and natural history. Arch Ophthalmol 62:566–579
126. Mehler MF (1988) The neuroophthalmologic septrum of the rostral basilar artery syndrome. Arch Neurol 45:966–971
127. Mizukami M, Takemae T, Tazawa T, Kawase T, Matsuzaki T (1980) Value of computed tomography in the prediction of cerebral vasospasm after aneurysmal rupture. Neurosurgery 7:583–586
128. Mohr G, Ferguson G, Khan M et al (1983) Intraventricular hemorrhage from ruptured aneurysms. Retrospective analysis of 91 cases. J Neurosurg 58:482–487
129. Moniz E (1927) L'encephalographie arterielle, son importance dans la localisation des tumeurs cerebrales. Rev Neurol 2:72–90

130. Moniz E (1933) Aneurisme intra-craniem de la carotid interne droit rendu visible pur l'arteriographie cerebrale. Rev Oto Neuro Ophthal 11:746–748
131. Morgagni JB (1769) De sedibus et causis morborum per anatomen indagatis, book 1, letters 3 and 4. Venetis, ex typog. Remodiniana. [Translated by Alexander B (1960) The seats and causes of diseases investigated by anatomy. Hafner, New York, pp 42–43, 77–78]
132. Muller PJ, Deck JHN (1974) Intraocular and optic nerve sheath hemorrhage in cases of sudden intracranial hypertension. J Neurosurg 41:160–166
133. Nehls DG, Flom RA, Carter LP, Spetzler RF (1985) Multiple intracranial aneurysms determining the site of rupture. J Neurosurg 63:342–348
134. Nelson PB, Seif BM, Maroon JC, Robinson AG (1981) Hyponatraemia in intracranial disease, prehaps not the syndrome of inappropriate secretion of antidiuretic hormone (SIADH). J Neurosurg 55:938–941
135. Nelson PB, Seif SM, Gutal J, Robinson A (1984) Hyponatremia and natriuresis following subarachnoid hemorrhage in a monkey model. J Neurosurg 60:233–237
136. Nibbelink BW, Torner JC, Henderson WC (1977) Intracranial aneurysm and SAH. A report on a radomised treatment study. Stroke 8:200–218
137. Nishioka H (1916) Evaluation of the conservative management of ruptured intracranial aneurysm. J Neurosurg 25:574–592
138. Nornes H (1973) The role of intracranial pressure in the arrest of hemorrhage in patients with ruptured intracranial aneurysm. J Neurosurg 39:226–234
139. Öhman J (1990) Hypertension as a risk factor for epilepsy after aneurysmal subarachnoid hemorrhage and surgery. Neurosurgery 27:578–581
140. Okawara SH (1973) Warning signs prior to rupture of an intracranial aneurysm. J Neurosurg 38:575–580
141. Osaka K (1977) Prolonged vasopasm produced by the breakdown products of erythrocytes. J Neurosurg 47:403–411
142. Osler W (1877) Aneurism of second bifurcation of the right middle cerebral artery: rupture: extrasation of blood into the Sylvian fissure and laceration of substance of the temporo-sphenoidal lobe: death in 36 hours. Clin Pathol Rep Montreal Hosp 1:30
143. Ozaki N, Mullan S (1979) Possible role of the erythrocyte in causing prolonged cerebral vasospasm. J Neurosurg 51:773–778
144. Pakarinen S (1967) Incidence, aetiology and prognosis of primary subarachnoid haemorrhage. Acta Neurol Scand [Suppl] 29:1–128
145. Papazian M, Pararella M, Hames E, Frisk I (1993) Aneurysms of the temporal bone. Ear Nose Throat J 72:474–484
146. Park BE (1979) Spontaneous subarachnoid hemorrhage complicated by communicating hydrocephalus. Epsilon amino-caproic acid as a possible predisposing factor. Surg Neurol 11:73–80
147. Pfausler B, Belcl R, Metzler R et al (1996) Terson's syndrome in spontaneous subarachnoid hemorrhage: a prospective study in 60 consecutive patients. J Neurosurg 85:392–394
148. Philips LH, Whisnant JP, O'Fallon WM, Sundt TM Jr (1980) The unchanging pattern of subarachnoid haemorrhage in a community. Neurology 30:1034–1040
149. Pla HW, Zierski J (1982) Giant cerebral aneurysms. Neurosurg Rev 5:117–148
150. Piepgras DG (1989) Management of incidental intracranial aneurysms. Clin Neurosurg 35:511–518
151. Pool J (1958) Cerebral vasopasm. N Engl J Med 259:1259–1264
152. Quincke H (1891) Die Lumbarpunktion des Hydrocephalus. Berlin Klin Wochenschr 28:929–965
153. Raga IA (1972) Aneurysm induced third nerve palsy. J Neurosurg 36:548–551
154. Rajshekhar V, Harbough RE (1992) Results of routine ventriculostomy with external drainage for acute hydrocephalus following subarachnoid hemorrhage. Acta Neurochir (Wien) 115:8–14
155. Raps EC, Rogers JD, Galetta SL et al (1993) The clinical spectrum of unruptured intracranial aneurysms. Arch Neurol 50:265–268
156. Rawlinson J, Colquhoun IR (1990) Aneurysms involving the intrapetrous internal carotid artery a rare cause of Horner's syndrome. Br J Radiol 63:69–72
157. Reunanen A, Aho K, Aromaa A, Knekt P (1986) Incidence of stroke in a Finnish prospective population study. Stroke 17:675–681
158. Robertson EG (1949) Cerebral lesions due to intracranial aneurysms. Brain 72:150–185

159. Rose FC, Sarner M (1965) Epilepsy after ruptured intracranial aneurysm. Br Med J 1:18–21
160. Rosenfeld JV, Barnett GH, Sila CA et al (1989) The effect of SAH on blood and CSF atrial natriuretic factor. J Neurosurg 71:32–37
161. Sahs AL, Perett GE, Lockley HB, Nishioka H (1966) Intracranial aneurysms and SAH. A co-operative study. Lippincott, Philadelphia
162. Salcman M, Rigamonti D, Namaguchi Y, Sadato N (1990) Aneurysms of the posterior inferior cerebellar artery-vertebral artery complex- variations on a theme. Neurosurgery 27:12–21
163. Sano K, Takakura K, Kassell NF, Sasaki T (eds) (1990) Cerebral vasopasm. Proceedings of the IVth international conference on cerebral vasospasm, Tokyo, 1990. University of Tokyo Press, Tokyo
164. Schievink WI, Wijdicks EFM, Parisi JE et al (1995) Sudden death from aneurysm subarachnoid hemorrhage. Neurology 45:871–874
165. Schultz PN, Sobol WM, Weingeist TA (1991) Long-term visual outcome in Terson syndrome. Ophthalmology 98:1814–1819
166. Seiler RW, Grolimund P, Aaslid R et al (1986) Cerebral vasospasm evaluated by transcranial ultrasound correlated with clinical grade and CT-visualized subarachnoid hemorrhage. J Neurosurg 64:594–600
167. Sengupta RP, McAllister VL (1986) Subarachnoid haemorrhage. Springer Verlag, Berlin Heidelberg New York, Tokyo
168. Sengupta RP, Chiu JSP, Brierley H (1975) Quality of survival following direct surgery for anterior communicating artery aneurysms. J Neurosurg 43:58–64
169. Sengupta RP, Gryspeerdt GL, Hankinson J (1976) Carotid ophthalmic aneurysms. J Neurol Neurosurg Psychatry 39:837–853
170. Shantharam VV, Clift GV (1974) Suprasellar aneurysm. An unusual cause of hypopituitarism. JAMA 229:1473
171. Shaw HE, Landers MB, Sydnor CF (1977) The significance of intraocular haemorrhage due to subarachnoid haemorrhage. Ann Ophthalmol 9:1403–1405
172. Shulman K, Martin BF, Popoff N, Ransohoff J (1963) Recognition and treatment of hydrocephalus following spontaneous subarachnoid hemorrhage. J Neurosurg 20: 1040–1049
173. Simon RP, Bayne LL (1984) Pulmonary lymphatic flow alterations during intracranial hypertension in sleep. Ann Neurol 15:188–194
174. Smith RR, Robertson JT (eds) (1975) Subarachnoid hemorrhage and cerebrovascular spasm. The first 'international' workshop. Thomas, Springfield
175. Smith RR, Zubkov YN, Tarassoli Y (1994) Cerebral aneurysms. Microvascular and endovascular management. Springer, Berlin Heidelberg New York, pp 90–104
176. Solenski NJ, Haley C, Kassel NF et al (1995) Medical complications of aneurysmal subarachnoid hemorrhage A report of the multicenter cooperative aneurysm study. Crit Care Med 23:1007–1117
177. Solomon RA, Fink ME, Pile-Spellman J (1994) Surgical management of unruptured intracranial aneurysms. J Neurosurg 80:440–446
178. Soni SR (1974) Aneurysms of the posterior communicating artery and oculomotor paresis. J Neurol Neurosurg Psychiatry 37:475–484
179. Stark RJ (1979) Supranuclear ophthalmoplegia with basilar artery aneurysms. Surg Neurol 12:447–452
180. Staub NC (1981) Pulmonary edema due to increased microvascular permeability. Annu Rev Med 32:291–312
181. Sundaram MBM, Chow F (1986) Seizures associated with spontaneous subarachnoid hemorrhage. Can J Neurol Sci 13:229–231
182. Sundt TM Jr (1990) Results of surgical management. In: Sundt TM Jr (ed) Surgical techniques for saccular and giant intracranial aneurysms. Williams and Wilkins, Baltimore, pp 19–23
183. Sundt TM, Kobayashi S, Fode NC et al (1982) Results and complications of surgical management of 809 intracranial aneurysms in 722 cases. J Neurosurg 56:753–765
184. Yoshimoto T, Uchida K, Kaneko U et al. (1979) An analysis of follow-up results of 1000 intracranial saccular aneurysms with definitive surgical treatment. J Neurosurg 50: 152–157
185. Symonds CF (1923) Contribution to the clinical study of intracranial aneurysm. Guy's Hosp Rep 4th Ser 73:139–158
186. Symonds CP (1924) Spontaneous subarachnoid haemorrhage. Q J Med 18:93–122

187. Takatu A, Shindo K, Tanaka S et al (1979) Fluid and electrolyte disturbances in patients with intracranial aneurysms. Surg Neurol 11:349–356
188. Takemae T, Mizukami M, Kim H et al (1978) Computed tomography of ruptured intracranial aneurysms in the acute stage – relationship between vasospasm and high density on CT scan. Brain Nerve 30:861–866
189. Tanaka H, Ueda Y, Date C et al (1981) Incidence of stroke in Shibata, Japan: 1976–1978. Stroke 12:460–466
190. Tanishma T (1980) Cerebral vasospasm. Contractile activity of hemoglobin in isolated canine basilar arteries. J Neurosurg 53:787–793
191. Teasdale G. Jennett B (1974) Assessment of coma and impaired consciousness. A practical scale. Lancet 2:81–84
192. Terson A (1900) De l'hemorragie dans le corps vitre au cours d'une hemorragie cerebrale. Clin Ophthalmol 6:309–312
193. Touho H, Karasawa J, Shishido H et al (1989) Neurogenic pulmonary edema in the acute state of hemorrhagic cerebrovascular disease. Neurosurgery 26:762–768
194. Tulleken CA (1976) Giant aneurysms of the posterior fossa presenting as space occupying lesions. Clin Neurosurg 79:161–186
195. Turnbull HM (1918) Intracranial aneurysms. Brain 41:50–56
196. van Gijn J. Bromberg JEC, Lindsay KW et al (1994) Definitions of initial grading, specific events, and overall outcome in patients with aneurysmal subarachnoid hemorrhage. A survey. Stroke 25:1623–1627
197. Van Swieten JC, Koudstaal PJ, Visser MC et al (1988) Interobserver agreement for the assessment of handicap in stroke patients. Stroke 19:604–607
198. Vassilouthis J, Richardson AE (1979) Ventricular dilation and communicating hydrocephalus following spontaneous subarachnoid hemorrhage. J Neurosurg 51:341–351
199. Vidal BE, Dergal EB, Cesarman E et al (1979) Cardiac arrhythmias associated with subarachnoid hemorrhage Prospective study. Neurosurgery 5:675–680
200. Volby B, Enevoldsen EM (1982) Intracranial pressure changes following aneurysm rupture. Part 1: clinical and angiographic correlation. J Neurosurg 56:186–196
201. Waga S, Ohtsubo K, Handa H (1975) Warning signs in intracranial aneurysm. Surg Neurol 3:15–20
202. Walter P, Neil-Dwyer G, Cruikshank JM (1982) Beneficial effect of adrenergic blockage in patients with subarachnoid haemorrhage. Br Med J 284:1661–1664
203. Walton JN (1956) Subarachnoid haemorrhage. Livingston, Edinburgh, pp 1–6
204. Wascher TM, Spetzler RF (1995) Saccular aneurysms of the basilar bifurcation. In: Carter LP, Spetzler RF (eds) Neurovascular surgery. McGraw-Hill, New York, pp 729–734
205. Weibers DO, Whisnant JP, Sundt TM Jr, O'Fallon WM (1987) The significance of unruptured intracranial saccular aneurysms. J Neurosurg 66:23–29
206. Weidler DJ (1974) Myocardial damage and cardiac arrhythmias after intracranial hemorrhage. A critical review. Stroke 5:759–764
207. Weinand ME, O'Boynick P, Goetz K (1989) A study of serum antidiuretic hormone and atrial natriuretic peptide levels in a series of patients with intracranial disease and hyponatremia. Neurosurgery 25:781–785
208. Weir B, Grace M, Hansen J, Rothberg C (1978) Time course of vasospasm in man. J Neurosurg 48:173–178
209. Weir BK (1978) Pulmonary oedema following fatal aneurysm rupture. J Neurosurg 49:502–507
210. Widal F (1903) Le diagnose de l'hemorragie meningee. Presse Med 2:413
211. Wijdicks EFM, Vermeulen MD, Hijdra A, van Gijn J (1985) Hyponatremia and cerebral infarction in patients with ruptured intracranial aneurysms: Is fluid restriction harmful? Ann Neurol 17:137–140
212. Wijdicks EFM, Vermeulen M, Ten Haaf JA et al (1985) Volume depletion and natriuresis in patients with a ruptured intracranial aneurysm. Ann Neurol 18:211–216
213. Wijdicks EFM, Vandongen KJ, van Gijn J et al (1988) Enlargement of the third ventricle and hyponatraemia in aneurysmal subarachnoid haemorrhage. J Neurol Neurosurg Psychiatry 51:516–520
214. Wijdicks EFM, Ropper AH, Hannicutt EJ et al (1991) Atrial natriuretic factor and salt wasting after aneurysmal subarachnoid hemorrhage. Stroke 22:1519–1524
215. Wilkins RH (ed) (1980) Cerebral vasopasm. Proceedings of the 2nd international workshop, Amsterdam, The Netherlands, 1979. Williams and Wilkins, Baltimore
216. Wilkins RH (ed) (1988) Cerebral vasospasm. Proceedings of the IIIrd international symposium in Charlottesville. Raven, New York

217. Winn HR, Richardson AE, Jane JA (1977) The long-term prognosis in untreated cerebral aneurysms. 1. Incidence of late hemorrhage in cerebral aneurysms: a 10 year evaluation of 364 patients. Ann Neurol 1:358–370
218. Winn HR, Almaani WS, Berga SL et al (1983) The long-term outcome in patients with multiple aneurysms Incidence of late hemorrhage and implications for treatment of incidental aneurysms. J Neurosurg 59:642–651
219. Wirth FP, Laws ER Jr, Piepgras D et al (1983) Surgical treatment of incidental intracranial aneurysms. Neurosurgery 12:507–511
220. Yasagil MG, Gasser JG, Hodosh RM, Rankin TV (1977) Carotid-ophthalmic aneurysms: direct microsurgical approach. Surg Neurol 8:155–165
221. Yasargil ME, Yonekawa T, Zumstein B, Stahl HJ (1973) Hydrocephalus following spontaneous subarachnoid hemorrhage. J Neurosurg 39:474–479

CHAPTER 3

Imaging for Intracranial Aneurysms

3.1 Introduction

Endovascular treatments, like other forms of less invasive neurosurgery, depend on accurate in vivo imaging. Imaging involves the detection of intracranial aneurysms, the diagnosis of any associated complications and assessment of their treatment (pre-procedure, peri-procedure and follow-up). The diagnosis of symptomatic aneurysms, either following rupture or at the onset of compression symptoms, is generally made by physical examination and the role of imaging is to confirm and refine the diagnosis. Asymptomatic aneurysms may be co-incidental to symptomatic lesions, and once a single aneurysm or pathology associated with intracranial aneurysms has been discovered, the exclusion of co-incidental aneurysms requires comprehensive imaging of the intracranial arteries. Screening individuals at risk of aneurysms, e.g. close relatives of patients, involves balancing the risk of morbidity due to the imaging against the risk a discovered aneurysm poses to that person's health. Imaging, therefore, has different roles in the management of patients with intracranial aneurysms, and the neuroradiologist is charged with choosing the modality most appropriate to the situation. In this chapter, the imaging of intracranial aneurysms will be discussed with these objectives in mind. The technical aspects of available imaging modalities are described in general neuroradiology texts and will not be reviewed here, but it is our intention to consider the role of different modalities in endovascular therapy and to concentrate on how they may be used in planning and performing aneurysm treatments.

Crucial to endovascular navigation and embolisation is angiography. Intra-arterial angiography remains the best available technique for imaging patent cerebral vessels. However, planar scanning offers additional information about aneurysms and their surrounding structures, e.g. the external dimensions of an aneurysm sac and the presence of mural calcification. Techniques of image enhancement by electronic post-processing are now available and both magnetic resonance (MR) and computed tomography (CT) scanning can be used for angiography. Physiological assessments are necessary to predict the effects of cerebral blood flow diversion performed in the management of some aneurysms. Data on cerebral blood flow and perfusion can be obtained using angiography, as well as ultrasound and nuclear medicine techniques. The different perspectives, provided by static and dynamic imaging and data from functional assessments, are important elements in the management of complex aneurysms. They will be considered in regard to the planning and monitoring of endovascular procedures and in the prevention of complications.

3.2 Detection of Bleeding Due to Intracranial Aneurysm Rupture

3.2.1 Computed Tomography

The clinical diagnosis of spontaneous intracranial haemorrhage due to aneurysm rupture has been discussed in Chap. 2. The ability of computed tomography (CT) to demonstrate acute intracranial haemorrhage and confirm the clinical diagnosis of subarachnoid haemorrhage (SAH) was appreciated soon after its introduction in the 1970s [74]. The high density of recently clotted blood (Fig. 3.1) makes the technique particularly suited for the detection of acute intracranial haemorrhage [46, 55, 91]. Imaging by CT not only confirms the diagnosis but will, in addition, demonstrate the distribution (intracerebral, intraventricular, subarachnoid or subdural) and volume of intracranial haemorrhage. The distribution of SAH may be helpful in predicting its cause and the volume in predicting the likely severity of the resulting illness [12, 25, 27, 61, 72]. The location of the ruptured aneurysm can frequently be inferred from the distribution of SAH (Fig. 3.2) [92]. In patients with suspected SAH, CSF sampling should be performed by lumbar puncture if scanning fails to demonstrate haemorrhage or any other cause of symptoms. It is unnecessary to obtain CSF following a positive scan except as a therapeutic manoeuvre to reduce intrathecal pressure, i.e. relief of hydrocephalus due to failure of CSF absorption. However, false negative results can occur with both CSF sampling and planar scanning.

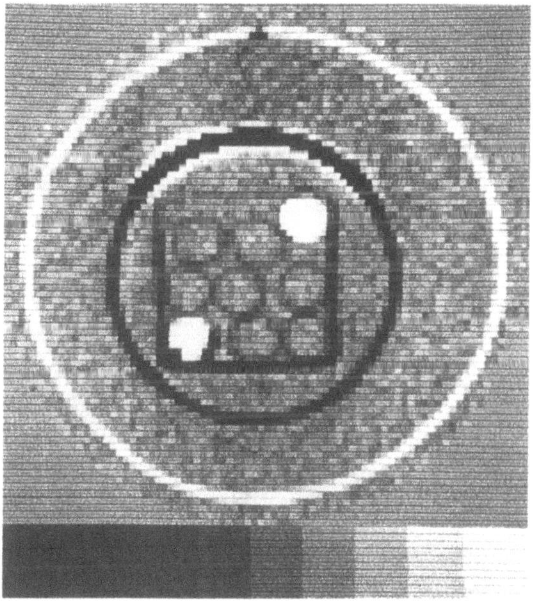

Fig. 3.1. Axial image obtained on the first clinical computed tomography scanner in the world, which was installed at Atkinson Morley's Hospital, London. This scan was performed prior to scanning patients. It shows a nine-chamber test phantom containing various biological fluids. The high density samples (*upper right* and *lower left*) were fresh clotted blood and haematoma fluid aspirated from a patient with acute subdural haematoma. (Courtesy of Dr J. Ambrose)

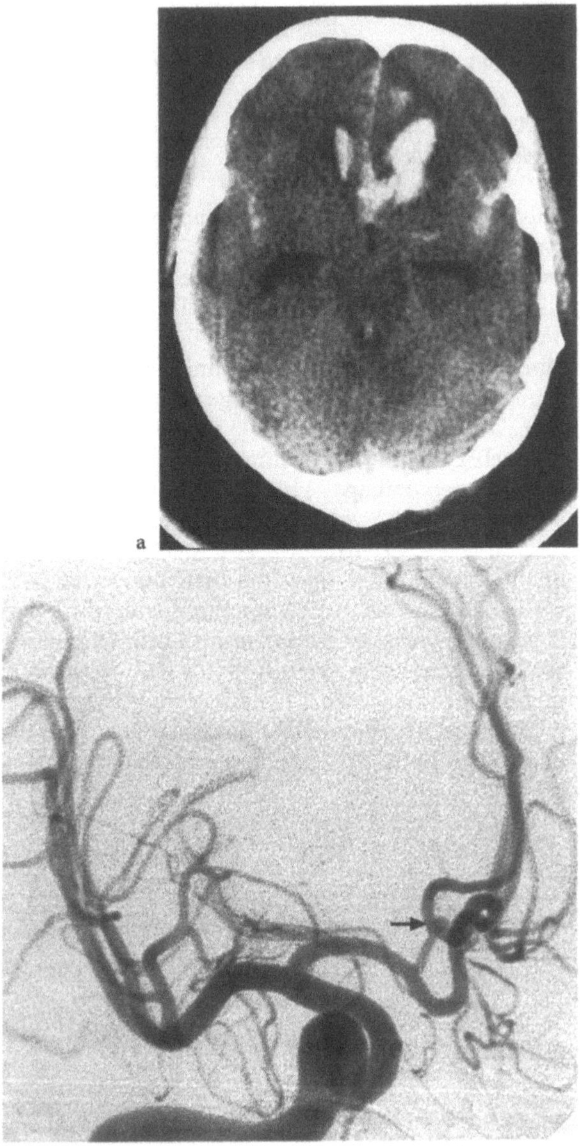

a

b

Fig. 3.2.
a Axial computed tomography scan showing acute subarachnoid haemorrhage with intraparenchymal and intraventricular haemorrhage.
b, c Intra-arterial digital subtraction angiography by right (**b**) and left (**c**) internal carotid artery injection 2 days after the haemorrhage shows no evidence of vasospasm and only faint filling of a small saccular aneurysm of the anterior communicating artery on **b** (*arrow*). **d, e** A repeat study was performed 4 days later and shows the aneurysm filling from the left side (**e**), and intense vasospasm of right (**d**) and left (**e**) anterior cerebral arteries.
(c–e see p. 79)

Currently CT is the most widely used imaging technique for the initial assessment of patients with suspected aneurysmal SAH. Its sensitivity depends on the amount of SAH and, since whole blood is rapidly cleared from the subarachnoid space, the timing of the scan is important. CT is most sensitive to recently clotted blood and its sensitivity decreases with time following aneurysm rupture. False negative scans in the first 2 days following rupture are rare and occur when aneurysm rupture causes very small volumes of haemorrhage. False negative scans also result from poor quality imaging due

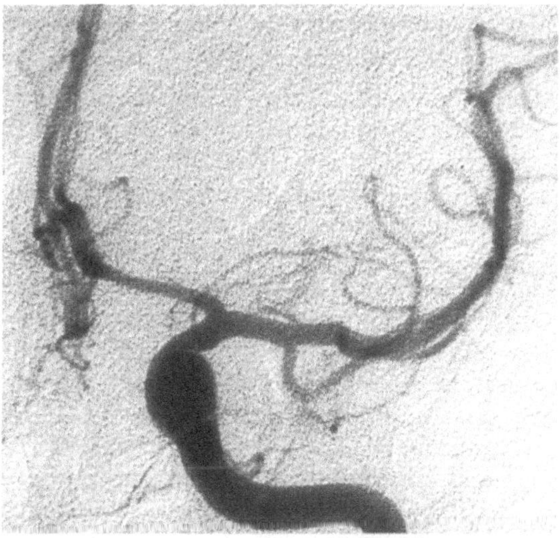

c

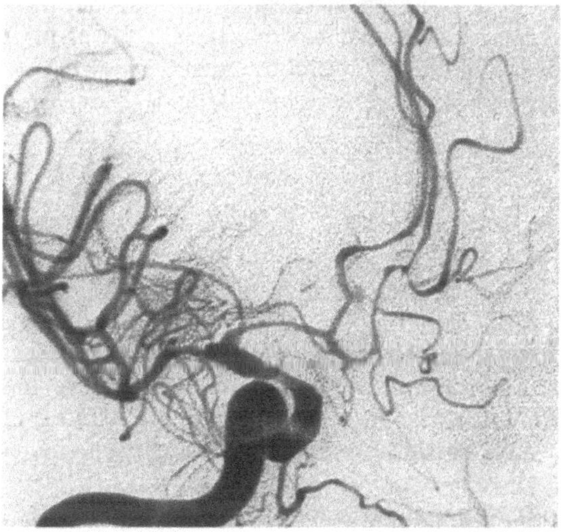

d

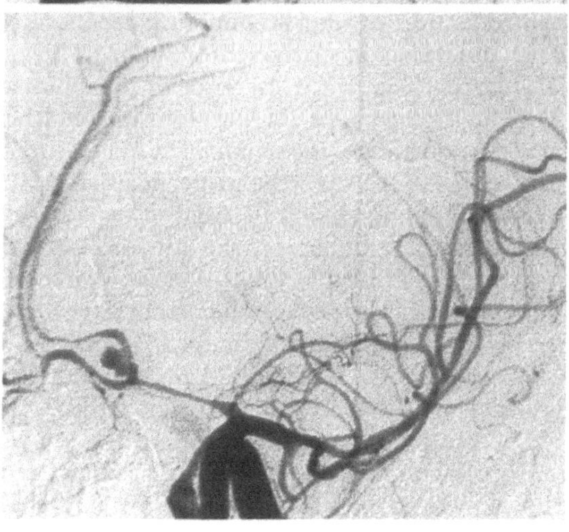

e

to inadequate scanners, artefacts caused by patients' movements or inaccurate interpretation by inexperienced radiologists. Haemorrhage in the posterior fossa and close to the skull base is more likely to be missed than supratentorial or intraventricular haemorrhage [3].

The chances of CT detection of haemorrhage reduce with time over the first 2 weeks following aneurysm rupture; positive scans were reported in 50% of SAH patients at 7 days but in only 20% after 9 days by van Gijn and van Dongen [105]. The clearance of high density haemorrhage from the subarachnoid space is accompanied by the appearance of free haemoglobin and subsequently bilirubin in CSF. Intraparenchymal haematomas are more slowly absorbed and CT evidence of haemorrhage may be present for weeks. The diagnosis of massive or major haemorrhage by CT is generally obvious and the need for confirmatory CSF sampling is reserved for patients with minor haemorrhage and false negative CT. Van der Wee et al. [104] reported sensitivity and specificity rates of 100% and 98%, respectively, for CT performed within 12 h of the onset of sudden headache, in a series of 175 patients. This left a small number (in this series 2%) of patients with negative CT scans whose symptoms were subsequently shown (by lumbar puncture and angiography) to be due to aneurysmal SAH.

3.2.2 Cerebrospinal Fluid Sampling

Cerebrospinal fluid sampling is therefore necessary to identify the small number of patients presenting with minor haemorrhages and negative CT scans (once any contraindication to lumbar puncture has been excluded). The major difficulty with this test is that blood staining of CSF may be due to aneurysmal SAH or to the lumbar puncture itself (i.e. so-called traumatic tap).

The discolouration of CSF caused by haemolysis of SAH was observed soon after the introduction of lumbar puncture by Quinke in 1891 [53] and the yellow colour described as xanthochromia by Milian and Chiray [60]. Xanthochromia is largely due to the presence of bilirubin and develops within hours of SAH but it takes time for the products of haemolysis to appear after intracranial haemorrhage in samples obtained by lumbar puncture. Lumbar puncture is therefore unlikely to be positive in the first few hours after SAH [107] and sampling should be delayed for at least 12 h.

There have been several studies on the rate of clearance of intracranial SAH; Strong [95], in a critical appraisal of the practice of repeated lumbar punctures as a therapeutic manoeuvre after traumatic SAH, showed that red cells were cleared from the lumbar CSF within 5–6 days. Adam and Prawirohardjo [2], studied the fate of ^{51}Cr-labelled red blood cells injected intracisternally in dogs and found that 75% of the radioactivity remained enmeshed in arachnoid trabeculae. Both studies concluded that lumbar puncture is not an effective means of removing the debris of haemolysis. However, xanthochromia of CSF can persist for several weeks [8]. Vermeulen et al. [109] reported that 70% of samples were still xanthochromic at 3 weeks and 40%, for 4 weeks after SAH.

Appropriately timed lumbar puncture and CSF sampling is, therefore, the best available method of excluding SAH as the cause of acute-onset headache. The practical problem remains that of distinguishing blood stained samples due to bleeding during sampling from aneurysmal SAH, and several methods have been proposed to cope with this difficulty. One time-honoured technique is to obtain three sequential samples and count the red cells in each. If the numbers of red cells fall over the sampling period the sample is judged to have been traumatic, on the basis that red cells originating from rupture of an intracranial aneurysm would be evenly mixed in lumbar CSF. However, this technique is not reliable if traumatic bleeding persists during sampling [20], and it is generally considered better to base diagnosis on the presence of xanthochromia. But the reliability of even this estimation is controversial. The absence of xanthochromia on visual inspection or spectrophotometry was considered sufficient to exclude spontaneous SAH by Vermeulen et al. [108] but not by MacDonald and Mendelow [57]. In order to distinguish between blood staining of CSF caused by aneurysm rupture from traumatic sampling, additional estimations of ferritin [35, 114], and more recently D-dimer [51] (a cross-linked fibrin derivative), have been proposed. Though useful in most instances, both additional measurements have been shown to be dependent on the timing of lumbar puncture after SAH and false negative results have been reported [71].

In the management of CT negative patients with equivocal results from CSF sampling, the decision to proceed to angiography will depend on a careful interpretation of the history and physical examination. By and large, given the potentially dire consequences of aneurysm re-rupture, angiography should be performed. The role of CT and MR angiography in this situation will be discussed in sects. 3.3.2 and 3.3.3 below. One final point to consider when interpreting the results of CSF sampling is that lumbar puncture is an uncertain method of diagnosing aneurysm rebleeding, because haemolytic products can persist in CSF for weeks [109].

3.2.3
Magnetic Resonance Imaging

Magnetic resonance imaging (MRI) has been advocated for the acute investigation of patients after aneurysmal SAH [43, 67, 88], but it is generally accepted that acute SAH is difficult to detect on spin-echo MRI because it is masked by the high signal returned by CSF [7, 117]. Use of a fluid-attenuated inversion recovery sequence (FLAIR), which negates the signal of CSF, can demonstrate acute SAH [67], but requires a relatively long scanning time which limits the usefulness of this sequence in practice. However, the conspicuity of SAH on MRI using T1-weighted and proton density-weighted images improves with time after bleeding, because the concentration of paramagnetic methaemoglobin increases. Ogawa et al. [69] reported detection rates for examinations using T1-weighted and proton density-weighted se-

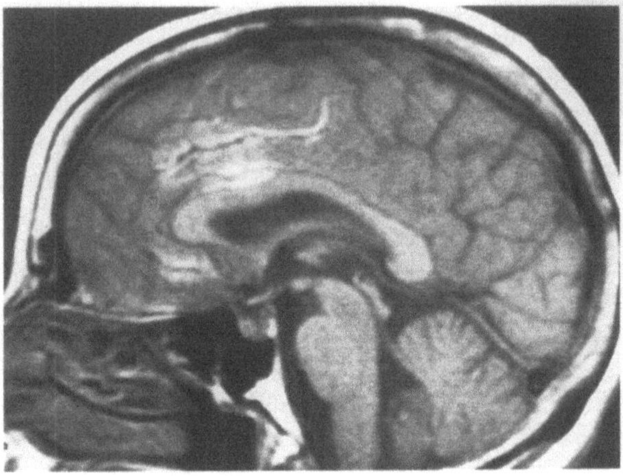

Fig. 3.3.
Sagittal T1-weighted magnetic resonance imaging of a patient who presented 8 days after onset of headache. High signal due to subarachnoid methaemoglobin is evident around the pericallosal and callosal marginal arteries in this unenhanced image. An anterior communicating artery aneurysm was demonstrated on intra-arterial digital subtraction angiography

quences of 52% and 86%, respectively (4–14 days post-ictus), and 90% and 100% for chronic examinations (more that 14 days post-ictus). MRI is therefore potentially the best method of demonstrating SAH in patients presenting late after aneurysm rupture (Fig. 3.3) and may be positive for SAH when CT is normal [88].

3.2.4 Complications of Subarachnoid Haemorrhage

The complications associated with aneurysmal SAH have been described in Chap. 2. These cause delayed deterioration in patients' neurological state which may occur abruptly or insidiously. Imaging by CT scan is the principle arbiter of the cause of rapid clinical deterioration since hydrocephalus or rehaemorrhage can usually be easily distinguished. Ready access to CT is therefore mandatory in centres caring for patients in the acute period after SAH. A gradual deterioration in the patient's neurological condition may be due to various causes such as hydrocephalus, vasospasm and cerebral ischaemia, or electrolyte disturbances.

CT scanning will exclude hydrocephalus and diagnose established cerebral infarction but not early ischaemia or infarction, nor cerebral vasospasm. Direct imaging of vasospasm requires intra-arterial digital subtraction angiography (IA-DSA), though non-invasive techniques such as MRA and transcranial Doppler ultrasound [1, 28, 101] can provide indirect data about its severity and consequence (see sect. 3.3.3).

A correlation between the severity of angiographic and symptomatic vasospasm was demonstrated by Fisher et al. [28]. Severe vasospasm, though not invariably symptomatic, was associated with delayed ischaemic deficits in 80% of their patients. The relative importance of large or small artery vasospasm to the development of ischaemic symptoms is unknown but it is hardly surprising, given the variability of collateral cerebral blood flow, that not all patients with severely narrowed basal arteries are symptomatic. However, a strong correlation exists between the location and size of SAH, as demonstrated by early CT scanning, and angiographic vasospasm [28, 48, 72, 86, 98, 99]. Saito et al. [86] showed that angiographic vasospasm was commonest in arteries close to subarachnoid clot. The amount of SAH on CT, severity of angiographic vasospasm and symptoms all correlate [48, 98]. Fisher et al. [28] classified CT scans performed within 5 days of ictus into four grades: (1) no SAH, (2) diffuse SAH less than 1 mm thick, (3) localised clots or layers of haemorrhage 1 mm or thicker and (4) intraventricular or intracerebral haemorrhage with or without SAH. Angiographic spasm was demonstrated in only one of 18 patients in groups 1 and 2, but in 23 of 24 patients in groups 3 and 4. All the patients with severe vasospasm showed symptoms and signs of ischaemia or infarction [28]. Thus a patient's liability to develop delayed ischaemia can be predicted from the early CT scan findings [72].

CT scanning, in addition to predicting patients at risk of developing cerebral vasospasm, will demonstrate established infarction. There may be a role for MRI in the evaluation of such patients (Fig. 3.4) since it has been reported to be more sensitive to early ischaemic changes than CT [19]. But in a larger prospective comparative study of CT and MRI in acute stroke, Mohr et al. [62] found both techniques equally accurate and CT better at predicting whether neurological deficits would be permanent or not. Planar scanning (we currently use CT) should always be performed immediately prior to angioplasty for symptomatic vasospasm in order to exclude the presence of established cerebral infarction and/or haemorrhage.

3.3 Detection of Intracranial Aneurysms Acutely After Subarachnoid Haemorrhage

3.3.1 Intra-arterial Angiography

Angiography is indicated following the diagnosis of spontaneous SAH to identify its cause. When aneurysmal SAH is suspected, angiography should be performed by IA-DSA since this method is currently the most reliable means of aneurysm detection or exclusion [33]. As will be discussed below, planar scanning can demonstrate aneurysms with a sensitivity that increases in proportion to aneurysm size, but both CT and MR techniques can miss small ruptured intracranial aneurysms. That is not to say that IA-DSA is 100% reliable, and its relatively invasive nature is a deficit, but it is the most sensitive method available [22, 83].

Angiography is performed to identify the aneurysm site, to obtain an anatomical assessment of its vascular geometry (in particular the size of the osteum and lumen, and their relationship to adjacent arteries) and to assess the presence of collateral blood flow. Since intracranial aneurysms are multiple in 20%–25% of patients all the intracranial arteries must be assessed following the diagnosis of an aneurysm. It is no longer tenable to argue that

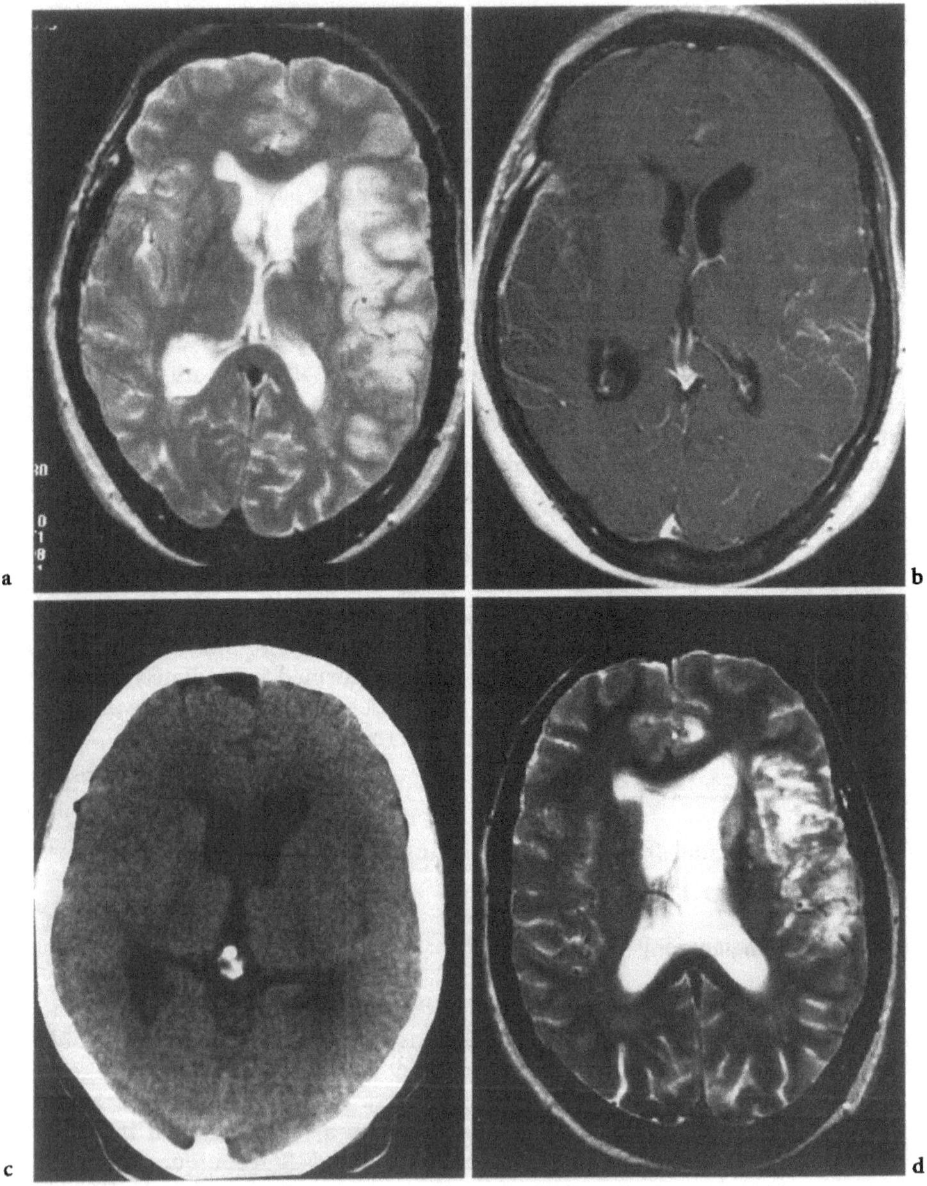

Fig. 3.4. a, b Axial T2-weighted (**a**) and gadolinium enhanced T1-weighted (**b**) magnetic resonance imaging (MRI) 2 weeks after subarachnoid haemorrhage caused by rupture of a left middle cerebral artery (MCA) aneurysm when the patient developed symptoms of vasospasm. **c** Ten days later, with persistent hemiparesis axial computed tomography (**c**) shows only small focal areas of low attenuation in the region of the head of the left caudate nucleus. **d, e** However, repeat T2-weighted (**d**) and gadolinium enhanced T1-weighted (**e**) MRI shows more extensive signal change and enhancement in the left MCA territory consistent with infarction. (**e** see p. 85)

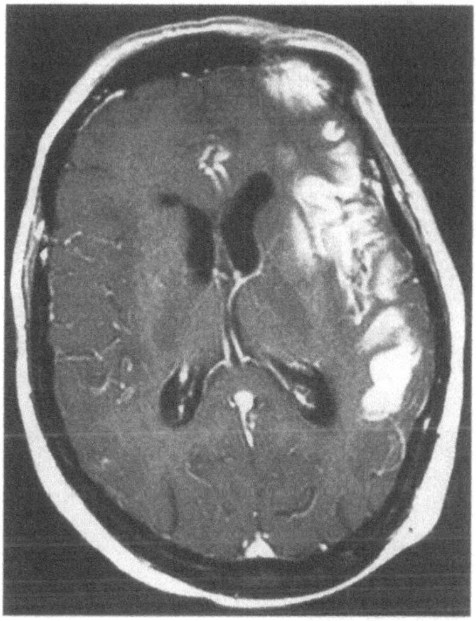

Fig. 3.4 e

vertebral artery injections should not be performed in older patients because a posterior circulation aneurysm would not be considered for surgical treatment since coil embolisation is now often possible in such patients [82], although, obviously, the presence of atherosclerotic stenosis may preclude safe selective catheterisation. Furthermore, angiography needs to be performed with regard to the patient's condition. In this respect, the examinations following SAH should be planned in the light of CT or MRI findings regarding the likely site of a ruptured aneurysm (the most likely aneurysm bearing artery being studied first) since, if the patient's condition deteriorates and prevents a complete study, identification of the ruptured aneurysm allows its acute treatment. The diagnosis of coincidental aneurysms can wait until the patient is well enough to undergo further angiography.

In addition to the detection of aneurysm(s), IA DSA will demonstrate vasospasm, vascular displacements due to haematoma or hydrocephalus and other vascular pathologies. Our protocol consists of transfemoral carotid and vertebral catheterisation, with angiography by hand injections of non-ionic contrast media under local anaesthesia. In most instances after SAH, angiography is performed without sedation since, provided adequate analgesia is given, patients recovering from acute SAH are usually able to remain sufficiently still and sedation may confuse the interpretation of the neurological examination. Excessive restlessness or irritability usually implies some degree of cerebral dysfunction and hydrocephalus or metabolic causes such as hyponatraemia and hypercarbia should be excluded before angiography. A series of standard projections are obtained with lateral, frontal and oblique views of the anterior circulation and lateral, frontal (Towne's projection) and oblique (intermastoid oblique projection) views of the posterior circulation. To this repertoire, supplementary projections should be made to ensure ade-

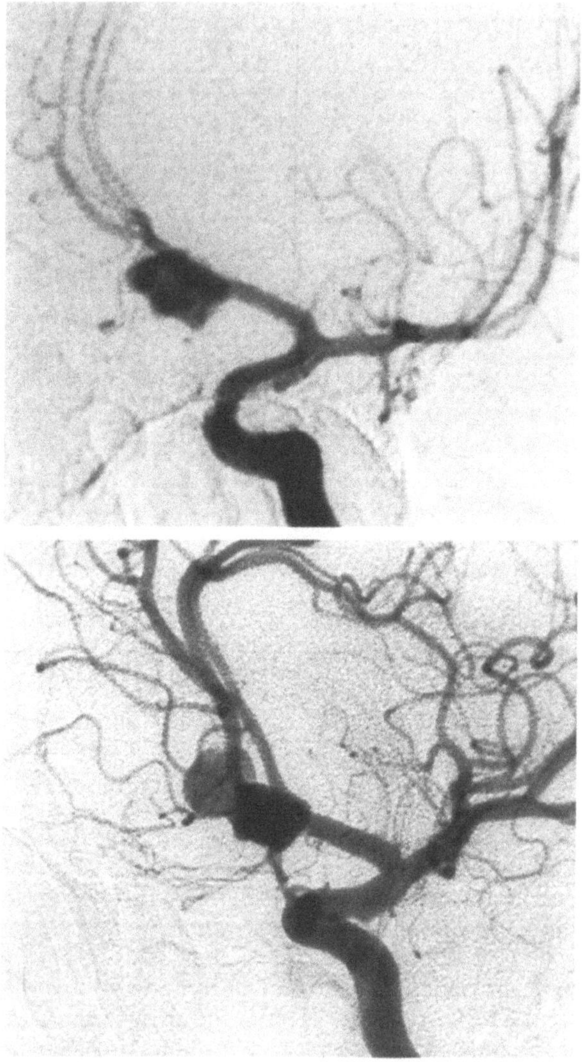
a

b

Fig. 3.5.
a Left carotid intra-arterial digital subtraction angiography showing a saccular anterior communicating artery aneurysm 24 h after rupture. **b** The aneurysm rebleed before treatment and a second angiogram 8 days later (immediately prior to coil embolisation) shows a daughter lobule at the fundus

quate visualisation of likely aneurysm sites, such as the anterior communicating artery (ACoA) and the middle cerebral artery (MCA) bifurcation. Cross compression of the contralateral cervical carotid artery or the ipsilateral carotid artery during vertebral artery (VA) injections to improve contrast filling of the anterior and posterior communicating arteries should be performed judiciously [116]. In the acute situation, angiography should be sufficiently detailed to decide if endovascular treatment is appropriate, but not excessively prolonged, by the addition of non-standard projections and techniques, such as rotational angiography, since these can be better obtained during endovascular treatment with the patient under general anaesthesia.

There are few contraindications to performing angiography as soon as practically possible after SAH (Fig. 3.5). While there are no absolute contraindications, the risk posed by relative contraindications such as a history of a severe hypersensitivity reaction to contrast media, cardiac or pulmonary disease and bleeding diathesis must be considered. Angiography should be performed once the patient's condition is stable. The heart rate and rhythm, systemic blood pressure and oxygen saturation should be monitored during the procedure. Maintenance of an adequate airway and supervision of the patient may well require the assistance of an anaesthetist. Though it is our routine practice not to perform diagnostic angiography under general anaesthesia, this may be warranted in patients unable to cooperate or maintain adequate blood oxygen levels. Signs of raised intracranial pressure due to intracerebral haematoma is an indication for limited cerebral angiography under general anaesthesia prior to emergency neurosurgical drainage.

Aneurysm re-rupture during cerebral angiography is rare [54, 100]; it occurred only once amongst the 5484 SAH patients of the cooperative study [85]. It is debatable whether transcatheter injections of contrast media in normal cervical arteries increases the intra-arterial pressure of the intracranial arteries. Greitz [32] found that the carotid intra-arterial pressure did not increase after rapid injections of large contrast media volumes but rises in systemic blood pressures of up to 30 mmHg have been observed [63]. However, Hilal [38] postulated that excessive rises in intra-arterial pressure were possible in pathological states such as vasospasm. It is statistically probable that aneurysms are more likely to re-rupture when angiography is performed in the acute period. A causal link is difficult to prove, but factors that could contribute to aneurysm rupture during angiography were considered by Liliequist et al. [54]. They reviewd 25 reported cases of aneurysm rupture during angiography and concluded that contrast injection rates above 6 ml/min and manoeuvres leading to excessive spontaneous cross circulation should be avoided. Applying such precautions seems prudent when performing angiography after aneurysmal SAH, but the risks are small and should not be a reason for delaying the investigation given that patients are at risk of spontaneous re-bleeding.

Cerebral angiography by IA-DSA is the gold standard against which other methods of imaging intracranial aneurysms are compared (see below). After spontaneous SAH, intra-arterial angiography fails to identify any structural cause for bleeding in 2%–27% of patients [11, 13, 29, 44, 45, 66, 94, 96, 97, 113]. The prognosis in this group of patients is better than those with aneurysmal SAH [18, 26, 77] and it is therefore assumed that in most instances bleeding was due to a different cause and not simply an unidentified aneurysm. A perimesencephalic distribution of SAH is characteristic in patients without aneurysms on angiography [78, 106]. However, IA-DSA is subject to a small false negative rate for structural causes of SAH, estimated at less than 2% by Foster et al. [29]. Aneurysms are likely to be missed because of poor quality images or inadequate vessel opascification by contrast media in the acute period after SAH (see Fig. 3.2). Failure of aneurysms to fill on contrast angiography is usually due to local vasospasm, but occasionally aneurysms are not visualised despite normal opascification of parent arteries

[75]. It is our practice to perform repeat angiography in patients with a clinical diagnosis of SAH when: (a) the diagnosis was confirmed by CT or CSF sampling and the distribution of SAH on CT was not confined to the perimesencephalic cisterns, or (b) the first angiogram was not comprehensive, or (c) the first angiogram was inadequate because opascification of vessels was poor and/or vasospasm was present. In all patients with angiogram-negative spontaneous SAH and prior to a second angiogram, MR scanning is performed since this may identify an aneurysm that failed to opascify on IA-DSA [24, 75]. Repeat intra-arterial angiography should be performed under optimum conditions and include injections of internal and external carotid arteries as well as both vertebral arteries.

3.3.2
CT Angiography

Angiography by CT scanning has a potentially important role in the acute investigation of spontaneous SAH since IA-DSA is associated with a small risk of causing additional morbidity. In a recent report of 1095 patients examined by Gryzska et al. [33] using IA-DSA, the rate of morbidity due to neurological deficits was 0.09%, with transient deficits occurring in 0.45% of patients. Avoiding such risks would be of obvious benefit and planar scanning may allow a rapid non-invasive method of identifying recently ruptured aneurysms. Such management is particularly attractive to the endovascular therapist since, once the cause of aneurysmal SAH has been identified, treatment can be planned and IA-DSA performed under general anaesthesia, immediately prior to embolisation (see sect. 3.4.1).

Several centres have reported experience with CT angiography in the acute period after SAH [36, 70, 91, 110]. CT scanning during infusions of radiographic contrast [65] may show intracranial aneurysms, but it has not been widely adopted in the initial assessment of spontaneous SAH because it does not provide an adequate preoperative demonstration of aneurysms to replace IA-DSA and therefore simply increases the time and cost of the examination. CT angiography [36, 70], however, especially if performed with helical CT [91] can produce computer-generated 3D images of blood vessels. These are currently being evaluated in the acute management of aneurysmal SAH and potentially provide all the data needed to plan endovascular treatment or microvascular surgery (Fig. 3.6). Vieco et al. [110] reported sensitivity rates for CT angiography of 77%–97% and specificity rates of 87%–100% for the detection of ruptured aneurysm in 30 SAH patients. The examinations required an intravenous pump injection of 100 ml of radiographic contrast media at a rate of 2 ml/s.

3.3.3
Magnetic Resonance Angiography

A less invasive alternative is MR angiography (MRA) but the claustrophobic nature of current machines and the relatively long scanning times during

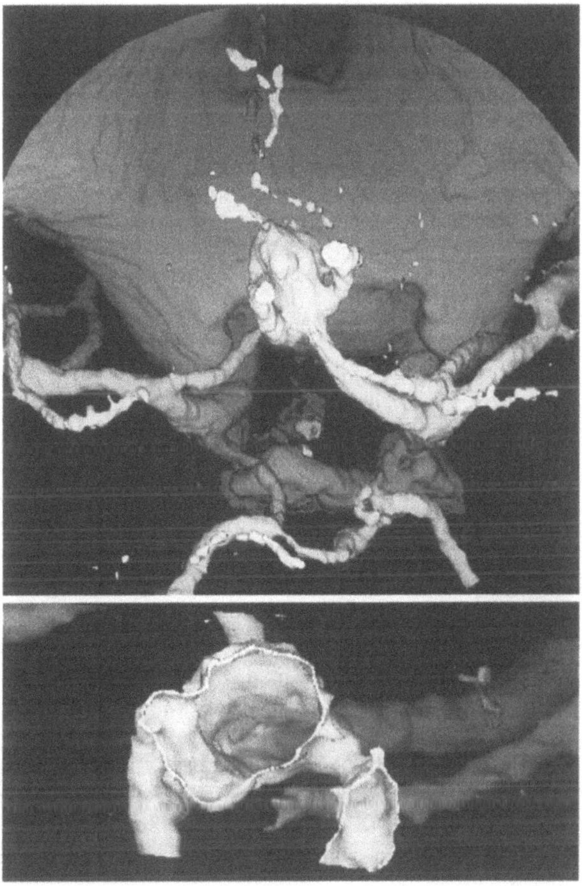
a
b

Fig. 3.6.
a Three-dimensional computed tomography angiogram with volume rendering showing a dominant right anterior cerebral artery and an anterior communicating artery aneurysm. **b** The data has been processed to give an endoscopic view of the aneurysm lumen. This examination was performed prior to endosaccular emobolisation and after acute subarachnoid haemorrhage. (Courtesy of Dr. K. Fukasaku)

which patients are largely inaccessible to their attendants are seen as practical difficulties restricting the technique's general use. Nevertheless, there have been encouraging reports of MRA after SAH which have shown that imaging is possible with sensitivity and specificity rates similar to those obtainable in patients examined with unruptured aneurysms [31, 115]. Two small studies compared the ability of MRA and IA-DSA to detect intracranial aneurysms in the acute period after SAH. Gouliamos et al. [31] reported one false negative examination each for MRA and IA-DSA in 14 patients and Wilcox et al. [115] reported sensitivity of 81% and specificity of 100% for aneurysms on MRA compared to IA-DSA in 39 SAH patients. Sankhla et al. [87] used a 3D time-of-flight (TOF) technique in the assessment of 51 SAH patients, 25 of whom were scanned within 48 h of ictus. They obtained satisfactory images in 75% of patients and 20 patients underwent craniotomy and clipping of 22 aneurysms without additional imaging. All patients were subsequently assessed by IA-DSA. Misinterpretation of MRA in four patients was attributed to poor quality imaging but none of these patients were subjected to inappropriate craniotomy.

The same group subsequently reported on the use of MRA for anterior midline aneurysms [47]. In this study of 30 patients there were no false negative MRA examinations. Problems of interpretation may be caused by the presence of chemical shift artefacts on MRA due to haematoma adjacent to a ruptured aneurysm, but in this situation spin-echo MRI can be diagnostic [115]. Although MRA may be less sensitive than IA-DSA in the diagnosis of acutely ruptured aneurysms, it is reassuring that the specificity is high and there have been no reports of patients undergoing craniotomy following a false positive scan [87, 115]. Keogh and Sankhla's [47] proposal that surgical treatment can be planned on the basis of good quality positive MRA examinations seems reasonable if IA-DSA is performed after negative examinations and postoperatively; the later to assess the operative result and to exclude the presence of coincidental aneurysms.

The accuracy of MRA was assessed by Aprile et al. [5], who collected 496 patient studies from a review of 16 reports published between 1990 and 1996. The sensitivity was calculated at 89.4% and specificity at 97.8% in this heterogeneous group of patients, most of whom presented following SAH. The risk of false negative examinations is highest for small aneurysms, i.e. less than 5 mm in diameter [42, 56]. Within this constraint, however, the accuracy of angiography by planar scanning in the detection of intracranial aneurysms is high enough to advocate its use as the first-line investigation of patients symptomatic of intracranial aneurysms outside the acute period after aneurysm rupture. It is probable that future advances will increase the acceptability of MRA for the acute assessment of patients with spontaneous SAH and reduce the need for pre-treatment diagnostic IA-DSA. The more difficult question to answer, particularly for those planning the provision of imaging services, is which modality CT or MR is the better method for non-invasive angiography.

3.3.4 Ultrasound

The use of transcranial Doppler (TCD) ultrasound to measure blood flow velocities and to image the basal cerebral artery, as well as to monitor vasospasm after aneurysmal SAH is well established [1, 101]. Colour-coded TCD ultrasound has also been employed to identify intracranial aneurysm after SAH [9, 10]. Wardlaw and Cannon [111] reported being able to identify 30 of 33 aneurysms demonstrated by IA-DSA in a group of 35 selected patients. They employed a modified Doppler ultrasound technique called "color Doppler energy" to improve the technique's sensitivity for intracranial vascular imaging. Like TCD examinations, imaging depended on obtaining a satisfactory bone window and in five patients (12.5%) they were unable to obtain satisfactory images because of obscuring bone.

3.4 Imaging for Symptomatic Unruptured and Asymptomatic Aneurysms

3.4.1 Computed Tomography

Symptomatic unruptured intracranial aneurysms are generally larger than ruptured aneurysms at the time of presentation. They are therefore more likely to be detected on planar scans. On unenhanced CT, calcification in the aneurysm wall or partial thrombosis of the lumen may be visible as areas of high attenuation, but generally only larger aneurysms, or those serendipitously included in the scan plane, can be diagnosed. The patent lumen of an aneurysm will enhance following administration of intravenous contrast. Early attempts to use CT in the diagnosis of unruptured aneurysms relied on the use of multiple scans with narrow slice widths and contrast enhancement (CECT) to demonstrate small aneurysms [6, 90]. More recently the addition of 3D-reconstruction techniques [4] and helical CT scanning [91] has improved the accuracy of the technique (see Fig. 3.6). Aoki et al. [4] reported 100% sensitivity for the technique in a small series of patients compared with intra-arterial angiography. Schwartz et al. [91] compared intra-arterial angiography, helical CT angiography and MRA in 21 patients with 30 aneurysms. There were no false negatives for aneurysms larger than 3 mm on CT or MR angiograms, and the two techniques were rated similar in their ability to detect and delineate aneurysms.

3.4.2 Magnetic Resonance Angiography

There have been several studies of different MRA techniques for the detection of intracranial aneurysms [15, 17, 39, 40, 50, 58, 73, 80, 91, 93]. The overall sensitivity and specificity of MRA for intracranial aneurysms range from 79%–100% and 92%–100%, respectively, when compared to intra-arterial angiography [27, 39, 73]. Aneurysms not detected tended to occur close to the skull base, particularly at the posterior inferior cerebellar artery (PICA) origin [80, 115]. Ross et al. [80], using 3D TOF MRA combined with spin-echo MRI, reported 95% sensitivity and 100% specificity for detecting at least one aneurysm greater than 3 mm in diameter. Huston et al. found 3D phase contrast to be superior to TOF in a comparative study [40]. Most observers advocate the need for an inspection of the individual partitions and/or MRI images [80, 115]. The conspicuity of aneurysm may also be improved by multiple overlapping thin-slice techniques [15], contrast enhancement by intravenous administration of gadolinium [50] and advanced post-processing using surface-rendering algorithms to reformat images [17] (Fig. 3.7).

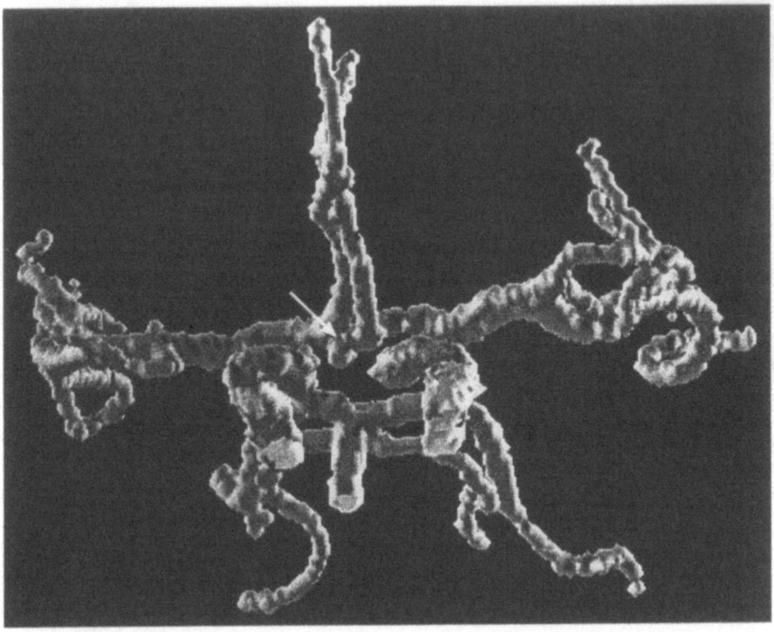

Fig. 3.7. Three-dimensional magnetic resonance angiogram of the basal cerebral arteries using a surface rendering algorithm showing a small anterior communicating artery aneurysm (*arrow*)

3.4.3 Screening for Asymptomatic Aneurysms

There is no doubt that preemptive treatment of asymptomatic intracranial aneurysms could prevent the morbidity associated with their growth and/or rupture. Before adopting such a health care policy we need, firstly, an accurate and safe way of diagnosing intracranial aneurysms and, secondly, a comprehensive understanding of their natural history so that the risks and benefits of such a policy can be properly assessed. At the moment, the morbidity of aneurysm rupture can be predicted with reasonable accuracy but we still do not know the risk of future rupture posed by an unruptured aneurysm. The natural history of unruptured aneurysms was discussed in Chap. 2 and is currently the subject of an international study of unruptured aneurysms being organised by the Mayo Clinic. This study may provide accurate data on the natural history of unruptured aneurysms, but until it reports, it is difficult to make an objective evaluation of the risks and benefits of a screening program for the general population.

Screening has been advocated amongst groups of people with an increased risk of developing aneurysms, e.g. patients with polycystic renal disease [41, 52, 84] and those with a strong family history of intracranial aneurysms [14, 89]. In these two subgroups, the prevalence of aneurysm has been estimated at 7%–22% [23, 41, 64, 84]. The imaging modality chosen by most investigators has been MRA because of the absence of ionising radiation and the small (but in this situation very relevant) risk of morbidity associated with the alternatives, i.e. intra-arterial angiography and contrast-enhanced CT scanning [36, 70]. Despite the ability of MRA [41, 84] and CT angiography [23] to detect asymptomatic aneurysms in patients with polycystic renal disease (Ruggieri et al. [84] reported finding 13 aneurysms in 93 polycystic patients), the logic of screening these patients has been questioned. Black [14] reviewed the arguments for screening families with polycystic renal disease for aneurysms and concluded that it could not be justified because of current uncertainties about their natural history, the risks of surgery, and the accuracy of current imaging techniques. Conversely, Schievink et al. [89] have advocated screening individuals from families in which two or more members have aneurysms. They argue that the operative risks of elective surgery are low [37, 76] and that members of such families are naturally concerned and often actively seek the reassurance of screening [79].

Accepting that MRA is currently the most appropriate means of screening patients; is the technique sufficiently accurate in the detection of asymptomatic aneurysms to justify the costs of a screening programme? Ronkainen et al. [79] performed MRA on 400 members of 68 families. Unlike examinations done acutely after SAH, all the images were adequate for diagnosis. They found 43 aneurysms in 37 patients, 32 of whom were then studied by IA-DSA. There were four false positive MRAs in this subgroup – a specificity of 87.5%. The IA-DSA demonstrated four aneurysms undiagnosed by MRA. An assessment of the sensitivity of MRA compared to IA-DSA was obviously not possible since IA-DSA was only performed after positive MRA studies. Nakagawa et al. [64] screened 400 volunteers with IA-DSA but MRA studies were obtained in only 30 subjects. The reason for performing MRA was not stated and it is therefore difficult to deduce its sensitivity from this study. However, it is likely that MRA performed in well and cooperative subjects will be at least as accurate as studies performed in symptomatic patients.

Determining the efficiency of screening is complex. Central to the argument is the likelihood of aneurysm rupture; if aneurysms rupture soon after they develop and before they can be detected, then screening is useless [14]. Alternatively, if a stable state develops in which future rupture is unlikely, again detecting and treating such lesions is a waste of resources. Obuchowski et al. [68] recently reviewed the efficacy of screening individuals with a family history of aneurysm and concluded that non-invasive screening was only justified in those 30 years old or younger. They estimated that a screening program would actually reduce life expectancy if all patients with unruptured aneurysms were diagnosed and underwent surgery. Their recommendation for screening in young people depended on an assumed constant risk rate of aneurysm rupture. Such assumptions highlight the uncertainties in our understanding of the behaviour of intracranial aneurysm. The non-invasive imaging now available provides the means for studies into the natural history of intracranial aneurysm. Screening of the general population is currently not justified, but the arguments for its use in high-risk groups are finely balanced [21] and may be of benefit if undertaken on a selective basis.

3.5 Imaging for Endovascular Treatment

3.5.1 Pre-procedural Evaluation

Once referred for endovascular therapy, the patient harbouring intracranial aneurysm(s) is assessed by physical examination and neuroradiological imaging. The endovascular therapist requires data about the site, size and geometry of the aneurysm as well as the presence of other pathologies and the overall state of the cerebral vasculature (particularly collateral support by the circle of Willis). In most instances the decision to recommend endovascular therapy is based on the IA-DSA since it provides all or most of the required data. Additional pre-treatment imaging can help to evaluate the relationship of the aneurysm neck to adjacent structures, to demonstrate its effect on the adjacent brain and to exclude complications following SAH.

Planar scanning with CT or MRI should be performed prior to endovascular treatment to confirm SAH, exclude complications such as cerebral infarction or hydrocephalus and provide a baseline scan for patients presenting with symptomatic unruptured aneurysms causing mass effect. MRI is particularly useful for evaluating very large and giant aneurysms before and after treatment by endosaccular packing or parent artery occlusion. The overall aneurysm size can be determined and the wall thickness assessed (see Chap. 1, Fig. 1.7). Pre-treatment MRI may also show signal changes due to compression of the surrounding brain [34] and flow-sensitive MR sequences with cine-loop display will demonstrate volume changes in larger aneurysms due to pulsatile blood flow [59, 102]. Pre-treatment baseline imaging is therefore helpful to assess the effect of treatment on aneurysm size and the surrounding structures [34, 103].

Most pertinent to the pre-treatment evaluation is an assessment of the aneurysm neck size since this will determine the feasibility of endosaccular packing. Several authors have reported initial experiences with 3D imaging techniques to measure aneurysms and to analyse the size of the osteum and its orientation to parent and adjacent arteries using CT [4, 30] or MR scanning [16, 50]. Theoretically, imaging is best performed by helical CT scanning since turbulence of blood flow at the aneurysm neck and slow flow within large and giant aneurysms may reduce the signal available for MRA. For imaging larger aneurysms, 3D MRI with contrast enhancement (gadolinium) can help to overcome this problem [50]. A refinement to standard 3D imaging is the use of surface-rendering algorithms in post-processing to improve image quality. This technique, applicable to CT or MR angiography, allows the display of endovascular anatomy simulating that of intravascular endoscopy [17, 49]. Sophisticated pre-procedural imaging is of benefit in some complex aneurysms and can help in patient selection and treatment planning (see Figs. 3.6 and 3.7).

3.5.2 Imaging During Endovascular Treatments

Endovascular treatments of all types require high quality fluoroscopy, road-mapping and digitised imaging. For endosaccular packing of aneurysms bi-plane angiography has the advantages of speed and safety in the placement of coils or other embolic devices. During treatment by occlusion of the parent artery, angiography by injection of collateral cerebral arteries and cerebral blood flow estimations help to predict those patients unable to tolerate permanent artery occlusion. These latter techniques will be discussed in the next chapter (Sects. 4.3.4, 4.3.5).

In all types of endovascular therapies the navigation and placement of embolic agents and materials is monitored by IA-DSA. An angiographic assessment is made prior to embolisation to confirm the findings of pre-treatment imaging and to exclude new features such as the development of vasospasm or aneurysm enlargement (Figs. 3.2 and 3.5) and as a baseline for identifying any complication such as distal embolism during treatment. The preliminary angiogram should be carefully inspected to exclude fresh thrombus in the aneurysm lumen (see Chap. 4, Fig. 4.9). If the circle of Willis had not previously been demonstrated, the patency of potential collateral arteries should be assessed. Prior to endosaccular packing, the operator should determine the optimum angiographic projections that clearly demonstrate the aneurysm neck and obtain an estimation of the aneurysm sac size in order to choose the most appropriate coils. Rotational angiography may help to identify the best projection.

The aneurysm neck may be difficult to image because of overlapping arterial branches, eg. at the MCA bifurcation or in complex aneurysm associated with fenestrations, and intra-aneurysmal angiography may help to define the neck and its relationship to parent arteries. However, the technique is often of limited value since contrast media generally outlines only the outflow of the aneurysm sac. If performed, contrast injections should be made with great care since any rise in pressure within the aneurysm sac could provoke rupture. Blood flow is turbulent around wide necked aneurysms and frequently radiographic contrast initially underfills the neck region, presumably because of poor mixing with unopascified blood. This effect makes estimation of the neck size from IA-DSA difficult. Once coils have been placed, blood flow in and out of the aneurysm is reduced and contrast media mixing is more even, making it easier to estimate the true neck size.

Periprocedural monitoring of cerebral arterial blood velocities can be performed by TCD [81], but maintaining the ultrasound probe position is difficult. During treatments with temporary or permanent arterial occlusion, physiological monitoring is required. The techniques and their rationale will be discussed in Chap. 4. Following endovascular treatment, control angiography should be repeated to ensure that thromboembolism has not occurred and to document the patency of parent arteries, for comparison with subsequent angiography should the patient's condition deteriorate.

3.5.3 Follow-up Imaging

In the 1–2 days following endosaccular coil embolisation or treatment by occlusion of the parent artery, complications may develop which require imaging. Occult rupture of a treated aneurysm can occur during endosaccular packing or in the immediate post-procedural period. CT scanning should be readily available and performed if there is any deterioration in the patient's neurological state on recovery from general anaesthesia, to exclude bleeding or the development of another complication such as acute hydrocephalus. If unconscious patients are treated and remain inaccessible to examination because of the need for sedation to maintain mechanical ventilation, then it can be argued that CT scanning should be routinely performed, even after apparently uncomplicated embolisation. The principles of neurosurgical post-operative management apply to endovascular therapies, i.e. the cause of any deterioration must be determined, usually by imaging.

Early repeat IA-DSA and monitoring of intracranial arterial velocities by transcranial Doppler are employed to assess the severity of delayed cerebral vasospasm and monitor its treatment. Imaging techniques, particularly non-invasive modalities such as perfusion and diffusion MRI, are being evaluated as potential methods of monitoring cerebral blood supply after aneurysmal SAH or treatment by parent artery occlusion. For patients presenting with compression symptoms from unruptured aneurysms, the findings on clinical examination dictate the need for follow-up imaging. Worsening of a patient's symptoms or signs, or simply their failure to improve after satisfactory endovascular treatment, is an indication for a re-evaluation by planar scanning or IA-DSA. Comparison with a pre-treatment baseline scan or post-embolisation angiogram can be helpful in this situation (see Fig. 3.8; see also Chap. 7, Fig. 7.10).

There is general agreement that aneurysms treated by endovascular techniques, and particularly after endosaccular coil embolisation, need to be followed up in order to document the security of the embolisation. For small aneurysms this requires IA-DSA since intra-aneurysmal metal coils cause artefacts on both CT and MR scans. However, useful follow-up information about the size and filling of giant and large aneurysms can be obtained using MRI/MRA, which are generally superior to CT for follow-up assessments [105]. In order to overcome the problem of coil-induced MR artefacts, Watson [112] proposed reversal of the phase encoding direction for MRA, but neither MRI nor MRA are currently able to detect the small changes in the neck region that may predate aneurysm regrowth.

Follow-up IA-DSA should be based on procedural imaging and the same "working projection" used to image the neck region, since this is the likely site of residual or recurrent filling of the aneurysm. Neck remnants or "rests" are liable to enlarge due to aneurysm regrowth or following compaction of the coil mass (see Chap. 7, Figs. 7.7, 7.8). No firm recommendation on intervals between treatment and follow-up angiograms can be made on the basis of our current understanding of the endovascular healing process.

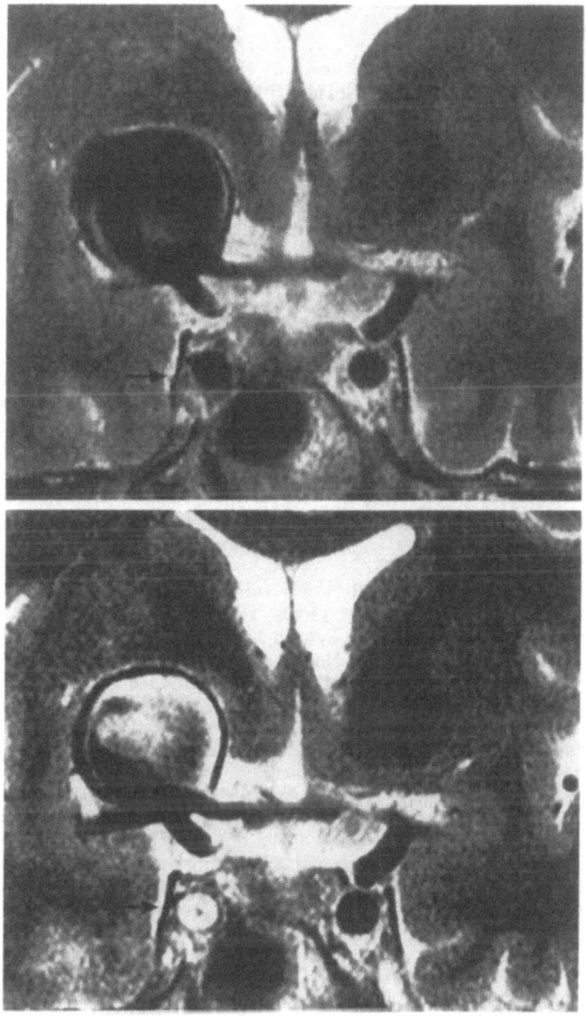

a

b

Fig. 3.8.
a Coronal T2-weighted magnetic resonance imaging (MRI) showing a large aneurysm of the terminal internal carotid artery (ICA). The wide neck includes the origins of the anterior cerebral artery and middle cerebral artery. Endovascular treatment was performed by balloon occlusion of the proximal ICA (*arrows*). **b** Follow-up MRI shows residual flow in the lateral portion of the aneurysm sac, probably due to collateral blood flow via the anterior communicating artery

A variety of protocols are therefore practised by endovascular treatment centres; these generally include an early follow-up study at 3–6 months and then a late follow-up at 1–3 years (see Chap. 5, Sect. 5.4.3). Some therapists prefer to obtain a follow-up study very soon after embolisation, particularly when treating ruptured aneurysms to ensure that the aneurysm has been occluded and to reassure patients that they are protected against re-haemorrhage.

References

1. Aaslid R, Huber P, Nornes H (1984) Evaluation of cerebrovascular spasm with transcranial Doppler ultrasound. J Neurosurg 60:37–41
2. Adam JE, Prawirohardjo S (1959) Fate of red blood cells injected into cerebrospinal fluid pathways. Neurology 9:561–564
3. Adams HP, Kassell NF, Torner JC, Sahs AL (1983) CT and clinical correlations in recent aneurysmal subarachnoid hemorrhage: a preliminary report of the Cooperative Aneurysm Study. Neurology 33:981–988
4. Aoki S, Sasaki Y, Machida T et al (1992) Cerebral aneurysms: detection and delineation using 3-D-CT angiography. AJNR Am J Neuroradiol 13:1115–1120
5. Aprile I, Biasizzo A, Lavaroni R et al (1996) Valutazione degli aneurismi cerebrali con angio-Rm. Riv Neuroradiol 9:541–550
6. Asari S, Satoh T, Sakurai M et al (1982) Delineation of unruptured cerebral aneurysms by computerised angiotomography. J Neurosurg 57:527–534
7. Atlas SW (1993) MR imaging is highly sensitive for acute subarachnoid hemorrhage... not! Radiology 186:319–332
8. Barrows LJ, Hunter FT, Banker BQ (1955) The nature and clinical significance of pigments in the cerebrospinal fluid. Brain 78:59–80
9. Baumgartner RW, Mattle HP, Kothbauer K, Schroth G (1994) Transcranial color-coded duplex sonography in cerebral aneurysms. Stroke 25:2429–2434
10. Becker G, Greiner K, Kaune B et al (1991) Diagnosis and monitoring of subarachnoid hemorrhage by transcranial color-coded real-time sonography. Neurosurgery 28:814–820
11. Beguelin C, Seiler R (1983) Subarachnoid hemorrhage with normal cerebral panangiography. Neurosurgery 13:409–411
12. Bell BA, Kendall BE, Symon L (1980) Computed tomography in aneurysmal subarachnoid haemorrhage. J Neurol Neurosurg Psychiatry 43:522–524
13. Bjorkesten G, Halonen V (1965) Incidence of intracranial vascular lesions in patients with subarachnoid hemorrhage investigated by four-vessel angiography. J Neurosurg 23:29–32
14. Black WC (1994) Intracranial aneurysm in adult polycystic kidney disease: is screening with MR angiography indicated? Radiology 191:18–20
15. Bladder DD, Parker DL, Ahn SS et al (1992) Cerebral MR angiography with multiple overlapping slab acquisition. Part II. Early clinical experience. Radiology 183:379–389
16. Bontozoglou N, Spanos H, Lasjaunias P, Zarifis G (1994) Three-dimensional display of the orifice of intracranial aneurysms: a new potential application for magnetic resonance angiography. Neuroradiology 36:346–349
17. Bontozoglou NP, Spanos H, Lasjaunias P, Zarifis G (1995) Intracranial aneurysms: endovascular evaluation with three-dimensional-display MR angiography. Radiology 197:876–879
18. Brismar J, Sundbarg G (1985) Subarachnoid hemorrhage of unknown origin: prognosis and prognostic factors. J Neurosurg 63:349–354
19. Bryan RN, Levy LM, Whitlow WD et al (1991) Diagnosis of acute cerebral infarction: comparison of CT and MR imaging. AJNR 12:611–620
20. Burama OJS, Janson HLF, Den Bergh FAJTM, Bots GTHAM (1981) Blood-stained cerebrospinal fluid: traumatic puncture or haemorrhage. J Neurol Neurosurg Psychiatry 44:144–147
21. Butler WE, Barker FG II, Crowell RM (1996) Patients with polycystic kidney disease would benefit from routine magnetic resonance angiographic screening for intracerebral aneurysms: a decision analysis. Neurosurgery 38:506–516
22. Caplan LR, Wolpert SM (1991) Angiography in patients with occlusive cerebrovascular disease: views of a stroke neurologist and neuroradiologist. AJNR 12:593–601
23. Chapman AB, Rubinstein D, Hughes R et al (1992) Intracranial aneurysms in autosomal dominant polycystic kidney disease. N Engl J Med 327:916–920
24. Curnes JT, Shogry MEC, Clark DC, Elsner HJ (1993) MR angiographic demonstration of an intracranial aneurysm not seen on conventional angiography. AJNR 14:971–973
25. Davis JM, Davis KR, Crowell RM (1980) Subarachnoid hemorrhage secondary to ruptured intracranial aneurysm: prognostic significance of cranial CT. AJR 134:711–715
26. Eskesen V, Sorensen EB, Rosenørn J, Schmidt K (1984) The prognosis in subarachnoid hemorrhage of unknown etiology. J Neurosurg 61:1029–1031

27. Fisher CM, Kistler JP, Davis JM (1980) Relation of cerebral vasospasm to subarachnoid hemorrhage visualised by computerised tomographic scanning. Neurosurgery 6:1–9
28. Fisher CM, Roberson GH, Ojemann RG (1977) Cerebral vasospasm with ruptured saccular aneurysms: the clinical manifestations. Neurosurgery 1:245–248
29. Forster DM, Steiner L, Hakanson S, Bergvall U (1978) The value of repeat panangiography in cases of unexplained subarachnoid hemorrhage. J Neurosurg 48:712–716
30. Fukasaku K (1996) 3D CT Angiography (3D CTA) as pre-embolization study for embolization of cerebral aneurysm. Presented at the 12th Annual Meeting Jap Soc Intravasc Neurosurg, Nagoya, 28–29 November
31. Gouliamos A, Gotsis E, Vlahos L et al (1992) Magnetic resonance angiography compared with intra-arterial digital subtraction angiography in patients with subarachnoid haemorrhage. Neuroradiology 35:46–49
32. Greitz T (1956) A radiologic study of the brain circulation by rapid serial angiography of the carotid artery. Acta Radiol Suppl 140
33. Grzyska U, Freitag J, Zeumer H (1990) Selective cerebral intraarterial DSA: complication rate and control of risk factors. Neuroradiology 32:296–299
34. Halbach VV, Higashida RT, Dowd CR et al (1994) The efficacy of endosaccular aneurysm occlusion in alleviating neurological deficits produced by mass effect. J Neurosurg 80:659–666
35. Halgren R, Terent A, Wide L et al (1980) Cerebrospinal fluid ferritin in patients with cerebral infarction or bleed. Acta Neurol Scand 61:384–392
36. Harbaugh RE, Schlusselberg DS, Jeffery RR (1992) Three-dimensional computerised angiography in the diagnosis of cerebrovascular disease. J Neurosurg 76:408–414
37. Heiskanen O, Poranen A (1987) Surgery of incidental intracranial aneurysms. Surg Neurol 28:432–436
38. Hilal SK (1966) Hemodynamic changes associated with the intraarterial injection of contrast media. New toxicity test and a new experimental contrast medium. Radiology 86:615–633
39. Horikoshi T, Fukamachi A, Nishi H, Fukasawa I (1994) Detection of intracranial aneurysms by three-dimensional time-of-flight magnetic resonance angiography. Neuroradiology 36:203–207
40. Huston J III, Rufenacht DA, Ehman RL, Wiebers DO (1991) Intracranial aneurysms and vascular malformations: comparison of time-of-flight and phase-contrast MR angiography. Radiology 181:721–730
41. Huston J III, Torres VE, Sullivan PP et al (1993) Value of magnetic resonance angiography for the detection of intracranial aneurysms in autosomal dominant polycystic renal disease. J Am Soc Nephrol 3:1871–1877
42. Huston J III, Nichols DA, Leutmer PH et al (1994) Blinded prospective evaluation of sensitivity of MR angiography to known intracranial aneurysms: importance of aneurysm size. AJNR Am J Neuroradiol 15:1607–1614
43. Jenkins A, Hadley DM, Teasdale GM et al (1988) Magnetic resonance imaging of acute subarachnoid hemorrhage. J Neurosurg 68:731–736
44. Juul R, Fredriksen TA, Ringkjob R (1986) Prognosis in subarachnoid hemorrhage of unknown etiology. J Neurosurg 64:359–362
45. Kassell NF, Turner JC, Jane JA et al (1990) The international cooperative study on the timing of aneurysm surgery. Part 2, surgical results. J Neurosurg 73:37–47
46. Kendall BE, Lee BCP, Claveria E (1976) Computerised tomography and angiography in subarachnoid haemorrhage. Br J Radiol 49:483–501
47. Keogh AJ, Sankhla SK (1996) Magnetic resonance angiography for anterior midline aneurysms. Br J Neurosurg 10:143–147
48. Kistler JP, Crowell RM, Davis KR et al (1983) The relation of cerebral vasospasm to the extent and location of subarachnoid blood visualized by CT scan: a prospective study. Neurology 33:424–436
49. Kollias S, Samara C, Valavanis A (1996) Surface rendering and endoscopic postprocessing of 3D MR angiography in the work-up of intracranial aneurysms. Proc 34th Meeting Am Soc Neuroradiol, Seattle 23–27 June, p143
50. Kurihara N, Takahashi S, Higano S et al (1995) Evaluation of large intracranial aneurysm with three-dimensional MRI. J Comput Assist Tomogr 19:707–712
51. Lang DT, Berberian LB, Lee S, Autt M (1990) Rapid differentiation of subarachnoid hemorrhage from traumatic lumbar puncture using D-dimer assay. Am J Clin Pathol 93:403–405
52. Levey AS (1990) Screening for occult intracranial aneurysms in polycystic renal disease: interim guidelines. J Am Soc Nephrol 1:9–12

53. Levinson A (1919) Cerebrospinal fluid in health and in disease. C.V. Mosby, St Louis, pp 17–30
54. Liliequist B, Lindqvist M, Probst F (1976) Rupture of intracranial aneurysm during carotid angiography. Neuroradiology 11:185–190
55. Liliequist B, Lindqvist M, Valdimarsson E (1977) Computed tomography and subarachnoid haemorrhage. Neuroradiology 14:21–26
56. Litt AW (1994) MR angiography of intracranial aneurysms: proceed, but with caution. AJNR 15:1615–1616
57. MacDonald A, Mendelow AD (1988) Xanthochromia revisited: a re-evaluation of lumbar puncture and CT-scanning in the diagnosis of subarachnoid haemorrhage. J Neurol Neurosurg Psychiatry 51:342–344
58. Marchal G, Bosmans H, Van Fraeyenhoven L et al (1990) Intracranial vascular lesions: optimization and clinical evaluation of three-dimensional time-of-flight MR angiography. Radiology 175:443–448
59. Meyer FB, Huston J III, Riederer SS (1993) Pulsatility increases in aneurysm size determined by cine phase-contrast MR angiography. J Neurosurg 78:879–883
60. Milian G, Chiray S (1902) Bull Soc Anat 4:550
61. Mizukami M, Takemae T, Tazawa T et al (1980) Value of computed tomography in the prediction of cerebral vasospasm after aneurysm rupture. Neurosurgery 7:583–586
62. Mohr JP, Biller J, Hilal SK et al (1995) Magnetic resonance versus computed tomographic imaging in acute stroke. Stroke 26:807–812
63. Nadjmi M, Braun H, Cavallini L, Nippert M (1968) Hämodynamische und physikalische Aspekte der retrograden Brachialis-angiographie. Dtsch Z Nervenheilkd 194:328–343
64. Nakagawa T, Hashi K (1994) The incidence and treatment of asymptomatic, unruptured cerebral aneurysms. J Neurosurg 80:217–223
65. Newell DW, Le Roux PD, Dacey RG et al (1989) CT infusion scanning for the detection of cerebral aneurysms. J Neurosurg 71:175–179
66. Nishioka H, Torner JC, Graf CJ (1984) Cooperative study of intracranial aneurysms and subarachnoid hemorrhage: a long term prognostic study. III. Subarachnoid hemorrhage of undetermined origin. Arch Neurol. 41:1147–1151
67. Noguchi K, Ogawa T, Inugami A et al (1995) Acute subarachnoid hemorrhage: MR imaging with fluid-attenuated inversion recovery pulse sequences. Radiology 196:773–777
68. Obuchowski NA, Modic MT, Magdinec M (1995) Current inplications for the efficacy of noninvasive screening for occult intracranial aneurysms in patients with a family history of aneurysms. J Neurosurg 83:42–49
69. Ogawa T, Inugumi A, Hatazawa J et al (1995) MR diagnosis of subacute and chronic subarachnoid hemorrhage: comparison with CT. AJR 165:1257–1262
70. Okuno T, Moriwaki H, Miyamato K et al (1988) Usefulness of CT angiography for demonstrating cerebral aneurysms. Neurol Surg 16:249–257
71. Page KB, Howell SJ, Smith CML et al (1990) Bilirubin, ferritin, D-dimers and erythrophages in the cerebrospinal fluid of patients with suspected subarachnoid haemorrhage but negative computed tomography scans. J Clin Pathol 47:986–989
72. Pasqualin A, Rosta L, Da Pian R et al (1984) Role of computed tomography in the management of vasospasm after subarachnoid hemorrhage. Neurosurgery 15:344–353
73. Patrux B, Laissy JP, Jouini S et al (1994) Magnetic resonance angiography (MRA) of the circle of Willis: a prospective comparison with conventional angiography in 54 subjects. Neuroradiology 36:193–197
74. Paxton R, Ambrose J (1974) The EMI scanner. A brief review of the first 650 patients. Br J Radiol 47:530–565
75. Renowden SA, Molyneux AJ, Anslow P, Byrne JV (1994) The value of MRI in angiogram-negative intracranial haemorrhage. Neuroradiology 36:422–425
76. Rice BJ, Peerless SJ, Drake CG (1990) Surgical treatment of unruptured aneurysms of the posterior circulation. J Neurosurg 73:165–173
77. Rinkel GJE, Wijdicks EFM, Vermeulen M et al (1990) Outcome in perimesencephalic (non-aneurysmal) subarachnoid hemorrhage. Neurology 40:1130–1132
78. Rinkel GJE, Wijdicks EFM, Vermeulen M et al (1991) Nonaneurysmal perimesencephalic subarachnoid hemorrhage: CT and MR patterns that differ from aneurysmal rupture. AJNR 12:829–834
79. Ronkainen A, Puranen MI, Hernesniemi JA (1995) Intracranial aneurysms: MR angiographic screening in 400 asymptomatic individuals with increased familial risk. Radiology 195:35–40
80. Ross JS, Masaryk TJ, Modic MT et al (1989) Intracranial aneurysms: evaluation by MR angiography. AJNR 11:449–456

81. Rowe JG, Byrne JV, Molyneux A, Rajagopalan (1995) Haemodynamic consequences of embolizing aneurysms: a transcranial Doppler study. Br J Neurosurg 9:749–757
82. Rowe JG, Molyneux AJ, Byrne JV et al (1996) Endovascular treatment of intracranial aneurysms: a minimally invasive approach with advantages for elderly patients. Age Ageing 25:372–376
83. Ruggieri PM, Masaryk TJ, Ross JF (1992) Magnetic resonance angiography. Cerebrovascular applications. Stroke 23:774–780
84. Ruggieri PM, Poulas N, Masaryk TJ et al (1994) Occult intracranial aneurysms in polycystic kidney disease: screening with MR angiography. Radiology 199:33–39
85. Sahs AL, Perret GE, Locksley GB, Nishioka H (eds) (1969) Intracranial aneurysms and subarachnoid hemorrhage. A cooperative study. Lippincott, Philadelphia
86. Saito I, Shigeno T, Aritake K et al (1979) Vasospasm assessed by angiography and computerized tomography. J Neurosurg 51:466–475
87. Sankhla SK, Gunawardena WJ, Coutinho CMA et al (1996) Magnetic resonance angiography in the management of aneurysmal subarachnoid haemorrhage: a study of 51 cases. Neuroradiology 38:724–729
88. Satoh S, Kadoya S (1988) Magnetic resonance imaging of subarachnoid hemorrhage. Neuroradiology 30:361–366
89. Schievink WI, Limburg M, Dreissen JJR et al (1991) Screening for unruptured familial intracranial aneurysms: subarachnoid hemorrhage 2 years after angiography negative for aneurysms. Neurosurgery 29:434–438
90. Schmid UD, Steiger HJ, Huber P (1987) Accuracy of high resolution computed tomography in direct diagnosis of cerebral aneurysms. Neuroradiology 29:152–159
91. Schwartz RB, Tice HM, Hooten SM et al (1994) Evaluation of cerebral aneurysms with helical CT: correlation with conventional angiography and MR angiography. Radiology 192:712–722
92. Scotti G, Ethier R, Melancon D et al (1977) Computed tomography in the evaluation of intracranial aneurysms and subarachnoid hemorrhage. Radiology 123:85–90
93. Sevick RJ, Tsurada JS, Schmalbrock P (1990) Three dimensional time-of-flight MR angiography in the evaluation of cerebral aneurysms. J Comput Assist Tomogr 14:874–881
94. Shephard RD (1984) Prognosis of spontaneous (non-traumatic) subarachnoid hemorrhage of unknown cause. Lancet I:777–779
95. Strong W (1934) The disappearance of blood from the cerebrospinal fluid in traumatic subarachnoid haemorrhage. Surg Obstet Gynecol 58:705–710
96. Susuki S, Kayama T, Sakurai Y (1987) Subarachnoid hemorrhage of unknown cause. Neurosurgery 21:310–313
97. Sutton D (1962) Arteriography. Livingstone, Edinburgh, pp 8, 321
98. Suzuki J, Komatsu S, Sato T, Sakurai Y (1980) Correlation between CT findings and subsequent development of cerebral infarction due to vasospasm in subarachnoid haemorrhage. Acta Neurochir (Wien) 55:63–70
99. Tazawa T, Mizukami M, Kawase T et al (1983) Relationship between CT enhancement on computed tomography and cerebral vasospasm in patients with subarachnoid hemorrhage. Neurosurgery 12:643–648
100. Teal JS, Wade PJ, Bergeron RT et al (1973) Ventricular opacification during carotid angiography secondary to rupture of intracranial aneurysm. Case report. Radiology 106:581–583
101. Tsuchiya T, Yasaka M, Yamaguchi T et al (1991) Imaging of the basal cerebral arteries and measurement of blood velocity in adults by using transcranial real-time color-flow Doppler sonography. AJNR Am J Neuroradiol 12:497–502
102. Tsuruda JS, Halbach VV, Higashida RT et al (1988) MR evaluation of large intracranial aneurysms using cine low flip angle gradient-refocused imaging. AJR 151:153–156
103. Tsuruda JS, Serick RJ, Halbach VV (1991) Three-dimensional time-of-flight MR angiography in the evaluation of aneurysms treated by endovascular balloon occlusion. AJNR 13:1129–1136
104. van der Wee N, Rinkel GJE, Hasan D, van Gijn J (1995) Detection of subarachnoid haemorrhage on early CT: is lumbar puncture still needed after a negative scan? J Neurol Neurosurg Psychiatry 58:357–359
105. van Gijn J, van Dongen KJ (1982) The time course of aneurysmal haemorrhage on computed tomograms. Neuroradiology 23:153–156
106. Van Gijn J, van Dongen KJ, Vermeulen M, Hijdra A (1985) Perimesencephalic hemorrhage: a nonaneurysmal and benign form of subarachnoid hemorrhage. Neurology 35:493–497

107. Vermeulen M, van Gijn J (1990) The diagnosis of subarachnoid haemorrhage. J Neurol Neurosurg Psychiatry 53:365–372
108. Vermeulen M, Hasan O, Blijenberg BG et al (1989) Xanthochromia after subarachnoid haemorrhage needs no revisitation. J Neurol Neurosurg Psychiatry 52:826–828
109. Vermeulen M, van Gijn J, Blijenberg BG (1983) Spectrophotometric analysis of CSF after subarachnoid haemorrhage: limitations in the diagnosis of rebleeding. Neurology 33:112–114
110. Vieco PT, Shuman WP, Alsofrom GF, Gross CE (1995) Detection of circle of Willis aneurysms in patients with acute subarachnoid hemorrhage: a comparison of CT angiography and digital subtraction angiography. AJR 165:425–430
111. Wardlaw JM, Cannon JC (1996) Color transcranial "power" Doppler ultrasound of intracranial arteries. J Neurosurg 84:459–461
112. Watson V (1993) Use of MRA after GDC embolisation. Working Group in Interventional Neuroradiology, 13th Meeting, Val D'Isere, 17th to 22nd January
113. West HH, Mani RL, Eisenberg RL (1977) Normal cerebral arteriography in patients with spontaneous subarachnoid hemorrhage. Neurology 27:592–594
114. Wick M, Fink W, Pfister W et al (1988) Ferritin in cerebrospinal fluid differentiation between central nervous system haemorrhage and traumatic spinal puncture. J Clin Pathol 41:809–814
115. Wilcox D, Jaspan T, Holland I et al (1996) Comparison of magnetic resonance angiography with conventional angiography in the detection of intracranial aneurysms in patients presenting with subarachnoid haemorrhage. Clin Radiol 51:330–334
116. Wright RL (1962) Pressure considerations in carotid compression during angiography. J Neurosurg 19:375–377
117. Zimmerman RD, Heier LA, Snow RB et al (1988) Acute intracranial hemorrhage: intensity on sequential MR scans at 0,5T. AJR 150:651–661

Chapter 4

Endovascular Treatments

4.1 Development of Treatments

The idea of using blood vessels as natural access channels to reach and treat intracranial vascular lesions has stimulated the development of various delivery systems (i.e. microcatheters) and devices. The tortuosity, narrowness, delicacy and irregularity of intracranial arteries, as well as the presence of the carotid syphon, are obstacles to intracranial catheter navigation. Furthermore, since intracranial arteries are surrounded by and nourish the noblest biological tissue on earth, the consequences of their damage or perforation are potentially catastrophic. Several pioneer investigators have, in the past, directed their efforts to overcoming these formidable difficulties.

4.1.1 Intracranial Catheterisation

The history of endovascular navigation starts with the work of two neurosurgeons, Luessenhop and Velasquez [62] of Georgetown University Hospital (Washington, USA) who in 1964 reported the first catheterisation of intracranial vessels. They used a glass chamber, surgically connected to the external carotid artery, to deliver a length of silastic tubing into the internal carotid artery (ICA) and thereby into intracranial arteries. In one of several versions of what was effectively the first flow-directed catheter, the distal tip of the catheter was inflated, like a balloon, to temporarily occlude the neck of a large posterior communicating artery (PCoA) aneurysm. They stated that "intraluminal manipulation of the intracranial arteries about the circle of Willis is possible technically and is tolerated by these arteries when the forces involved are approximately the same as the systolic blood pressure." Furthermore, they prophetically wrote as follows: "catheterization as well as embolisation of the intracranial arteries may have therapeutic usefulness, particularly in the treatment of aneurysms and arteriovenous malformations." However, at the time catheterisation of cerebral arteries was generally considered exceedingly difficult and hazardous.

Developments in catheter technology were pioneered by Frei and colleagues from the Department of Electronics of the Weizman Institute of Science (Rehovoth, Israel). In 1966 [34] they published a description of a novel catheter which they called POD (para-operational device). This catheter was designed for superselective catheterisation with the minimum of vessel trauma. The proximal portion was made of polyethylene and the distal portion of soft silicone rubber. The distal section measured only 1.3 mm in outer diameter and was 7 cm in length. Embedded in the tip of the silicone tubing was a micromagnet 1 mm in diameter. External magnetic fields, both continuous and alternating, could be applied to pull the micromagnet-tipped microcatheter (by the continuous field) and to cause it to vibrate (by the alternating magnetic field). The effect was to induce the catheter to "swim" within the vessels by reducing friction between the catheter tip and the inner vessel wall. They also introduced the concepts of a guide catheter to support POD in the extracranial vasculature and a side-arm adapter (which they called the "plastic T") to introduce the microcatheter and to inject saline to flush the guide catheter. Today, 30 years later, we are still using tools developed for this system, including an inner stylet to push the flexible end of the microcatheter. Frei et al. [34] considered electrothrombosis a possible therapy for intracranial aneurysms and stated that "possibly the most dramatic application of the POD catheter is for the electrical obliteration of cerebral aneurysms and the selective treatment of other cerebral anomalies." They successfully tested the magnetically guided catheter in vitro using a glass model of the carotid artery syphon and were able to select and catheterise model aneurysms.

The concept of magnetic guidance became popular amongst investigators during the 1960s, much in the manner that balloon-tipped microcatheters, driven by blood flow, became popular in the 1970s and early 1980s. In 1967, Yodh and colleagues [110] from the Neurosurgery Service of the Massachusetts General Hospital, Boston, constructed a "magnet system for use in such areas as the treatment of intracranial aneurysms and other vascular malformations". Applying the same principles as Frei et al., the system used a large (5 kW) movable external electromagnet to propel and guide a 1.3-mm permanent magnet incorporated in the tip of a silastic microcatheter. Six different tips were made, in detachable and non-detachable versions. The detachable tip included a cavity at the rear of the micromagnet filled with paraffin wax in which a minute heating coil was embedded. Constructed of ten turns of 0.5-mm copper wire, the coil was connected to an external source of electricity via copper leads in the catheter and, when a current of 400 mA was applied, heating of the coil caused the wax to melt and the tip to detach. One non-detachable version was constructed with a central lumen in the tip magnet so that embolic materials could be injected. They predicted three uses for the catheters: (1) to block the feeding vessels of certain intracranial vascular malformations by implanting the detachable tip or by injecting congealable plastic, (2) to thrombose certain intracranial aneurysms by endosaccular injection of a congealable plastic, or by detaching a magnetic tip inside the sac and then injecting, through the catheter, iron particles which would adhere to the detached tip and (3) for superselective intra-arterial injections of chemotherapeutic drugs in high concentrations for the treatment of glioma. These concepts are only now being exploited, 30 years later.

Alksne [2], in 1968, developed a similar catheter capable of being directed into glass aneurysms by an external magnetic field. Iron microspheres could be injected via the microcatheter and kept in place by the externally applied magnetic field. One year later, the first report of magnetically guided intracranial navigation in man was made by Driller et al. [28]. They utilized a POD catheter, introduced by percutaneous carotid puncture, to perform the first ever catheterisation of the middle cerebral artery of a patient. In the same year, Molcho et al. [74] reported on the superselective injection, via a POD catheter, of a cytotoxic material into the middle cerebral artery of a patient suffering from a malignant tumor of the brain. In 1970, Montgomery et al. [76] described a modified version of POD which incorporated a small detachable balloon which could be inflated and detached. A rubber valve retained the solution used to inflate the balloon. This was the first report of a detachable balloon for endovascular use. In 1973, Cares et al. [14], from the Neurosurgery Service of Massachusetts General Hospital, Boston, and the Massachusetts Institute of Technology, Cambridge, Massachusetts, introduced the concept of endosaccular balloon occlusion of aneurysms. They published details of experimental work on a magnetically guided intravascular catheter that could deliver iron microspheres, isobutyl-2-cyanoacrylate, and detachable balloons for endovascular obliteration of aneurysms and arteriovenous malformations. The catheter, which was made of silicone, was flow-directed and the external magnetic field was utilized only to deflect its tip at critical arterial junctions. They developed a detachable balloon made of latex with a carbon steel cylinder in the collar used to mount the balloon on the catheter. To inflate and detach the balloon from the catheter, a solution containing 25% serum albumen was injected to fill the balloon and the carbon steel cylinder was heated by means of a remote (extracorporal) radiofrequency induction coil. When the temperature of the cylinder reached 55°C, the albumen coagulated and sealed the orifice of the balloon. Injection of an additional 0.1 cc of albumen solution expanded the delivery microcatheter and detached the balloon.

In 1974, 1 year later, Hilal et al. [48] reported on the clinical use of a slightly modified version of the POD catheter in 120 patients. They were able to perform percutaneous catheterisation of vessels such as the basilar, middle cerebral and lenticulostriate arteries. They injected embolic substances, including acrylics, into arteriovenous malformations, performed intracranial intravascular electroencephalography and, in one patient, performed endovascular electrothrombosis of a basilar artery aneurysm.

In spite of some success in negotiating intracranial vessels, POD did not become popular for three main reasons:

1. The apparatus, especially the external magnet, was cumbersome and the magnetic field disturbed the fluoroscopic images.
2. The distal silicone section of the catheter was able, in many instances, to selectively catheterise intracranial vessels without magnetic guidance.
3. It became apparent to most investigators that the best way of propelling a microcatheter was to mount a balloon on the tip and allow it to be carried by antigrade blood flow (as first practiced by Luessenhop and Velasquez in the early 1960s).

The most recent milestone in the history of neuro-endovascular navigation occurred in the mid-1980s. Erik Engelson, a 25-year-old bio-mechanical engineer working with a company in California (Target Therapeutics), had the idea of improving the microcatheter used in liver embolisation. He attached to the proximal polyethylene portion a short distal section which was softer than polyethylene but stiffer than the silicone tubing used in existing microcatheters. He also introduced a steerable microguide wire with a deformable tip to negotiate sharp vascular bends and engineered a small radiopaque marker at the tip of the catheter. By pushing the microcatheter over the microguide wire the system was capable of entering brain vessels and remaining steerable [30]. In 1985, Engelson started animal testing of his new catheter, which he called Tracker, with Choi and Berenstein at the Interventional Neuroradiology Section, New York University. The Tracker catheter was first used in patients in 1986, in the external carotid artery and subsequently in intracranial vessels. It allowed intracranial navigation simply by pushing the catheter and for the first time the operator did not have to rely on an external force, i.e. external magnets, nor antegrade blood flow to perform distal superselective catheterisation [55]. A range of such microcatheters are now availabe to the endovascular therapist, designed for endovascular navigation using a microguide wire. They are used to deliver balloons, coils and liquid agents [24, 81, 109].

4.1.2 Balloons

In 1970, Kessler and Wholey [54] and in 1971 Prolo and Hanbery [86] reported on their experience of percutaneous internal carotid occlusion with non-detachable balloon catheters in patients with intracranial aneurysms and carotid cavernous fistulae. In 1974, a report of the clinical use of balloon-tipped microcatheters and detachable balloons by Serbinenko of the Burdenko Neorosurgical Institute, Moscow [95], established the endovascular treatment of intracranial aneurysms. This report concerned the treatment of more than 300 patients with vascular lesions. It was the first to demonstrate the feasibility of endovascular closure of high-flow carotid cavernous fistulae with preservation of the carotid artery and endosaccular occlusion of intracranial aneurysms. This work had an exceptional influence on future investigators, forming the clinical basis for the new discipline of endovascular neurosurgery and interventional neuroradiology.

There followed a series of reports. Debrun et al. in 1975 [2 1], Laitinen and Servo in 1978 [58], Di Tullio et al. in 1978 [23], Taki et al. in 1979 [103] and Romodanov and Shcheglov in 1982 [88] reported clinical experiences with detachable balloons for embolisation of intracranial vascular lesions. The mechanisms used by these workers to detach a balloon from the delivery microcatheter varied, but the underlying concept was the same, i.e. to occlude a vascular cavity (artery, vein or aneurysm) by filling it with one or more balloons delivered via the endovascular route. The next decade saw the development of neuro-endovascular centres in which balloon occlusion of aneurysm-bearing arteries and endosaccular occlusion of intracranial aneurysms were practiced. These procedures, originally conceived by endovascular neurosurgeons, were applied by a new specialist: the interventional neuroradiologist. Investigators such as Debrun (University Hospital, London, Ontario) [22], Merland (Hopital Lariboisière, Paris), Berenstein (New York University, New York) [7] among other centres, treated patients with intracranial aneurysm by parent vessel occlusion. Shcheglov (Research Institute of Neurosurgery, Kiev), Hieshima (University of California, San Francisco) [45], and

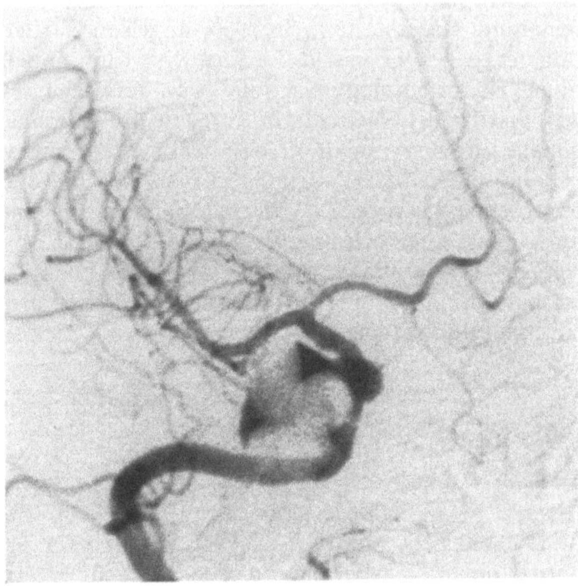

Fig. 4.1.
Oblique frontal intra-arterial digital subtraction angiography showing a large aneurysm of the right cavernous carotid artery packed with three balloons. The balloons, though filling the majority of the aneurysm, are unable to completely fill the lumen (unlike coils) because of their shape and rigidity

Moret (Institute Rothschild, Paris) [78] pioneered endosaccular balloon occlusion of intracranial aneurysms with preservation of the parent vessel [45, 88]. Their institutions attracted an entire generation of interventional neuroradiologists.

Parent vessel occlusion continues to be practiced for giant or fusiform aneurysms (see below), but endosaccular balloon occlusion has in the last 5 years been superceded by coil embolisation [39, 40]. The use of balloons for endosaccular occlusion of intracranial aneurysms was associated with a relatively high rate of complications which limited their clinical use. Higashida et al. [46] reported 18% mortality and 11% morbidity rates following balloon embolisation of inoperable intracranial aneurysm. Romodanov and Shcheglov [88] considered balloon embolisation to be contraindicated in small aneurysms, in aneurysms with a wide neck, and during the acute phase after subarachnoid haemorrhage, especially in the presence of vasospasm since the mortality amongst such patients was 22%. This high incidence of morbidity was the reason for the shift from balloons to coils for endosaccular embolisation of aneurysms. The greater safety of coils is probably due to their different physical structure. It is intuitive that balloons and coils behave differently when used as endosaccular packing materials. Intrasaccular balloons were filled with hydroxyethylmethacrylate (HEMA), a solidifying agent utilized to prevent balloon deflation. HEMA-filled balloons are stiff and more likely to transmit the energy of the systolic pulse to the walls of the aneurysm (Fig. 4.1). Intrasaccular coils appear to absorb part of this energy, buffering the transmitted blood pressure before the systolic pulse wave hits the wall of the aneurysm. This effect may explain the difference in early rehaemorrhage rates after the two treatments; aneurysm rebleeding rates are significantly lower when coils rather than balloons are used for endosaccular embolisation (see below).

4.1.3
Coils

In 1989, Hilal [50] reported the first use of thrombogenic coils for endosaccular packing of intracranial aneurysms, though coils had been used for occlusion of the carotid artery [8]. Coils were rapidly adopted for the endosaccular treatment of aneurysms because they can be deposited piecemeal so that aneurysms of differing size and shape can be completely filled (Fig. 4.2). The coils initially available were designed for embolisation of feeding arteries to tumours and proved too short and difficult to place accurately enough for aneurysm packing. There were a few reports of their use in clinical practice [15, 26, 57], but they were soon superceded by detachable coils, which are longer and allow the operator to control detachment from a delivery wire by mechanical or electrical means [16, 40].

In 1990 [40], a novel endovascular method with controllable and electrolytically detachable platinum coils (Guglielmi detachable coil (GDC), Target Therapeutics, Freemont, California) was developed to provide a less invasive and safer method of treating intracranial aneurysms. The coils are very soft in order not to damage the aneurysmal wall. They adapt to the shape of the aneurysm sac without causing significant distortion of the fragile wall, and are used to fill the aneurysm lumen as completely as possible. The ease with which they deform allows them to adapt to the effects of the systolic pulse, rather than opposing it.

4.2
Treatment Types

4.2.1
Introduction

The role of endovascular treatments in the management of patients with intracranial aneurysms has, until recently, been that of a second-line treatment confined to the management of those aneurysms unsuitable for clipping because of their size or location, or because craniotomy was contraindicated. A less invasive approach that avoids craniotomy, brain retraction, surgical vessel manipulation and potential complications such as wound infection, is particularly attractive in high surgical risk patients. It could be expected to reduce post-treatment hospital stay and recovery time. However, any alternative to conventional surgical clipping is only justified if it carries an advantage for the patient. Secondary considerations of the two treatment approaches are their relative costs; both social and financial. For comparisons to be made between extravascular and endovascular treatments, these factors should be considered, as well as the long-term security they provide against

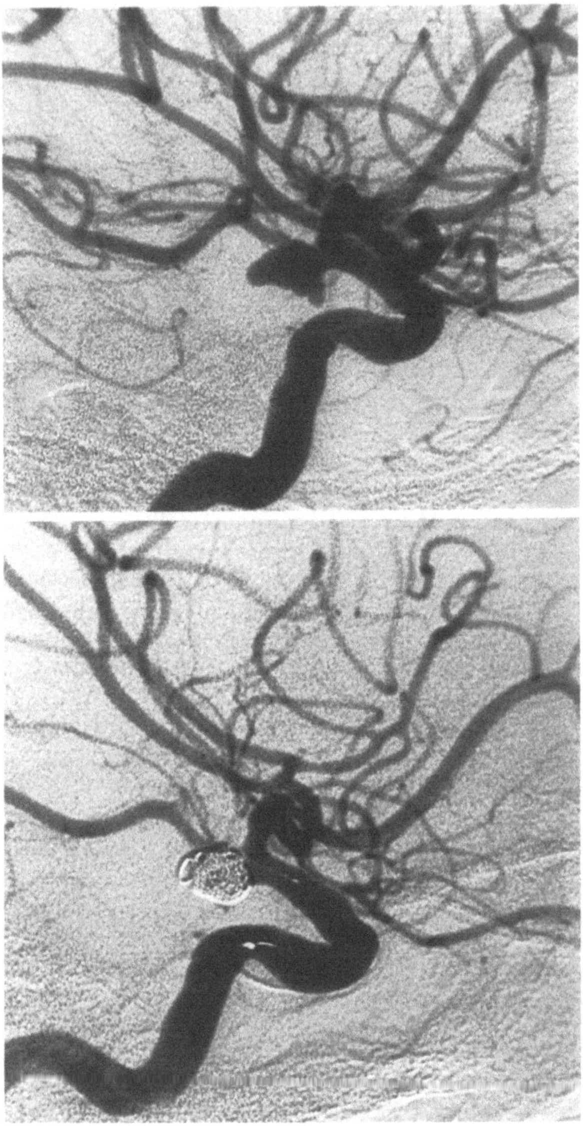

Fig. 4.2 a, b.
Lateral intra-arterial digital subtraction angiograms **a** before and **b** during coil embolisation with detachable coils. The aneurysm prior to embolisation has a concave inferior margin. After the introduction of a coil, the same margin is convex as the sac is filled with the occluding mass of coils

aneurysm enlargement and rupture. The endovascular and extravascular approaches have different constraints which in the long run will determine their roles in the management of intracranial aneurysms.

The current endovascular treatments of aneurysms may be divided into two broad categories: (1) occlusion of the arterial axis (parent vessel) harboring the aneurysm and (2) occlusion of the aneurysm alone, with preservation of the parent vessel. Treatment by parent artery occlusion is widely practised for inoperable fusiform and saccular aneurysms, and those with wide necks.

Treatment to occlude the lumen of saccular aneurysms, whilst preserving patency of the parent artery, involves endosaccular packing, generally with coils. This technique depends on the relative sizes of the aneurysm sac and neck since the neck must be small enough to contain the coils. These two endovascular techniques (endosaccular packing and parent artery occlusion) will now be considered separately.

4.2.2 Parent Artery Occlusion

4.2.2.1 Introduction

Occlusion of the parent artery proximal to an aneurysm was proposed and performed for popliteal aneurysms by John Hunter over 200 years ago [84]. The principle was extended to intracranial aneurysm by Victor Horsely who, in 1885 [53], ligated the common carotid artery to treat an intracranial aneurysm in a patient presenting with signs of optic chiasm compression. Carotid artery ligation was performed by other surgeons for aneurysms causing compression symptoms [80] or following their rupture during craniotomy [98]. Planned direct surgical treatment became possible after the introduction of cerebral angiography. Dott performed the first wrapping of an intracranial aneurysm in 1931 [25] and McConnell successfully packed an aneurysm with muscle in 1937 [72]. In 1938, Dandy clipped the neck of an aneurysm [18] preserving the parent artery and determining the direction of surgical effort for the last 50 years. Subsequent developments in neuroanaesthesia, aneurysm clip design and the introduction of the operating microscope have reduced the risks associated with extravascular clipping and extended its range. However, parent artery occlusion has continued to be practised throughout this century for unclippable aneurysms of the internal carotid [32, 83, 92, 97], the anterior cerebral [29], middle cerebral [27], vertebral and basilar arteries [102]. Surgical techniques for parent artery occlusion are either Hunterian ligation, i.e. occluding the parent artery proximal to the aneurysm neck or trapping, in which the aneurysm is isolated between proximal and distal arterial ligations [27, 102].

Over the last 20 years, endovascular balloon occlusion has replaced surgical ligation for aneurysm treatment by parent artery occlusion. This is largely due to the need for a period of temporary occlusion of the artery to be ligated in order to test the adequacy of collateral cerebral blood flow. Recognised by Matas and Allen [68] as early as 1911, this precaution is effective in predicting acute cerebral ischaemia but not delayed neurological deficits [67]. In order to prevent complications gradual carotid occlusion, over hours or days, was advocated in the past, rather than abrupt surgical ligation. Special carotid clamps were developed by Selverstone and White [94] and Crutchfield [17] in the 1950s and used until the introduction of balloons by Serbinenko [95] in 1974. These clamps were placed around the artery to be occluded and then closed when the patient was awake and accessible to neurological examination. Some allowed the surgeon to close the device by small

Fig. 4.3 a–c.
Lateral angiography by **a** superselective and **b,c** internal carotid contrast injections. There is a small aneurysm of the distal middle cerebral artery. **c** This was treated by endovascular occlusion of the artery proximal to the aneurysm using a pretzel shaped platinum coil (*arrow*). (**c** see p. 113)

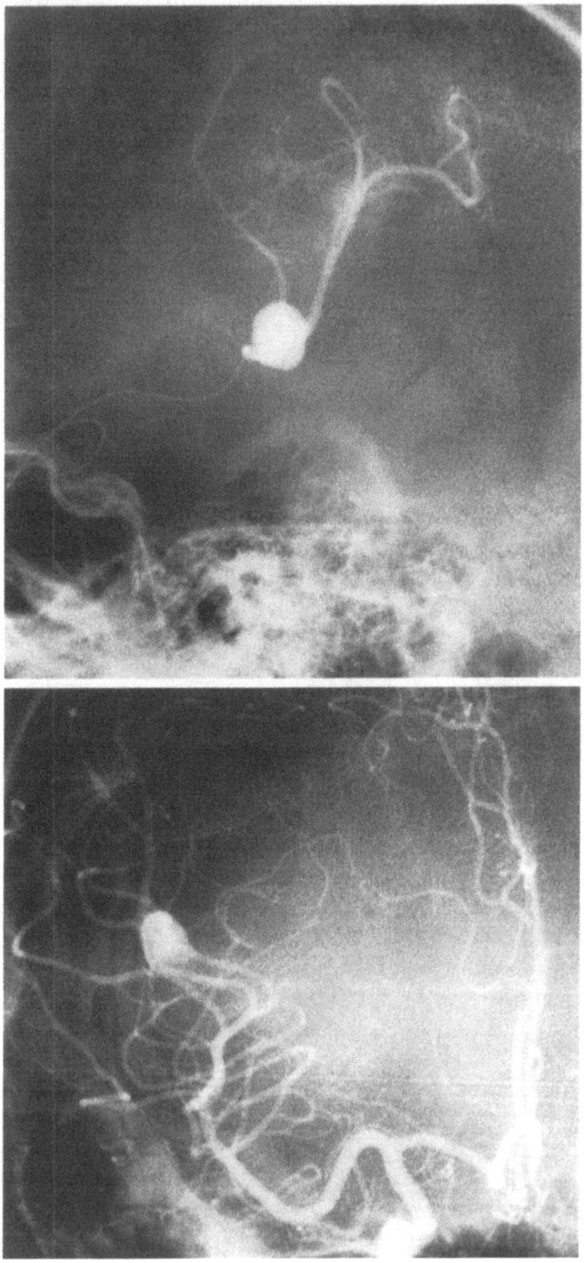

a

b

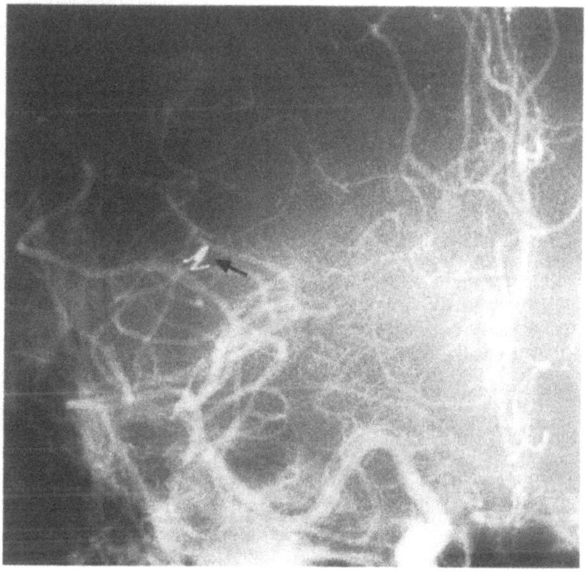

Fig. 4.3 c

increments over several days, in order to gradually reduce blood flow and stimulate the development of collateral blood supply. However, carotid blood flow is not significantly reduced until the cross-sectional area of the vessel is less than 2 mm^2, making staged clamping pointless, since blood flow is unaffected until the clamp is virtually closed [9]. Such procedures have now been completely superceded by balloon test occlusions which are performed both above and below the level of the circle of Willis in the awake patient. Test occlusion may be combined with provocative manoeuvres to stress the cerebral blood flow reserve but, though effective in anticipating and preventing acute cerebral ischaemia, they are, like their predecessors, not totally reliable at predicting the occurrence of delayed ischaemia [59, 73].

As a direct result permanent endovascular balloon occlusion has replaced surgical ligation because it can be combined with test occlusion which is easily performed on the awake patient, allowing continuous neurological examination, while concurrent angiography will demonstrate the degree of collateral support and obtain an accurate assessment of the effects of occlusion at any particular site on blood flow within the aneurysm [6, 33, 47]. Parent artery occlusion can also be performed with coils and novel endovascular ligature devices are being developed for use in vessels of different sizes (Fig. 4.3). Endovascular trapping can also be performed, whereby the aneurysm is isolated by placing balloons or coils in the parent artery proximal and distal to its neck.

An alternative technique, based on the Hunterian principle that aneurysm regression can be induced by altering flow in the parent artery, is to cause flow reversal in the basilar artery by occluding both vertebral arteries (Fig. 4.4). Originally proposed by Dandy [19], vertebral artery occlusions are performed for saccular or fusiform aneurysms of the basilar artery, collateral

Fig. 4.4.
a Lateral intra-arterial digital subtraction angiography by injection of the right internal carotid artery following balloon occlusion of both vertebral arteries. Retrograde flow is evident in the basilar artery and contrast faintly fills the sac of an aneurysm of the proximal basilar artery (*arrow*). **b** Sagittal T1-weighted magnetic resonance imaging showing high signal thrombosis of the aneurysm lumen

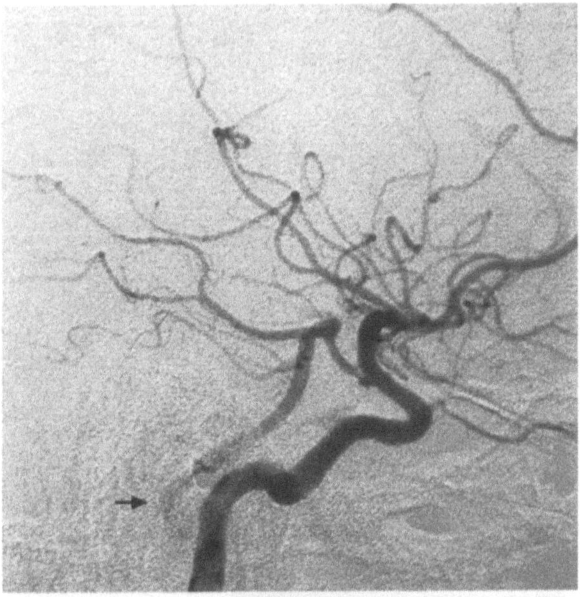

a

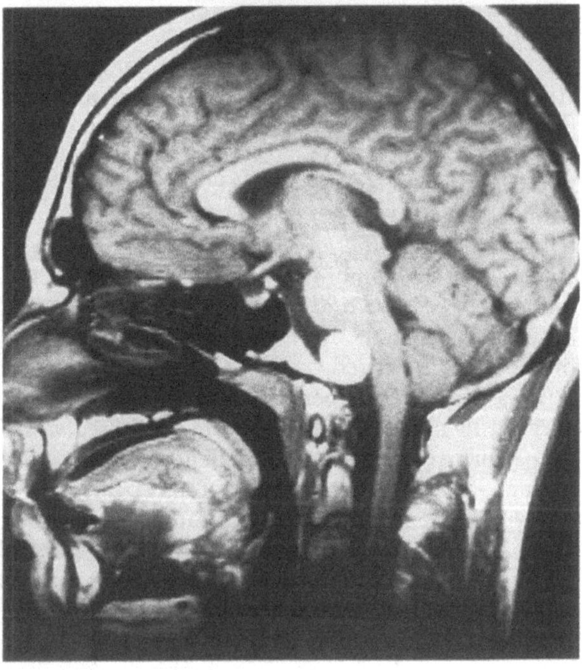

b

flow via the posterior communicating arteries maintaining the blood supply to the brainstem and cerebellum. Both surgical and endovascular techniques may be supplemented by prior revascularisation (by-pass) surgery in order to maintain adequate cerebral blood flow after occlusion of the aneurysm-bearing cranial arteries [60, 99].

4.2.2.2
Indications for Treatment

Sacrifice of the parent artery for the treatment of intracranial aneurysms should be considered in the following situations:

- *Giant saccular aneurysms (diameter greater than 25 mm), with wide necks and heavily calcified walls.* These aneurysms are difficult to treat by clipping or endosaccular packing because the aneurysm neck is wide and often obscured by the large aneurysm sac. The walls are thick, often calcified and rigid, making it difficult to apply clips and, in our experience, endosaccular packing with coils is associated with a high failure rate; aneurysm regrowth occured in nine of 11 (80%) giant aneurysms, 6 months after coil embolisation [10].
- *Wide-necked or fusiform aneurysms.* Wide-necked aneurysms may be unsuitable for clipping or endosaccular coil packing because of the proximity of adjacent vessels, lack of a neck capable of retaining coils or because of difficulties of surgical access. Aneurysms of the cavernous carotid artery are examples of such lesion; the aneurysm neck is often wide and relatively inaccessible for surgical exposure [7, 35]. Endovascular treatment of fusiform aneurysms inevitably involves occlusion of the parent artery whether proximal occlusion, endosaccular packing or trapping are performed.
- *Distal aneurysms above the circle of Willis on smaller arteries.* Such aneurysms may be difficult to locate during surgery and the small calibre of the parent vessel hinders endosaccular treatment.
- *Post-traumatic pseudoaneurysms and infectious aneurysms.* These aneurysms have fragile walls which may be perforated during endosaccular packing. They also generally occur on distal arteries and when collateral circulation is judged to be adequate, the endovascular route utilising balloons, acrylate glue or microcoils to occlude the parent artery is efficacious and avoids surgery in ill patients [43, 93].
- *Failed endosaccular embolisation.* Aneurysm regrowth after endosaccular coil embolisation may be managed by sacrifice of the parent artery as an alternative to repacking or clipping (Fig. 4.5).

4.2.2.3
Embolisation Devices for Endovascular Ligation

The ideal device for endovascular treatment of intracranial aneurysms by parent artery occlusion should cause temporary or permanent occlusion of the target vessel, allow blood flow to be rapidly re-established if needed and be completely reliable in its deployment. These attributes are obvious since, in most cases, the objective is to obtain a functional assessment of the effect

Fig. 4.5 a–c.
Frontal carotid intra-arterial digital subtraction angiography showing a giant carotid-ophthalmic aneurysm **a** before and **b** after endosaccular packing with coils. This patient presented with visual field loss which initially stabilised but later deteriorated, following recurrent filling of the aneurysm neck. **c** Balloon occlusion of the proximal internal carotid artery was performed and the patient's vision improved.
(c see p. 117)

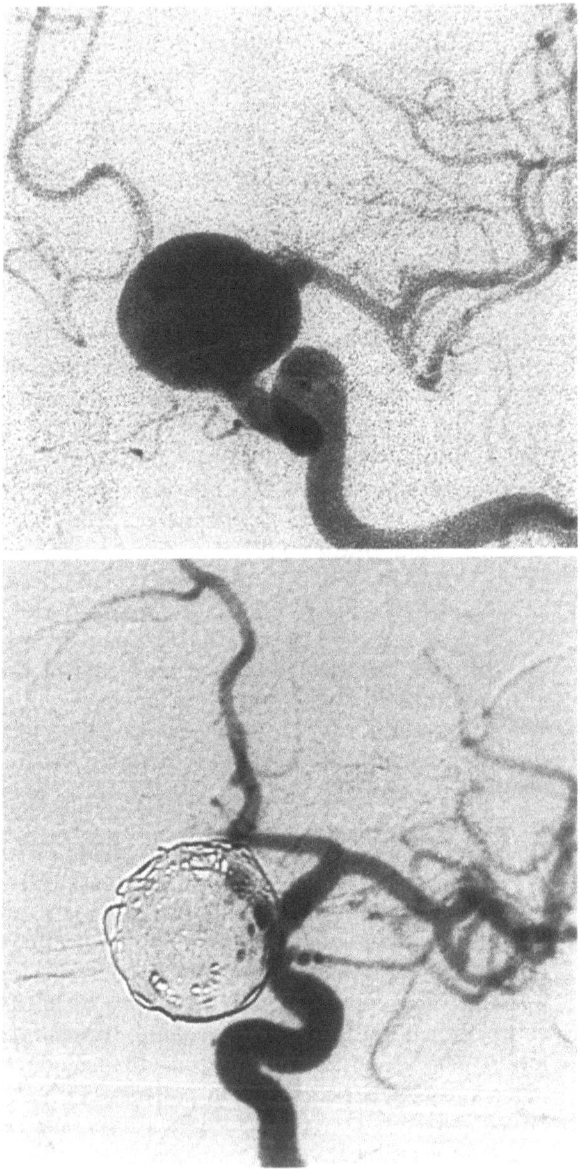

a

b

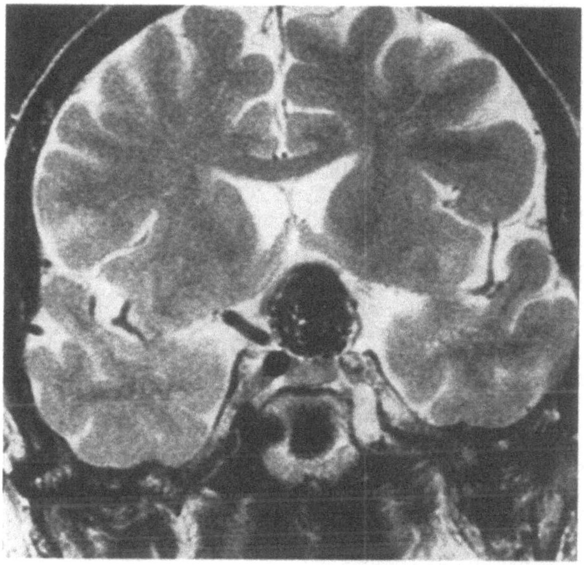

Fig. 4.5 c

of occlusion before the target artery is permanently occluded. Also important is the ability to reliably control the site and length of the ligation: devices, therefore, have to be navigable in the intracranial vasculature and be able to obstruct blood flow at a discrete point. For example, when it is necessary to occlude the middle cerebral artery in its M1 portion, a short occlusion device is less likely, than a long device, to obstruct the origins of lenticulostriate perforating arteries. Balloons or coils are used to perform endovascular arterial ligation; both have advantages and disadvantages.

Balloons are constructed of either latex or silicone [22, 45]. Silicone balloons have a higher expansion coefficient which makes them softer and more easily deformed than latex [52]. Silicone is more biologically stable than latex but, being semi-permeable, these balloons have to be filled with isotonic contrast media to prevent volume changes due to water moving across an osmotic gradient [44, 52]. There are a variety of techniques described for attaching them to catheters, but most are now manufactured with self-sealing valves, designed to hold the catheter tip and stop leakage after detachment. The currently available valved balloons are not totally reliable and are usually placed in tandem to ensure occlusion should one balloon deflate prematurely. Balloons are available in sizes small enough to reach arteries distal to the circle of Willis, but detachable balloons are to a greater or lesser extent liable to inadvertent detachment and require considerable skill for their safe intracranial navigation. They are available in different shapes since, in order to be stable in an artery, they have to be long and/or wide enough to obtain purchase on the vessel wall. They, therefore, tend to occlude a longer segment of artery than coils (Fig. 4.6).

Endovascular occlusion with coils is technically easier than balloons, but also depends on accurate sizing and control. Coils are manufactured in plati-

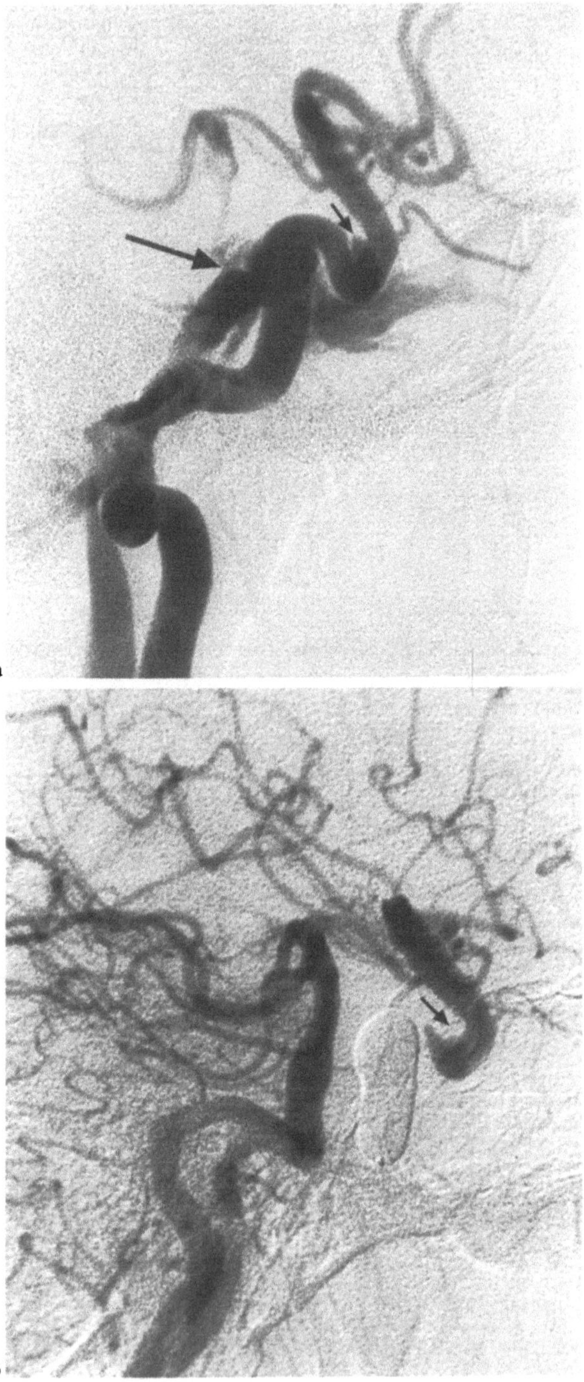

Fig. 4.6a,b.
Lateral intra-arterial digital subtraction angiography (IA-DSA) **a** before and **b** after balloon occlusion of the internal carotid artery (ICA). This patient presented with a spontaneous carotid-cavernous fistula. **a** The fistula is evident in the posterior portion (assumed to be due to rupture of an intracavernous aneurysm) of the cavernous sinus (*large arrow*). Contrast fills the cavernous sinus, inferior petrosal sinus and the superior ophthalmic vein. There is a small unruptured aneurysm at the mid-portion of the intracavernous ICA (*small arrow*). **b** IA-DSA has been performed by injection of the vertebral artery and retrograde filling of the supraclinoid ICA is seen. The fistula has been closed by parent artery occlusion in order to ensure regression of the coincidental aneurysm (*small arrow*)

a

b

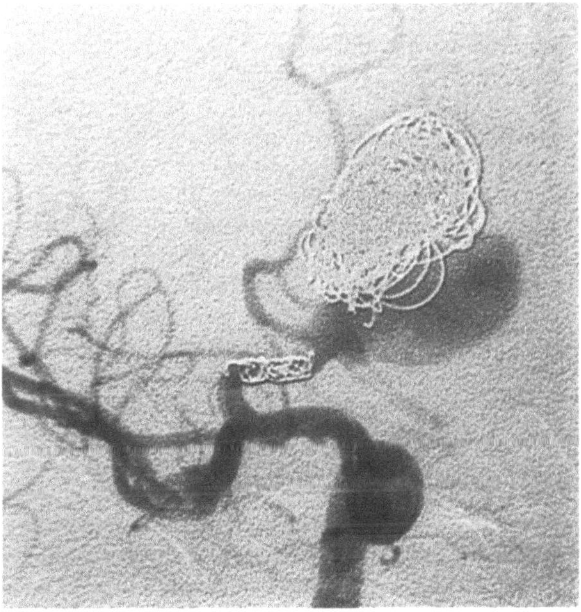

Fig. 4.7.
Oblique frontal intra-arterial digital subtraction angiography showing a giant anterior communicating artery aneurysm which has recurred following coil embolisation. Electrolytically detachable coils were used to occlude the anterior cerebral artery proximal to the wide aneurysm neck. Use of detachable coils in this situation is effective and allows preliminary assessment of collateral flow prior to their release

num, tungsten or steel and are similar, but smaller, to those used elsewhere in the body [8, 37]. They are available in various shapes and sizes and their thrombogenicity may be increased by the addition of fibres or special coatings. The simpler types are not attached to a control wire and are delivered by simply pushing or flushing through an appropriately sized catheter. Though less controllable, these are cheaper than controlled detachable coils, and therefore used in situations where positioning is not critical [49]. The controllable detachable coil represents a significant advance because it allows the operator to place, reposition, or exchange coils prior to their release. There are two methods for controlling coil detachment currently in clinical use: mechanical or electrolytic [39, 91]. The former uses a mechanical link to release the coil once it has been completely delivered from the microcatheter and the latter electrolysis. Thermal and other means of controlling detachment are being developed because, although electrolytic detachment is more reliable than mechanical separation, it is slower. Coils are generally easier to use in small distal arteries and detachable systems allow the operator to test a coil for size [87]in any particular vessel (Fig. 4.7).

4.2.2.4
Temporary Balloon Occlusion

4.2.2.4.1
Technique

Several authors have described protocols for temporary balloon occlusion (TBO) of cerebral arteries prior to endovascular or extravascular aneurysm surgery involving their permanent occlusion [4, 6, 7, 31, 33, 47, 49, 54, 69, 70, 75, 77, 85, 88, 96, 97]. In only two respects is there complete consensus; these are that patients should be anticoagulated and conscious (to be accessible for neurological examination) during the period of test occlusion. The technique practised by one of the authors (JVB) will be described and variations briefly outlined.

A silicone detachable balloon is placed at the proposed site of arterial occlusion and inflated for 20 min after anticoagulation by intravenous bolus injection of heparin sulphate. Prior to the test the patient is well hydrated, prepared with a mild sedative if required, and intravenous and intra-arterial access established for administration of fluids and monitoring. The adequacy of anticoagulation is assessed by estimation of the activated clotting time (ACT), and occlusion only performed when the ACT is three times baseline. The balloon is chosen following a complete intra-arterial angiogram of the cerebral circulation (including cross-compression studies) and sized according to the dimensions of the target artery. It is positioned at the site of proposed permanent occlusion, which is generally as close as practical to the aneurysm, i.e. immediately proximal to the neck. The site is usually determined by the need to obtain a stable balloon position. A road-map of the target artery is obtained and the balloon inflated with contrast (isotonic with saline) so as to just occlude flow in the artery. An assistant monitors the patient throughout the test period and collateral flow is demonstrated by angiography performed via a second catheter placed in the opposite carotid or vertebral artery. If the patient develops a neurological deficit the balloon is immediately deflated; if not and collateral blood flow on synchronous angiography appears adequate, then the balloon is detached in situ and a second balloon placed proximal to it in the same artery. The patient is then subjected to 48 h of intensive observation with continuous blood pressure monitoring and measures taken to prevent periods of hypotension.

Various aspects of the above procedure can be modified. The test may be performed with non-detachable balloons; these are constructed with a single or double lumen. The former, if attached to a flexible microcatheter, are easier to manoeuvre in tortuous arteries, but the latter allow a continuous saline flush to be provided into the vessel distal to the inflated balloon, the use of a guide wire for navigation and the measurement of intraarterial pressures [7, 70, 88, 101, 104]. However, using a detachable balloon for the test means it can be immediately deployed if collateral cerebral blood supply is adequate, which minimises the risk of emboli arising from static columns of blood proximal and distal to the occlusion balloon following deflation. The length of test occlusion times described vary from 15 min to over 1 h; in our experience ischaemic symptoms usually develop soon after balloon inflation and prolonged balloon inflation risks damaging the arterial wall [70, 75, 85, 96]. Some centres include electroencephalography in their protocol as an adjunct to neurological testing [85].

Provocative testing of the adequacy of collateral cerebral blood flow (CBF) can be performed by administration of the vasodilator acetazolamide [6] or sodium nitroprusside [100]. The induced hypotension undoubtedly identifies more patients unable to tolerate TBO than a normotensive test. In a group of 43 patients who tolerated TBO for 20 min, 21% developed neurological deficits following a reduction of systemic blood pressure to two thirds of baseline [100]. Inducing such deficits increases the sensitivity of TBO, but whether it increases the specificity is undetermined. Direct and indirect estimations of the effect of TBO on CBF can be made by stable xenon CT, ^{133}Xe single photon emission computed tomography (SPECT), ^{99m}Tc hexamethylpropylene-amine oxide (HMPAO) SPECT, H_2O^{15} positron emission tomography (PET) and transcranial Doppler ultrasound [4, 51, 70, 75, 85, 96, 101, 111]. Each method has its advocates but none, as yet, have been shown to accurately predict cerebral ischaemia after permenant artery occlusion [70, 111].

4.2.2.4.2
Risks and Benefits

The purpose of TBO is to identify patients at risk of stroke after parent artery sacrifice. The test is performed prior to carotid occlusion for a variety of indications but the majority of reports concerning the technique and its associated morbidity fail to differentiate underlying pathology which may contribute to immediate or delayed complications. For example, Standard et al. [100] quote rates for complications following clinically tolerated TBO of 5%–20%, but cite only those papers concerned with the surgical treatment of skull base neoplasms. Gonzalez and Moret [36] reported a complication rate of 10% for carotid balloon occlusion in patients with cervical lymphadenopathy due to cancer, whereas complications occurred in only 3% of patients treated for aneurysms.

Similarly, it is unreasonable to compare the incidence of delayed ischaemic symptoms following parent artery occlusion in aneurysm patients without distinguishing ruptured from unruptured aneurysm patients. Surgical ligation of the carotid artery was performed in 814 patients without preliminary TBO in the cooperative study, 82% of which were carried out within 3 weeks of aneurysm rupture [10]. Ischaemic symptoms and/or signs referable to the occlusion occured in 30% of those treated after SAH. A comparable figure for those treated for unruptured aneurysms can not be deduced from the presented data but Nishioka, in reporting outcomes, concludes that the incidence of ischaemic complications was highest in patients treated in the first few days after SAH and lowest in patients whose aneurysms had not ruptured [82].

Carotid ligation without preliminary test occlusion is undoubtably associated with an increased incidence of stroke. Linskey et al. [61] reviewed the literature and reported a cumulative incidence of stroke of 26%, whereas internal carotid artery occlusion performed after tolerance of TBO was complicated by permenant neurological deficits in only 4.7% of 192 patients repoted in five series [3, 4, 33, 47, 108], and in only 3% of their own patients.

The TBO test is therefore effective in preventing delayed stroke but two questions remain. Firstly, are some patients incorrectly excluded from treatment by the development of transient ischaemic symptoms. It would obviously be unethical to test this premise in practice since such patients are undoubtably at some considerable risk of stroke. Mathis et al. [70] reported that all their patients who, for one reason or another, had failed TBO and subsequently had carotid occlusion performed without by-pass grafts, experienced neurological deficits. Secondly, what is the additional morbidity associated with the performance of TBO? The reported incidence of complications resulting from TBO is 2.5%–8.3% for transient events and 0.4%–2.5% for permanent deficits [4, 33, 70, 96]. The largest reported series concerned 500 tests and reported complications in 3.2%; half were asymptomatic (mainly arterial dissections) and half associated with neurological deficits of which three quarters were transient [70]. Other complications reported due to TBO have been haematomas related to the anticoagulation employed during the test [100]. The test therefore carries a small risk of additional morbidity (in the order of that reported for intra-arterial angiography), but its general use has reduced the incidence of delayed cerebral ischaemia.

A controversy remains about the benefit of adding provocative tests and the need for measurements of CBF. The procedure, as described above, does not include a period of hypotension since there is as yet no evidence that it improves the specificity of TBO. The same concern restricts our use of CBF estimations by SPECT or xenon CT. It remains controversial which test is superior in predicting delayed ischaemia. Theoretically, the quantitative data concerning CBF provided by xenon CT is more objective and less dependent on interpretations of the relevance of asymmetric uptake of tracer than SPECT [112]. However, when quantitative (and qualitative) estimates of CBF are obtained they still require thresholds for determining the risk of a subsequent change in regional blood flow. Limits of absolute values of CBF set by various authors range from 30–40 ml/100 g per minute, below which patients are considered to have failed the test. The observed reduction in CBF (relative to baseline values) during temporary occlusion is also relevant and additional thresholds are described; both are somewhat arbitary recommendations [70, 73]. Furthermore, the problem remains that what is being attempted by such analyses is the prediction of morbidity due to different possible causes (i.e. hypoperfusion or thromboembolisation) and these predictions are based on changes induced by a non-physiological situation. Until consensus is reached about an optimum method of monitoring CBF changes during TBO, and such a method has been demonstrated to be of benefit, no logical recommendation on monitoring can be made. The results of permanent balloon occlusion, as with those of endosaccular GDC embolisation will be discussed in Chap. 7.

4.2.3 Endosaccular Packing (Coil Embolisation) with Parent Artery Preservation

4.2.3.1 Introduction

Endovascular treatment by endosaccular packing is the ideal method because, if the aneurysm sac is isolated from the arterial tree, the cerebral circulation is not compromised and the patient is protected against aneurysm rupture or regrowth. To compete with current microsurgical clipping techniques, endosaccular packing must reliably isolate the aneurysm which implies that the aneurysm is completely occluded. Endosaccular embolisation has been performed with balloons [46, 78, 88, 95], coils [5, 11, 13, 15, 40, 41, 50, 57] and various liquid agents [56, 64, 105]. Balloons are no longer generally used for the reasons outlined in Sect. 4.1.2 and because of the impossibility of completely filling an irregular shaped aneurysm with multiple balloons (Fig. 4.1).

Recent interest in the use of coils, which are more pliable and do conform to the shape of aneurysm lumens, has stimulated research into their efficacy. The long-term stability of coil embolisation has yet to be demonstrated, but in order to improve their thrombogenicity, various types of coils have been tested in experimental aneurysms [10, 37, 38, 39, 71]. Several workers have reported arterial wall repair with formation of a new endothelial layer over the ostea of embolised aneurysms [1, 20, 39, 71]. Liquid agents which theoretically can completely fill any shaped lumen, are also currently being tested [64]. Animal models have been used to demonstrate the feasibility of novel strategies to achieve occlusion of complex aneurysms, such as the use of a stent, placed in the parent artery to retain coils in the sac of wide-necked aneurysms or to redirect blood flow away from the neck [106, 107].

At the present time it has not been generally established which patients and which saccular intracranial aneurysms should be treated by either surgical clipping or by coil embolisation. Although data are now available on the efficacy of endovascular treatment with GDC for the prevention of rebleeding and relief of symptoms in the short to medium term [13, 63] and its effects on the incidence of symptomatic vasospasm after treatment of acutely ruptured aneurysms [79, 89], its long-term clinical efficacy has not yet been determined. Its role in the management of patients acutely after SAH is currently being evaluated [11]. Therefore, until such data are available it would seem advisable to select for treatment patients that are at high risk of morbidity if treated by craniotomy and those with aneurysms particularly suited for coil embolisation.

4.2.3.2 Indications

There is general consensus amongst endovascular therapists about the utility of GDC embolisation in the following circumstances:

- *Posterior circulation aneurysms.* Extravascular surgical treatment for most posterior circulation aneurysms is more difficult than for those of the anterior circulation and associated with higher rates of procedural complications [41]. The reported procedural morbidity associated with GDC embolisation is the same when aneurysms of the anterior or posterior circulations are treated [12].

- *Associated medical conditions.* Patients whose general state of health is a contraindication to craniotomy may be able to undergo endovascular treatment. For the same reason, elderly patients who, in the past would have been treated conservatively, should now be considered for coil embolisation [90].
- *Patients in poor condition following SAH.* Hunt and Hess grade IV and V patients and patients with post-SAH vasospasm are poor candidates for surgical clipping or endovascular treatment by parent artery occlusion and should be considered for coil endosaccular embolisation to prevent early rebleeding, in anticipation of recovery.
- *Patients with multiple aneurysms.* In order to avoid bilateral craniotomies [66] or those with moyamoya disease [65].
- *Surgical failure.* For the occlusion of aneurysms found to be unclippable at surgical exploration or after failure of surgical clipping or wrapping (Fig. 4.8).
- *Patients with symptoms of mass effect.* Small or large aneurysms should be considered for treatment since recent studies have shown remission of symptoms in this particular subset of patients [63].

Recommendations about whether a particular patient is to be treated by craniotomy and clipping or coil embolisation are based on clinical and angiographic assessments. As a general rule, small and large aneurysms with small necks (equal or less than 4 mm) are particularly suited to coil treat-

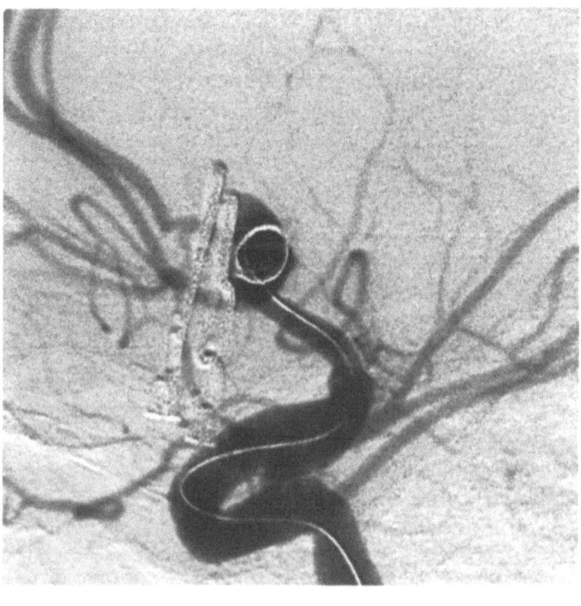

Fig. 4.8.
Oblique lateral carotid intra-arterial digital subtraction angiography showing a large, partially clipped aneurysm arising from the anterior communicating artery. This large post-operative residual sac was packed with Guglielmi detachable coils

ment [41, 113]. But the majority of such aneurysms are also ammenable to microsurgical clipping, so no firm recommendations about the selection of patients most suitable for coil embolisation can be made until the results of comparative clinical trails are known. However, if one accepts the premise that there are situations in which it is uncertain which approach is best, then it is legitimate to pose the question; what are the indications for microsurgical clipping? This question can be partially answered by indentifying the criteria that make aneurysms unsuitable for coil embolisation.

In assessing the suitability of aneurysms for endosaccular packing with coils there are several fundermental features of the angiogram helpful in deciding which aneurysms can or cannot be treated; these include:

- *Neck width.* Aneurysms with a neck greater than 4 mm in maximun diameter may be unable either to hold coils or to resist recurrence. They are better treated by surgical clipping or parent artery occlusion.
- *Aneurysm shape.* The shapes of saccular aneurysms can be defined by the ratio of neck to sac width. These dimensions are determined as the longest diameters visible on multi-projection angiography. If the neck is small relative to the size of the sac, then the neck:sac ratio will be in the order of 1:3 or greater and the aneurysm can be treated by coil embolisation. A broad-based or sessile aneurysm shape will have a neck:sac ratio in the order of 1:1 or 1:2 and be difficult to treat with coils (see below). However, this simple analysis does not take into consideration the shape of the sac nor the size of the neck relative to the size of the parent vessel.
- *Absolute aneurysm size.* Large and giant aneurysms generally have wide necks which involve a greater proportion of the circumference of the parent arterial wall than small aneurysms. They often incorporate the origins of adjacent branch arteries into the base of the sac which frustrates endosaccular packing since coils are likely to occlude the parent or these adjacent arteries. Such aneurysms are often sited at the basilar artery apex, the internal carotid artery bifurcation, the ophthalmic artery origin, the middle cerebral artery (MCA) bifurcation and the anterior communicating artery/anterior cerebral artery (ACoA/ACA) junctions (see Chap. 6).
- *Aneurysm location.* The relative ease of access to posterior circulation aneurysms via the endovascular route has been discussed and is reflected in the lower morbidity of coil embolisation compared with extravascular surgery in this situation. But other aneurysm locations are difficult to treat endovascularly because of the local anatomy, for example the MCA bifurcation where the position of eloquent branch arteries may be difficult to image and therefore preserve during coil embolisation. In this situation aneurysms are better explored at craniotomy and treated by microsurgical clipping.
- *Failed coil embolisation.* Clipping should be considered if coil embolisation proves impossible because of technical difficulties due to access or local anatomical constraints, and when aneurysms recur due to regrowth or coil compaction after initially successful treatment [42].
- *Unstable intraluminal thrombus.* The recognition of fresh and, therefore, unstable thrombus within the aneurysm sac is a contraindication to endosaccular packing (see Fig. 4.9).

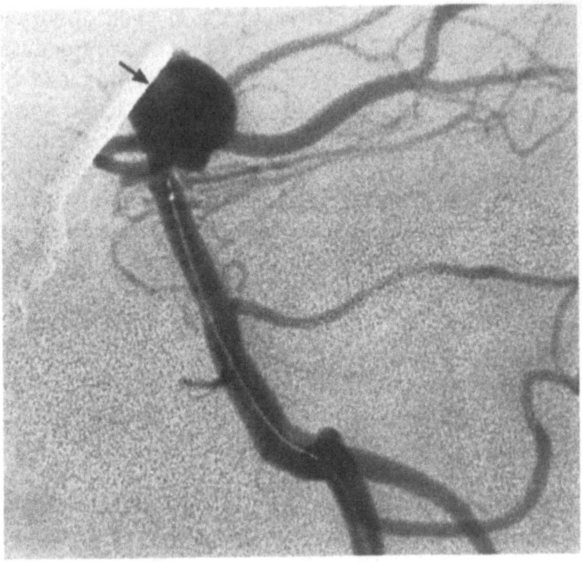

Fig. 4.9.
Oblique lateral vertebral intra-arterial digital subtraction angiography immediately prior to catheterisation of a basilar artery termination aneurysm. Surgical clipping had been attempted 3 weeks previously but the sac was only partially occluded. However, the aneurysm contains fresh thrombus (*arrow*) due to the distortion of its shape and intraluminal blood flow caused by the clip. Endosaccular packing with coils risks displacing such a thrombus, so treatment was postponed

The sucessful treatment of patients with intracranial aneurysm depends on close collaboration between the two approaches. The above analysis is an attempt to rationalise joint decision making, not a set of rules for two sides of a therapeutic divide. There are situations, such as the presence of intraparenchymal haemorrhage or hydrocephalus, when emergency surgical evacuation of haematoma or CSF drainage is life-saving. Conversely, there are situations when patients are too ill to undergo craniotomy and a less invasive procedure can protect them against fatal aneurysm rerupture. We therefore strongly advocate collaborative management.

4.2.3.3
Timing

Ideally, ruptured intracranial aneurysms should be excluded from the circulation as soon as possible to prevent rebleeding and allow aggressive treatment of complications such as vasospasm. For practical reasons, treatment may have to be postponed, e.g. until the following morning if the patient is admitted to hospital late in the evening. However, we believe that treatment should be performed as soon as possible and normally not delayed more than 24 h; the weekend should not be an obstacle to early aneurysm treatment.

While the timing of microsurgical clipping of aneurysms after rupture remains controversial, there is consensus that endovascular GDC treatment can be performed, and should be performed, acutely and that neither clinical grade, nor the presence of angiographic vasospasm are absolute contraindications to treatment. If parent vessel occlusion is the selected endovascular treatment for an acutely ruptured aneurysm, its effect on CBF have to be very carefully assessed. Since patients are liable to vasospasm and, if parent artery occlusion is performed early, its subsequent development may impare collateral blood flow, treatment should ideally be delayed until after the period when vasospasm occurs. A solution in this situation is to perform endosaccular packing with coils immediately after aneurysm rupture, so that definitive treatment by parent artery occlusion can be deferred for 2–3 months and the patient given time to recover from SAH and its complications.

4.2.3.4 Patient Management

The routine care of patients before, during and after coil embolisation as practiced by one of us (G.G.) will be outlined and this topic covered in depth in the next chapter. For patients presenting after aneurysm rupture, treatment is planned as soon as possible. If, for some reason, treatment has to be delayed, measures are taken to control systemic blood pressure (avoiding elevations above 160 mmHg) in the immediate post-haemorrhage period, provided there is no evidence of vasospasm. Anti-seizure medication is prescribed, as well as measures to prevent straining, such as during defecation. The patient should be nursed in a dark, quiet room and allowed a supportive companion. The intensive care unit is, typically, not designed for this, but high-dependency areas with "quiet rooms", if available, are ideal. If the patient is a smoker, access to cigarettes may be allowed. Analgesics and mild tranquilisers may be utilized to relieve pain or anxiety. Raised intracranial pressure due to acute hydrocephalus may be treated with cautious ventricular drainage, but since we feel that excessive drainage may precipitate rebleeding, we prefer to perform CSF drainage after the ruptured aneurysm has been secured by embolisation.

The endosaccular treatment of intracranial aneurysms should be performed with patients under general anaesthesia. This is particularly important in small, recently ruptured aneurysms where it is essential to have the patient perfectly still to perform safe aneurysm catheterisation and to manage possible complications (see Chap. 5). In some instances of large unruptured aneurysms, endosaccular treatment may be performed with the patient awake but sedated. It has been suggested that the systemic blood pressure should be judiciously lowered during endosaccular packing in order to reduce the mechanical stress on the wall of the aneurysm while coils are being delivered. We do not use this technique and see little to recommend it, since the endovascular therapist is able to control the speed and force with which coils are placed and should do this in such a way that only the minimum of pressure is applied to the sac wall. All patients are anticoagulated by administering heparin during the endovascular procedure (see Chap. 5).

After completion of the procedure an angiographic assessment of the embolisation is made and if there is a moderate degree of coil impingement upon the parent vessel or a significant amount of contrast stagnation within the coil mesh, systemic heparinisation is maintained until the next day. Otherwise, any residual anticoagulation effect of heparin is reversed by administering protamine sulphate. Following successful treatment patients are prescribed low doses of aspirin for 1 or 2 weeks. After endosaccular coil treatment of larger unruptured aneurysms which have been the cause of symptoms due to mass effect, patients are, in addition, given a short course of treatment with corticosteroids.

References

1. Ahuja AA, Hergenrother RW, Strother CM et al (1993) Platinum coil coatings to increase thrombogenicity: a preliminary study in rabbits. AJNR 14:794–798
2. Alksne JF (1968) Magnetically controlled intravascular catheter. Surgery 64:339–345
3. Andrews JC, Valvanis A, Fisch U (1989) Management of the internal carotid artery in surgery of the skull base. Laryngoscope 99:1224–1229
4. Anon VV, Aymard A, Gobin YP et al (1992) Balloon occlusion of the internal carotid artery in 40 cases of giant intracavernous aneurysm: technical aspects, cerebral monitoring and results. Neuroradiology 34:245–251
5. Apsimon T, Khangure M, Ives J et al (1995) The Guglielmi coil for transarterial occlusion of intracranial aneurysm: preliminary Western Australian experience. J Clin Neurosci 2:26–35
6. Aymard A, Gobin YP, Hodes JE et al (1991) Endovascular occlusion of vertebral arteries in the treatment of unclippable vertebrobasilar aneurysms. J Neurosurg 74:393–398
7. Berenstein A, Ransohoff J, Kupersmith M et al (1984) Transvascular treatment of giant aneurysms of the cavernous carotid and vertebral arteries. Functional investigation and embolization. Surg Neurol 21:3–12
8. Braun IS, Hoffman JC Jr, Casarella WJ, Davis PC (1985) Use of coils for transcatheter carotid occlusion. Am J Neuroradiol 6:953–956
9. Brice JG, Dowsett DJ, Lowe RD (1974) Haemodynamic effects of carotid artery stenosis. Br Med J 2:1363
10. Byrne JV, Hubbard N, Morris JH (1994) Endovascular coil occlusion of experimental aneurysms; Partial treatment does not prevent subsequent rupture. Neurol Res 16:425–427
11. Byrne JV, Molyneux AJ, Renowden SR (1994) Endosaccular coil embolisation of intracranial aneurysms. Neuroradiology 36:165
12. Byrne JV, Adams CBT, Kerr RSC et al (1995) Endosaccular treatment of inoperable intracranial aneurysms with platinum coils. Br J Neurosurg 9:585–592
13. Byrne JV, Molyneux AJ, Brennan RP et al (1995) Embolisation of recently ruptured intracranial aneurysms. J Neurol Neurosurg Psychiatry 59:616–620
14. Cares HL, Hale JR, Montgomery DB et al (1973) Laboratory experience with a magnetically guided intravascular catheter system. J Neurosurg 38:145–154
15. Casasco A, Aymard A, Gobin P et al (1993) Selective endovascular treatment of 71 intracranial aneurysms with platinum coils. J Neurosurg 79:3–10
16. Cekirge H, Saatci I, Firat M et al (1996) Interlocking detachable coil occlusion in the endovascular treatment of intracranial aneurysms: preliminary results. AJNR 17:1651–1657
17. Crutchfield WG (1959) Instruments for use in the treatment of certain intracranial vascular lesions. J Neurosurg 16:471–474
18. Dandy WE (1938) Intracranial aneurysm of the internal carotid artery, cured by operation. Ann Surg 107:654–657
19. Dandy WE (1944) Intracranial arterial aneurysms, Itheca, vol 8. Cromstock, New York, p 147
20. Dawson RC, Krisht AF, Barrow DL et al (1995) Treatment of experimental aneurysms using collagen-coated microcoils. Neurosurgery 36:133–140
21. Debrun G, Lacour P, Caron JP et al (1975) Inflatable and released balloon technique experimentation in dog-application in man. Neuroradiology 9:267–271
22. Debrun G, Fox A, Drake C et al (1981) Giant unclippable aneurysms: treatment with detachable balloons. AJNR 2:167–173
23. Di Tullio MV, Rand RW, Frisch BS (1978) Detachable balloon catheter. Its application in experimental arteriovenous fistulae. J Neurosurg 48:717–723
24. Dion JE, Duckweiler GR, Lylyk P et al (1989) Progressive suppleness pursil catheter; a new tool for superselective angiography and embolisation. Am J Neuroradiol 10: 1068–1070

25. Dott N (1933) Intracranial aneurysms. Cerebral arterioradiography: surgical treatment. Trans Med Chir Soc Edinb 40:219–236
26. Dowd C, Halbach V, Higashida R et al (1990) Endovascular coil embolization of unusual posterior inferior cerebellar artery aneurysm. Neurosurgery 27:954–961
27. Drake CG, Peerless SJ, Ferguson GG (1994) Hunterian proximal artery occlusion for giant aneurysms of the carotid circulation. J Neurosurg 81:656–665
28. Driller J, Hilal SK, Michelsen WJ et al (1969) Development and use of the POD catheter in the cerebral vascular system. Med Res Engin 8:11–16
29. Durity F, Logue V (1971) The effects of proximal anterior cerebral occlusion on anterior communicating artery aneurysms. Postoperative radiological survey of 43 cases. J Neurosurg 35:16–19
30. Engelson E (1988) United States patent n = 4739768. Catheter for guide-wire tracking
31. Erba SM, Horton JA, Latchaw RE et al (1988) Balloon test occlusion of the internal carotid artery with stable xenon/CT cerebral blood flow imaging. AJNR 9:533–538
32. Fincher EF (1939) An aneurysm of the internal carotid artery treated surgically. Yale J Biol Med 11:423–424
33. Fox AJ, Vinuela F, Pelz DM et al (1987) Use of detachable balloons for proximal artery occlusion in the treatment of unclippable cerebral aneurysms. J Neurosurg 66:40–46
34. Frei EH, Driller J, Neufeld HN et al (1966) The POD and its applications. Med Res Eng 5:11–18
35. Gobin P, Vinuela F, Gurian J et al (1996) Treatment of large and giant fusiform intracranial aneurysms with Guglielmi Detachable Coils. J Neurosci 84:55–62
36. Gonzalez CF, Moret J (1990) Balloon occlusion of the carotid artery prior to surgery for neck tumors. AJNR 11:649–652
37. Graves VB, Partington CR, Rufenacht DA et al (1990) Treatment of carotid artery aneurysms with platinum coils: an experimental study in dogs. AJNR 11(2):249–252
38. Graves VB, Strother CM, Rappe AH (1993) Treatment of experimental canine carotid aneurysms with platinum coils. AJNR 14:787–793
39. Guglielmi G, Vinuela F, Sepetka I et al (1991) Electrothrombosis of saccular aneurysms via endovascular approach. Part 1: electrochemical basis, technique and experimental results. J Neurosurg 75:1–7
40. Guglielmi G, Vinuela F, Dion J et al (1991) Electrothrombosis of saccular aneurysms via endovascular approach. Part 2: preliminary clinical experience. J Neurosurg 75:8–14
41. Guglielmi G, Vinuela F, Duckwiler G et al (1992) Endovascular treatment of posterior circulation aneurysms by electrothrombosis using electrically detachable coils. J Neurosurg 77:515–524
42. Gurian JH, Martin NA, King WA et al (1995) Neurosurgical management of cerebral aneurysms following unsuccessful or incomplete endovascular embolization. J Neurosurg 83:843–853
43. Halbach V, Higashida R, Dowd C et al (1993) Endovascular treatment of vertebral artery dissections and pseudoaneurysms. J Neurosci 79:183–191
44. Hawkins TD, Szaz KF (1987) The permeability of detachable latex rubber balloons. An in-vitro study. Invest Radiol 22:969–972
45. Hieshima GB, Grinnell VS, Mehringer CM (1981) A detachable balloon for transcatheter occlusions. Radiology 138:227–228
46. Higashida R, Halbach V, Barnwell S et al (1990) Treatment of intracranial aneurysms with preservation of the parent vessel: results of percutaneous balloon embolization in 84 patients. AJNR 11:633–640
47. Higashida RT, Halbach VV, Dowd C et al (1990) Endovascular detachable balloon embolization therapy of cavernous carotid artery aneurysms: results in 87 cases. J Neurosurg 72:857–863
48. Hilal SK, Michelsen WJ, Driller J et al (1974) Magnetically guided devices for vascular exploration and treatment. Laboratory and clinical investigations. Radiology 113:529–540
49. Hilal SK, Khandji AG, Chi TL et al (1988) Synthetic fibre-coated platinum coils successfully used for endovascular treatment of arteriovenous malformations, aneurysms and direct arteriovenous fistulas of CNS. Am J Neuroradiol 9:1030
50. Hilal SK, Khandji A, Solomon RW (1989) Obliteration of intracranial aneurysms with pre-shaped highly thrombogenic coils. Radiology 173:250–257
51. Johnson DW, Stringer WA, Marks MP et al (1991) Stable xenon CT cerebral blood flow imaging: rationale for and role in clinical decision making. AJNR 12:201–203
52. Kaufman SL, Strandberg JD, Barth KH et al (1979) Therapeutic embolization with detachable silicone balloons, long-term effects in swine. Invest Radiol 14:156–161

53. Keen WW (1890) Intracranial lesions. Med News 57:439–450
54. Kessler LA, Wholey MH (1970) Internal carotid occlusion for treatment of intracranial aneurysms: a new percutaneous technique. Radiology 95:581–583
55. Kikuchi Y, Strother CM, Boyer M (1987) New catheter for endovascular interventional procedures. Radiology 165:870–871
56. Kinugasa K, Mandai S, Terai Y et al (1992) Direct thrombosis of aneurysms with cellulose polymer. Part II: preliminary clinical experience. J Neurosurg 77:501–507
57. Knuckey NW, Haas R, Jenkins R et al (1992) Thrombosis of difficult intracranial aneurysms by the endovascular placement of platinum-Dacron microcoils. J Neurosurg 77:43–50
58. Laitinen L, Servo A (1978) Embolization of cerebral vessels with inflatable and detachable balloons. Technical note. J Neurosurg 48:307–308
59. Landolt AM, Millikan CH (1970) Pathogenesis of cerebral infarction secondary to mechanical carotid artery occlusion. Stroke 1:52–62
60. Lawton MT, Hamilton MG, Morcoa JJ et al (1995) Revascularization and aneurysm surgery: current techniques, indications and outcome. Neurosurgery 38:83–94
61. Linskey ME, Jungreis CA, Yonas H et al (1994) Stroke risk after abrupt internal carotid artery sacrifice: accuracy of preoperative assessment with balloon test occlusion and stable xenon-enhanced CT. AJNR 15:829–843
62. Luessenhop AJ, Velasquez AC (1964) Observations on the tolerance of the intracranial arteries to catheterization. J Neurosurg 21:85–91
63. Malisch T, Guglielmi G, Vinuela F et al Intracranial aneurysms treated with the Guglielmi detachable coil: midterm clinical results in 100 consecutive patients (submitted for publication)
64. Mandai S, Kinugasa K, Takashi O et al (1992) Direct thrombosis of aneurysms with cellulose polymer. Part I: results of thrombosis in experimental aneurysms. J Neurosurg 77:497–500
65. Massoud T, Guglielmi G, Vinuela F, Duckwiler G (1994) Saccular aneurysms in Moya Moya disease: Endovascular treatment using electrically detachable coils. Surg Neurol 41:452–467
66. Massoud T, Guglielmi G, Vinuela F, Duckwiler G (1996) Endovascular treatment of multiple aneurysms involving the posterior intracranial circulation. AJNR17:549–554
67. Matas R (1914) Testing of the efficiency of the collateral circulation as a preliminary to the occlusion of the great surgical arteries. JAMA 63:1441
68. Matas R, Allen CW (1911) Occlusion of large surgical arteries with removable metallic bands to test the efficiency of the collateral circulation. Experimental and clinical observations. JAMA 56:233
69. Mathis JM, Barr JD, Horton JA (1994) Physical characteristics of balloon catheter systems used in temporary cerebral artery occlusion. AJNR 15:1831–1836
70. Mathis JM, Barr JD, Jungreis CA et al (1995) Temporary balloon test occlusion of the internal carotid artery: experience in 500 cases. AJNR 16:749–754
71. Mawad ME, Mawad JK, Cartwright J et al (1995) Long-term histopathologic changes in canine aneurysms embolized with Guglielmi detachable coils. AJNR 16:7–13
72. McConnell AA (1937) Subchiasmal aneurysm, treatment by implantation of muscle. ZB Beurochir 2:269–274
73. Miller JD, Jawad K, Jennett B (1977) Safety of carotid ligation and its role in the management of intracranial aneurysms. J Neurol Neurosurg Psychiatry 40:64–72
74. Molcho J, Karny HZ, Frei EH et al (1970) Selective cerebral catheterization. IEEE Trans Biomed Eng 17:134–140
75. Monsein LH, Jeffery PJ, Van Heerden BB et al (1991) Assessing adequacy of collateral circulation during balloon test occlusion of the internal carotid artery with ^{99M}Tc-HMPAO SPECT. AJNR 12:1045–1051
76. Montgomery DB, Hale JR, Pierce NT et al (1970) A magnetically guided catheter system for intracranial use in man. IEEE Trans Magnet 6:374–375
77. Moody EB, Dawson RC, Sandler MD (1991) ^{99M}Tc-HMPAO SPECT imaging in interventional neuroradiology: validation of balloon test occlusion. AJNR 12:1043–1044
78. Moret J, Boulin A, Mawad M et al (1991) Endovascular therapy of berry aneurysms by endosaccular balloon occlusion. Neuroradiology 33 [Suppl]:135–136
79. Murayama Y, Malisch T, Guglielmi G et al The incidence of cerebral vasospasm following endovascular treatment of acutely ruptured aneurysms. Report on 69 patients treated with the Guglielmi Detachable Coils (submitted for publication)
80. Nattrass FJ (1928) Aneurysm of the carotid artery incavernous sinus-ligature of internal carotid artery: recovery. Edinb Med J 35:30–32

81. Nelson N (1990) A versatile, steerable, flow-guided catheter for delivery of detachable balloons. Am J Neuroradiol 11:657–658
82. Nishioka H (1966) Report on the cooperative study of intracranial aneurysms and subarachnoid hemorrhage. Section VIII, part 1. Results of the treatment on intracranial aneurysms by occlusion of the carotid artery in the neck. J Neurosurg 25:660–682
83. Odom GL, Tindall GT (1968) Carotid ligation in the treatment of certain intracranial aneurysms. Clin Neurosurg 23:101–116
84. Palmer JF (1835) The Works of John Hunter, FRS with notes, vol 1. Longmen, London, pp 543–551
85. Peterman SB, Taylor A, Hoffman JC (1991) Improved detection of cerebral hypoperfusion with internal carotid balloon test occlusion and ^{99M}Tc-HMPAO cerebral perfusion SPECT imaging. AJNR 12:1035–1041
86. Prolo DJ, Hanbery JW (1971) Intraluminal occlusion of a carotid-cavernous sinus fistula with a balloon catheter. J Neurosurg 237–242
87. Quintana F, Diez C, Gutierrez A et al. (1996) Traumatic aneurysm of the basilar artery. AJNR 17:283–285
88. Romodanov AP, Shcheglov VI (1982) Intravascular occlusion of saccular aneurysms of the cerebral arteries by means of a detachable balloon catheter. In: Krayenbuhl H (ed) Advances and technical standards in neurosurgery, vol 9. Springer, Berlin Heidelberg New York, pp 25–48
89. Rowe JG, Byrne JV, Molyneux A, Rajagopalan B (1995) Haemodynemic consequences of embolizing aneurysms: a transcranial doppler study. Br J Neurosurg 9:749–757
90. Rowe JG, Molyneux AJ, Byrne JV et al (1996) Endovascular treatment of intracranial aneurysms: a minimally invasive approach with advantages for elderly patients. Age Ageing 25:372–376
91. Sadato A, Taki W, Nishi S et al (1993) Treatment of a spontaneous carotid cavernous fistula using an electrodetachable microcoil. AJNR 14:334–336
92. Schorstein J (1940) Carotid ligation in saccular intracranial aneurysms. Br J Surg 28:50–70
93. Scotti G, Li MH, Righi C et al (1996) Endovascular treatment of bacterial intracranial aneurysms. Neuroradiology 38:186–189
94. Selverstone B, White JCS (1951) A new technique for gradual occlusion of the carotid artery. Arch Neurol Psychiatry (Chicago) 66:246
95. Serbinenko FA (1974) Balloon catheterization and occlusion of major cerebral vessels. J Neurosurg 41:125–145
96. Simonson TM, Ryals TJ, Yuh WTC et al (1992) MR imaging and HMPAO scintigraphy in conjunction with balloon test occlusion: value in predicting sequelae after permanent carotid occlusion. Am J Roentgenol 159:1063–1068
97. Skultery FM, Nishioka H (1966) The results of intracranial surgery in the treatment of aneurysms. J Neurosurg 25: 683–704
98. Sosman MC, Vogt EC (1926) Aneurysms of the internal carotid artery and the circle of Willis, from a roentgenological viewpoint. Am J Roentgenol 15:122–134
99. Spetzler RF, Schuster H, Roski RA (1980) Elective extracranial-intracranial arterial by pass in the treatment of inoperable giant aneurysms of the internal carotid artery. J Neurosurg 53:22–27
100. Standard SC, Ahuja A, Guterman LR et al (1995) Balloon test occlusion of the internal carotid artery with hypotensive challenge. AJNR 16:1453–1458
101. Steed DL, Webster MW, deVries EJ et al (1990) Clinical observations on the effect of carotid artery occlusion on cerebral blood flow mapped by xenon computed tomography and its correlation with carotid artery back pressure. J Vasc Surg 11:38–43
102. Steinberg GK, Drake CG, Peerless SJ (1993) Deliberate basilar or vertebral artery occlusion in the treatment of intracranial aneurysms. Immediate results and long-term outcome in 201 patients. J Neurosurg 79:161–173
103. Taki W, Handa H, Yamagata S et al (1979) Embolization and superselective angiography by means of balloon catheters. Surg Neurol 12:7–14
104. Tarr RW, Jungreis CA, Horton JA et al (1991) Complications of preoperative balloon test occlusion of the internal carotid arteries: experience in 300 cases. Skull Base Surg 1:240–244
105. Teng MM, Chen CC, Lirng JF et al (1994) N-butyl-2-cyanoacrylate for embolisation of carotid aneurysm. Neuroradiology 36:144–147
106. Turjman F, Acevedo G, Moll T et al (1993) Treatment of experimental carotid aneurysms by endoprosthesis implantation: preliminary report. Neurol Res 15:181–184

107. Turjman F, Massoud T, Ji C et al (1994) Combined stent implantation and endosaccular coil placement for treatment of experimental wide-necked aneurysms: a feasibility study in swine. AJNR 15:1087–1090
108. Weil SM, van Loveren HR, Tomsick TA et al (1987) Management of inoperable cerebral aneurysms by the navigational balloon technique. Neurosurgery 21:296–302
109. Wolpert SM. Kwan ESK, Heros D et al (1988) Selective delievery of chemotherapeutic agents with a new catheter system. Radiology 166:547–549
110. Yodh SB, Pierce NT, Weggel RJ et al (1968) A new magnet system for intravascular navigation. Med Biol Eng 6:143–147
111. Yonas H, Sekhar L, Johnson DW, Gur D (1989) Determination of irreversible ischemia by xenon-enhanced computed tomography monitoring of cerebral blood flow in patients with symptomatic vasospasm. Neurosurgery 24:368–372
112. Yonas H, Linskey M, Johnson DW et al (1992) Internal carotid balloon test occlusion does require quantitative CBF. AJNR 13:1147–1148
113. Zubillaga A, Guglielmi G, Vinuela F et al (1994) Endovascular occlusion of intracranial aneurysms with electrically detachable coils: correlation of aneurysm neck size and treatment results. AJNR 15:815–820

CHAPTER 5

Treatment by Endosaccular Packing with the Guglielmi Detachable Coil

5.1 Introduction

In 1989 [21], a new endovascular method was developed to offer patients (and their physicians) a less invasive and safer treatment for intracranial aneurysms. This method utilises controllable and electrolytically detachable platinum coils – the Guglielmi detachable coil (GDC, Target Therapeutics, Fremont, California) – designed to densely fill the aneurysm sac and thus to isolate saccular intracranial aneurysms from the rest of the cerebral circulation. GDCs are very soft and adapt to the aneurysm shape without causing significant distortion of its fragile wall. As discussed previously (Chap 4, Sect. 4.1.3), the softness of the coils allows them to absorb the systolic blood pulse pressure. The deployment and physical properties of coils are radically different from balloons, which transmit rather than absorb the "water-hammer" effect of pulsatile blood flow [20].

Since its first clinical use in early 1990 [22, 23] the GDC device has been utilized in many neuroendovascular centres [1, 5, 8, 10, 12–16, 19, 22, 25, 27–31, 33–35, 41, 42]. It is estimated that, by the end of 1996, more than 10 000 patients had been treated worldwide in over 250 centres. The technical characteristics of this type of coil will be discussed after a brief description of its background and the electrochemical principles involved in its development.

5.2 Electrothrombosis and the Electrolytic Process

5.2.1 Polarity of the Vessel Wall

In 1953, Sawyer and co-workers [38, 40] demonstrated that the intima of blood vessels has a constant negative charge of 3–5 mV, relative to the adventitia. As a result of this small charge, the negatively charged components of whole blood, i.e. white and red blood cells, platelets and fibrinogen, are repelled from the intima, which reduces the possibility of intravascular thrombosis. However, if the intima is injured, then the electrical polarity is reversed and the damaged intima becomes positively charged. In vitro migration of platelets to the anode (positively charged electrode) of an electrophoretic cell was shown by Bigelow and De Foyes [3] in 1952. The phenomenon causes post-traumatic vascular clotting by attracting the negatively charged particles, particularly platelets, to the site of injury.

5.2.2 Electrothrombosis

Electrothrombosis describes the process of thrombosis induced by an electric charge applied to whole blood. Sawyer and Pate [38, 39] applied a direct electric current to heparinised blood in vitro and caused blood components to aggregate at the anode; the components of blood attracted to the electrode were red blood cells, white blood cells, platelets and fibrinogen. The applied electric current varied between 2 mA and 10 mA and was applied for 30 min. The weight of thrombus formed was directly proportional to the product of current and length of time for which it was applied, i.e. coulombs of electricity. Several authors have performed similar experiments in vivo, confirming that a positive electrode attracts the negatively charged components of whole blood and causes thrombus formation. In 1961, Salazar [37] was able to completely occlude the coronary arteries of dogs by applying a 0.5 mA electric current for 2 h via an electrode positioned inside the artery. In 1965, Araki et al. [2] studied electrical thrombosis using internal (positive) and external (negative) electrodes and a 3-mA direct electric current applied for 1 h. They showed, using this technique, that thrombus could be induced in the carotid artery of dogs in 90% of cases. Thrombus formation was reduced if the artery was infused with heparin. Thompson et al. [44] developed a transcatheter technique to perform electrothrombosis of the aorta, femoral artery and common carotid artery in rabbits. They applied a 10-mA current to platinum and stainless steel endovascular electrodes.

Chen et al. (unpublished data) performed a series of in vitro experiments on heparinised blood of swine. They confirmed that the amount of thrombus was directly proportional to electrical charge (in coulombs). The following weights of thrombus was formed when the given current was applied for 3 min, using a platinum electrode: 1 mA=10 mg, 2 mA=12 mg, 3 mA=26 mg and 10 mA=85 mg. Miller et al. [32] applied 5–10 mA direct electric current to produce thrombosis of citrated blood of dogs using stainless steel or platinum electrodes. They found platinum to be three to four times more thrombogenic than stainless steel and that the size of the clot was the same with 0.25-mm or 0.9-mm diameter platinum electrodes.

Tenjin et al., in 1995 [43], published the results of treatment of experimental aneurysms in monkeys with GDC using a 1-mA current. The surfaces of the platinum coils were examined by scanning electron microscopy 1 h after the treatment and found to be covered with a thin layer of leukocytes, fibrin-like material and other proteins.

The in vitro and in vivo and experiments described above show that: (1) If a positive direct electric current is applied within a vessel, thrombus will precipitate on the positive electrode (anode); (2) the size and weight of the resulting thrombus is directly proportional to the coulombs (Ampere×second) of electric charge applied; and (3) platinum electrodes produce the maximum thrombosis and are not affected by electrolysis.

However, the small electric current (1 mA) used for detachment of GDC causes only minimal electrothrombus in vivo, especially if heparin is given. Increasing the electric current, to say 5 mA, would probably increase the amount of intra-aneurysmal thrombus generated by electrothrombosis.

5.2.3
Electrolysis

The process of electrolysis was described nearly 200 years ago by Alessandro Volta who made the first electric battery capable of producing a continuous current. When electrodes, connected to a battery, are placed in water, hydrogen gas is given off at the negative electrode and oxygen gas at the positive electrode. This process is called electrolysis. Electrolysis causes the anode of two iron electrodes to dissolve and the cathode to recruit ferrous ions. This process is used to detach the platinum GDC from stainless steel (iron) delivery wire since the coil is unaffected by electrolysis because it is a noble metal.

Piton et al. [36] tested the electrolytic properties of various metals in normal saline. These included silver, copper, platinum and stainless steel electrodes, all 0.5 mm in diameter. They applied a 10 mA direct electric current and showed that silver electrodes underwent electrolysis in 22 min, stainless steel electrodes in 12 min and copper electrodes were rapidly affected by oxidation. The platinum electrodes were unaffected.

5.3
The Guglielmi Detachable Coil

The GDC consists of a platinum coil soldered to a stainless steel delivery wire (Fig. 5.1).The platinum coil is deposited and detached from the delivery wire in the target aneurysm or vessel. It is more radiopaque than the delivery wire, from which it can be easily distinguished on fluoroscopy. The plati-

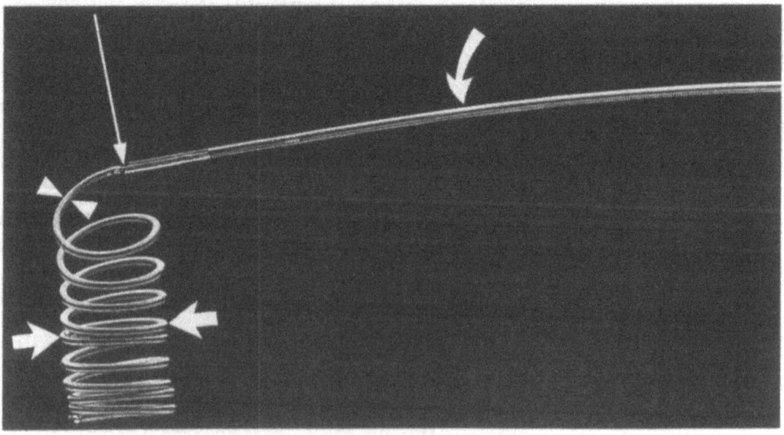

Fig. 5.1. Photograph of a Guglielmi detachable coil. The insulated, 0.010-in. stainless steel delivery wire is indicated by the *curved arrow*. The uninsulated junction between the platinum and the stainless steel components is indicated by the *long arrow*. The diameter of the circular memory of the platinum coil is between the *short arrows* and the primary diameter of the coil is between the *arrowheads*

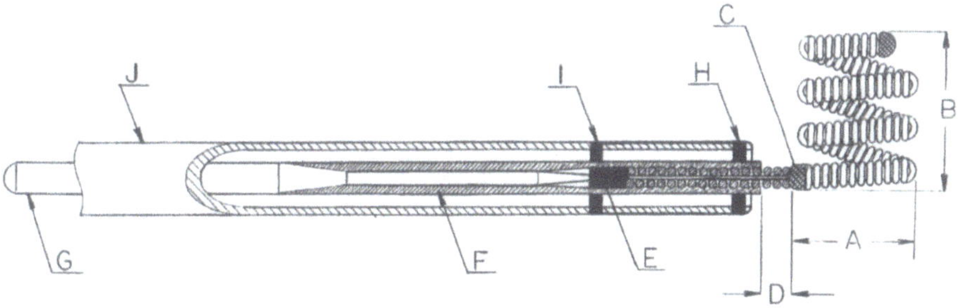

Fig. 5.2. Line drawing of the Guglielmi detachable coil (GDC). *A* Diameter of the circular memory; *B* the platinum component of the GDC; *C* junction between platinum and stainless steel; *D* the uninsulated portion of the delivery wire (this is the portion that undergoes electrolysis, detaching the coil in the aneurysm); *E* the proximal platinum marker on the delivery wire (see text); *F* the insulated delivery wire; *G* the proximal, uninsulated end of the delivery wire; *H* the distal radiopaque marker on the double marker microcatheter; *I* the proximal radiopaque marker on the double marker microcatheter; *J* the microcatheter

num portion is detached (typically in 1–3 min) from the delivery wire by electrolysis of the distal part of the steel delivery wire (Fig. 5.2). This is achieved by the passage of a 1 mA direct electric current. During passage of the current the platinum coil is positively charged which (as discussed above) may induce the formation of an "electrothrombus" in the aneurysm (Fig. 5.3).

The platinum portion of the GDC has been designed with different physical properties to allow the operator to select the appropriate coil for each aneurysm. The coils have to be soft enough not to rupture the fragile aneurysmal wall and stiff enough not to migrate out of the aneurysm. Softness and stiffness therefore have to be balanced. There are four parameters that characterise the platinum portion of a GDC: (1) circular memory, (2) diameter of the coil, (3) diameter of the platinum wire, and (4) length of the coil.

5.3.1 Circular Memory

Standard Guglielmi detachable coils are manufactured with a circular memory; this is the shape that the unrestrained coil takes. It is defined by the diameter of the coil loops or helical diameter (see Fig. 5.1). The memory is important in retaining the detached coil in the aneurysm sac. A straight coil would tend to migrate into the parent vessel. Currently, GDCs are available with circular memories of 2–20 mm; this diameter is uniform for all loops of the standard coil.

However, coils can be manufactured in different and more complex shapes. The so-called 2D-GDC are manufactured so that the circular memory of the first one and a half loops is smaller than the rest of the coil (Fig. 5.4). This design reduces the tendency of the first loop of coil to herniate out of the aneurysm (i.e. into the parent artery) during deployment. It is used, principally, at the start of endosaccular packing when such herniation most

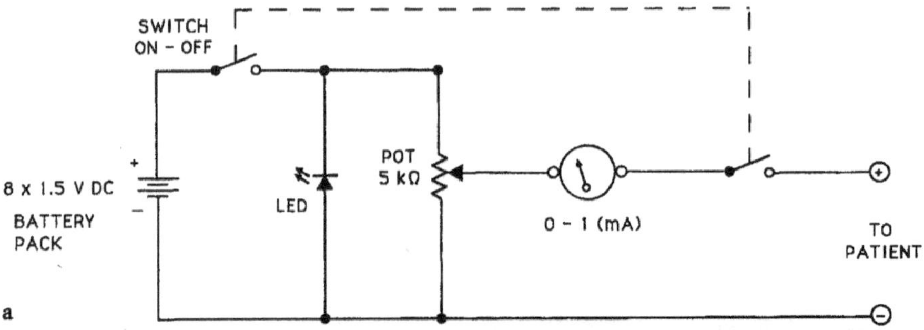

a

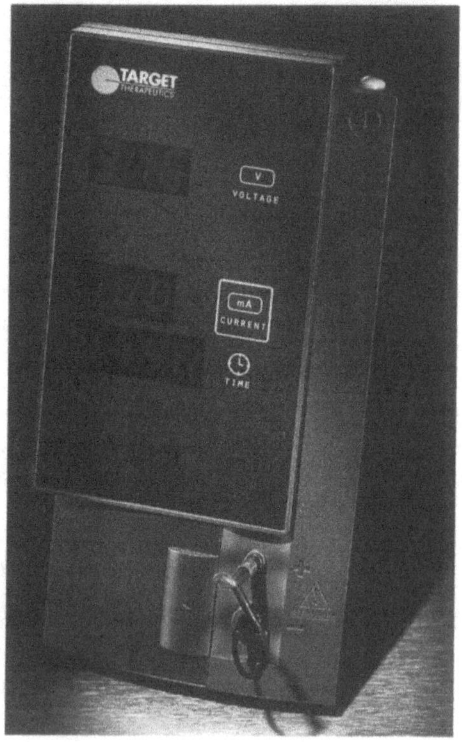

b

Fig. 5.3.
a, c Wiring diagrams of the first version (**a**) and latest version (**c**) of the Guglielmi detachable coil (GDC) generator (*LED*, light emitting diode; *POT*, potentiometer to regulate the electric current; *PCDC*, platinum coil detection circuit). **b** The latest version of the generator, which delivers a constant direct current of 1 mA until an intermittent tone signals coil detachment. GDC detachment typically occurs in 1–3 min. (**c** see p. 139)

commonly occurs. In addition, straight and "comma shaped" GDCs of between 4 and 10 mm in length are available to occlude small arteries. These coils can be used to perform parent artery occlusion for peripheral intracranial aneurysms, distal to the circle of Willis.

5.3.2 Diameter of the Coil

The primary diameter of the coil is the diameter of the wound platinum wire before the coil is shaped, i.e. given circular memory (see Fig. 5.1). This di-

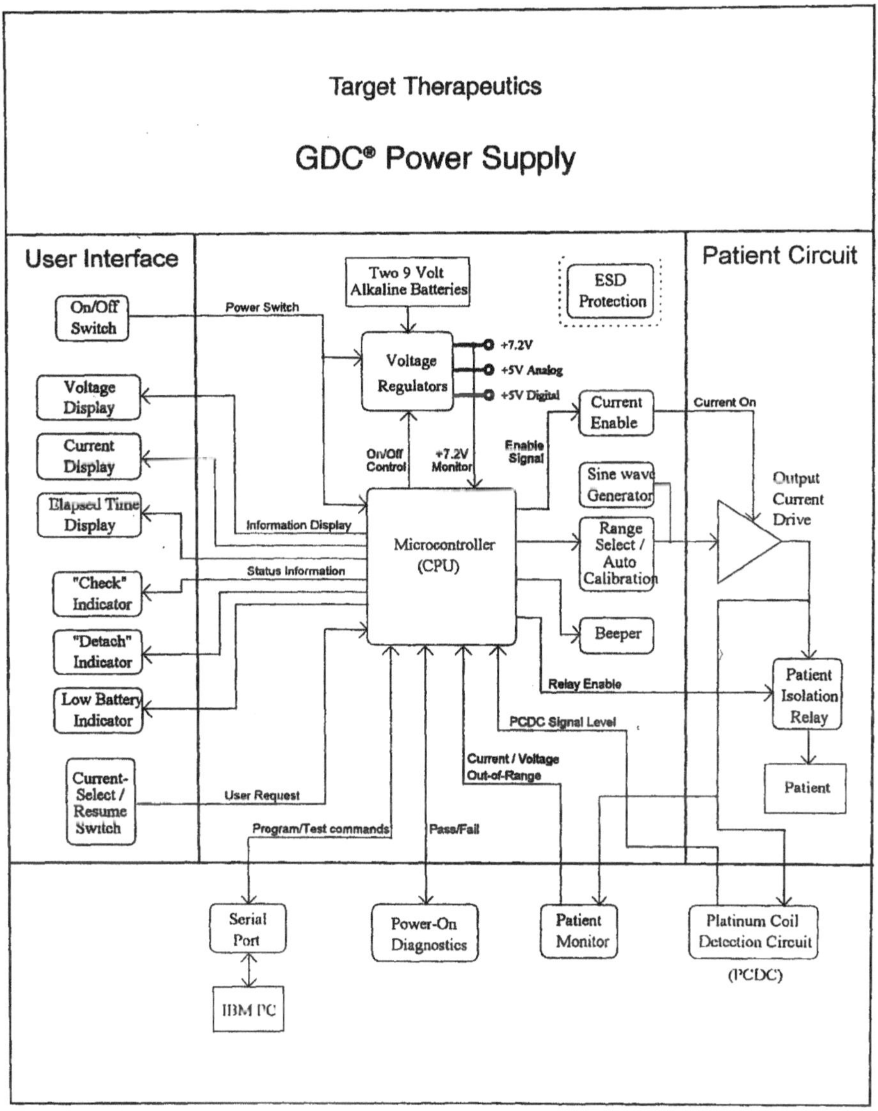

c

mension is important for matching coil with microcatheter and determines how easily it deforms, i.e. its softness. GDC-10, GDC–10 "soft", GDC-18, and GDC-18 "soft" are currently available. The primary diameter of the GDC-10 is 0.010 in. and of the GDC-10 "soft" 0.0095 in. They are more delicate than the GDC-18 and are used for treating small aneurysms. They can be delivered through both Tracker 10 and, carefully, through Tracker 18 catheters. The primary diameter of the GDC-18 is 0.015 in. and of the GDC-18 "soft" 0.0135 in. They are less malleable than the GDC-10 and are used for large and giant aneurysms. They can be delivered through the Tracker 18 only. The GDC-18 "soft" is approximately as deformable as the GDC-10.

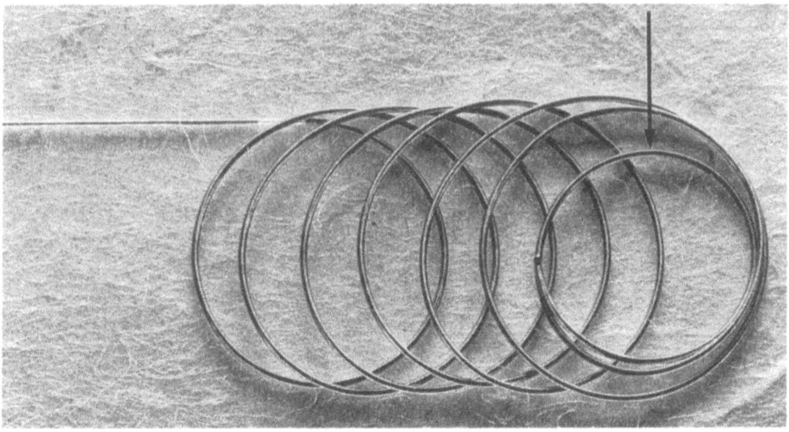

Fig. 5.4. A two-diameter Guglielmi detachable coil (GDC-2D). The distal loop (*arrow*) has a smaller circular memory than the rest of the coil; this helps to prevent herniation of the coil tip into the parent artery

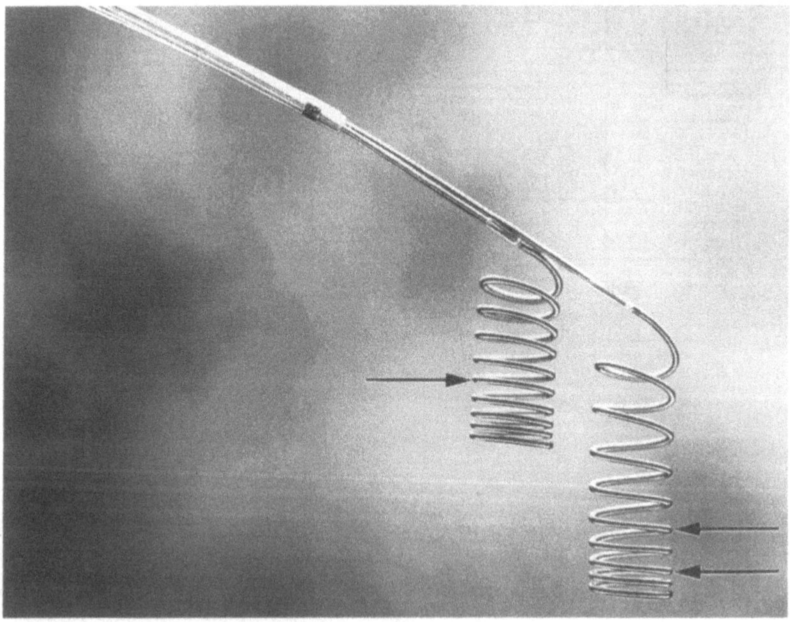

Fig. 5.5. A standard Guglielmi detachable coil (GDC)-10, 8 cm in length and 3 mm in circular memory (*single arrow*). A similar GDC-10 "soft" (*double arrow*) is softer. This increased softness is achieved by utilizing thinner platinum wire to construct the coil

5.3.3
Diameter of the Platinum Wire

The first step in the manufacture of GDCs is the winding of fine platinum wire to form a coil. Five different diameters of platinum wire are used in the construction of GDCs: (1) 0.002 in. for GDC-10, (2) 0.00175 in. for GDC-10 "soft", (3) 0.003 in. for GDC-18 (up to 14 mm in circular memory), (4) 0.004 in. for GDC-18 of larger circular memory, and finally (5) 0.00225 in. for the GDC-18 "soft". The thinner the platinum wire, the softer the coil. The primary diameter of the coils is determined by the winding process and not the diameter of the platinum wire (Fig. 5.5).

5.3.4
Coil Length

The length of a GDC refers to its length when straight, i.e. before it is given a circular or helical memory. Coils are manufactured from 2 to 30 cm in length. This length is not the same as the length of fine platinum wire used to make the coils. Each centimetre of a standard GDC-10 and GDC-18 weighs 5.6 mg and 12.6 mg, respectively. Thus, 180 cm of GDC-10 (or 80 cm of GDC-18) weighs 1.0 g.

5.4
Techniques of Coil Embolisation

5.4.1
Factors Influencing Endosaccular Packing

Endovascular therapy with preservation of the parent vessel using GDCs is appropriate for true saccular aneurysms, which represent the majority of intracranial aneurysms. Fusiform aneurysms can be cured by occlusion of the arterial axis with GDCs, if tolerated. Pseudoaneurysms and dissecting aneurysms should usually be treated as occlusion of the aneurysm and parent artery (Fig. 5.6). Pseudoaneurysms, or "false" aneurysms, are caused by traumatic damage to the entire arterial wall, whereas dissecting aneurysms are caused by arterial dissection, i.e. an intimal breach which may be spontaneous or post-traumatic (see Chap. 1, Sect. 1.4.4). In either situation the walls of the resulting aneurysms are disrupted and, even when they have a saccular appearance, they may not be able to retain coils. The use of GDCs to occlude parent arteries at or proximal to such aneurysm will not be considered further in this chapter.

Traditionally, the size of an aneurysm sac is classified as small (up to 15 mm), large (15–25 mm), or giant (larger than 25 mm). It is the authors' opinion, however, that a classification based on that of Yasargil [46] should be used, since this is more relevant to endosaccular packing with GDCs. In

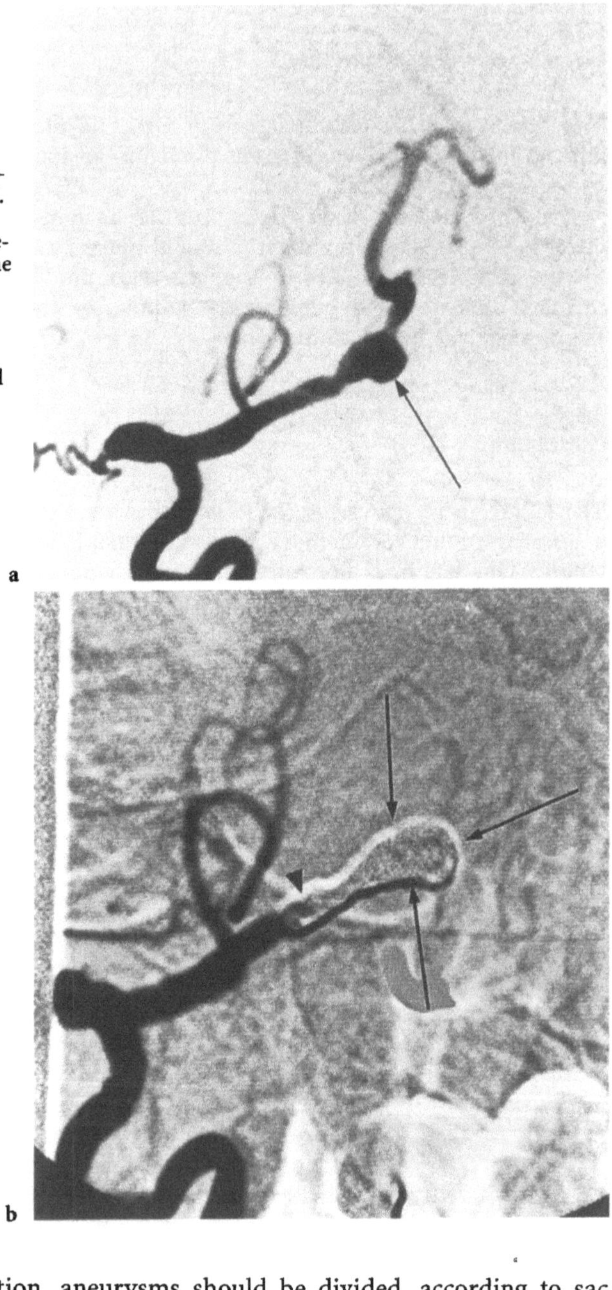

Fig. 5.6.
a Patient presenting with subarachnoid haemorrhage (SAH) due to rupture of a dissecting aneurysm of the right intracranial vertebral artery (VA) (*arrow*). This is a common site for a dissecting aneurysm to cause SAH. b Several Guglielmi detachable coils (GDC)-10 were delivered and detached into the aneurysm (*arrows*) and the VA between the aneurysm and the posterior inferior cerebellar artery (*arrowhead*), occluding the arterial axis. The posterior circulation was subsequently supplied solely by the contralateral VA (not shown)

our proposed modification, aneurysms should be divided, according to sac size, into six groups as follows: (1) "baby" (less than 2 mm), (2) small (2–6 mm), (3) medium (6–12 mm), (4) large (12–25 mm), (5) giant (25–35 mm), and (6) super giant (more than 35 mm). Treatment of very small (baby) and very large (super giant) aneurysms may not be possible with current endovascular devices, so it is helpful to identify them separately. An-

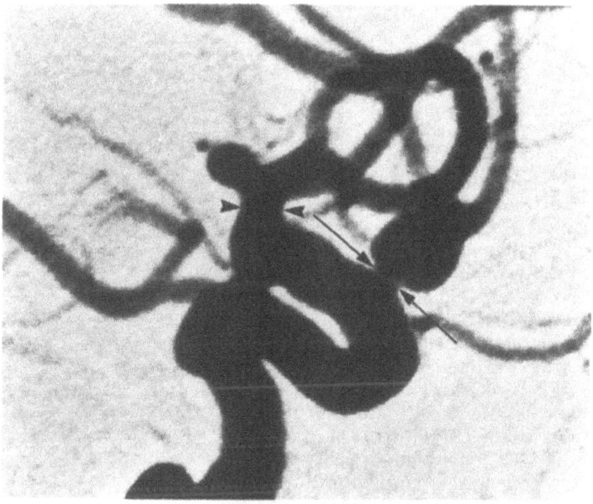

a

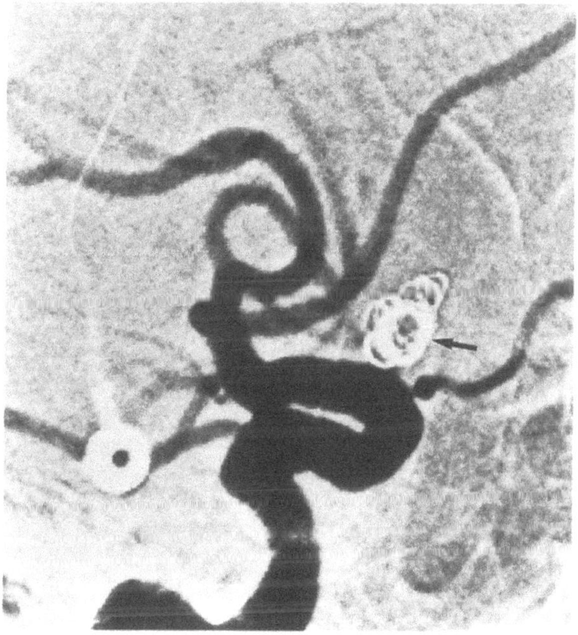

b

Fig. 5.7.
a Patient with a saccular carotid-ophthalmic aneurysm. The neck of the aneurysm is 2.3 mm. This value was obtained by comparing the average diameter of the internal carotid artery (3–5 mm proximal to the bifurcation this diameter is 3.5 mm, between *arrowheads*), with the aneurysm neck diameter (between *arrows*). **b** In spite of a loose coil packing (*arrow*) this aneurysm was completely excluded from the circulation due to the small size of the aneurysm neck

other advantage is that with so many GDC sizes available, four intermediate groups are now appropriate. In particular, it is helpful to distinguish small and medium aneurysms (which were all classed as small in the cooperative study) since the former are best treated with the GDC-10 system.

The opening (orifice or neck) of a saccular aneurysm can be small (1–3 mm) or large (4–10 mm) according to Yasargil [46]. For the purposes of endosaccular treatment, aneurysms should be classified as small-necked (less than 4 mm) or wide-necked (4 mm or more) [22, 24, 45, 47]. Aneurysm

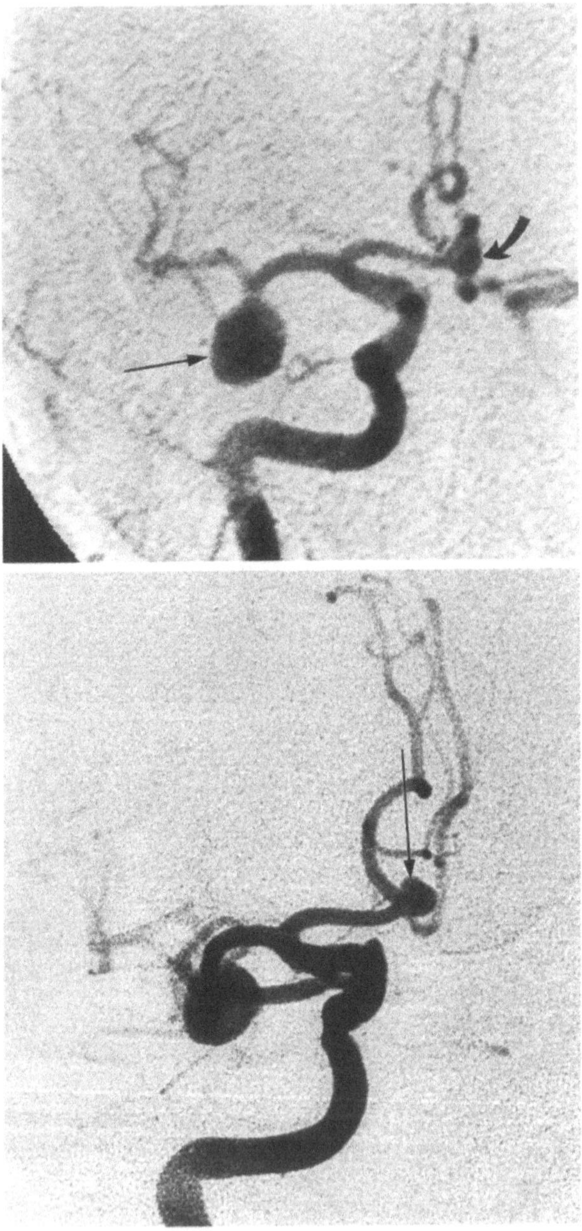

a

b

Fig. 5.8.
a Right carotid intra-arterial digital subtraction angiograpy of a patient with a small aneurysm of the anterior communicating artery (ACoA) (*curved arrow*) and a large aneurysm of the right middle cerebral artery (MCA; *arrow*). **b** With an appropriate oblique projection, the vascular anatomy of the ACoA aneurysm was accurately depicted (*arrow*). **c** The lumen of the ACoA aneurysm has been packed with Guglielmi detachable coils (GDCs). **d** In the same session, the tracker catheter was positioned in the sac of the MCA aneurysm and intra-aneurysmal angiography showed the fusiform nature of this aneurysm. The *single arrow* depicts the aneurysm inflow, while the two *arrowheads* show the two outflowing arteries. Endovascular treatment was not performed. (**c** and **d** see p. 145)

dimensions can be measured from the diagnostic angiogram either using an internal or external reference (Fig. 5.7). The former technique consists of comparing the (known) size of the internal carotid or basilar artery with the size of the aneurysm sac or neck [4, 47]. Alternatively an external reference (such as a coil) is taped to the patients' skin and included in the angiographic projection. With the possible exception of 1–2 mm orifices, it seems

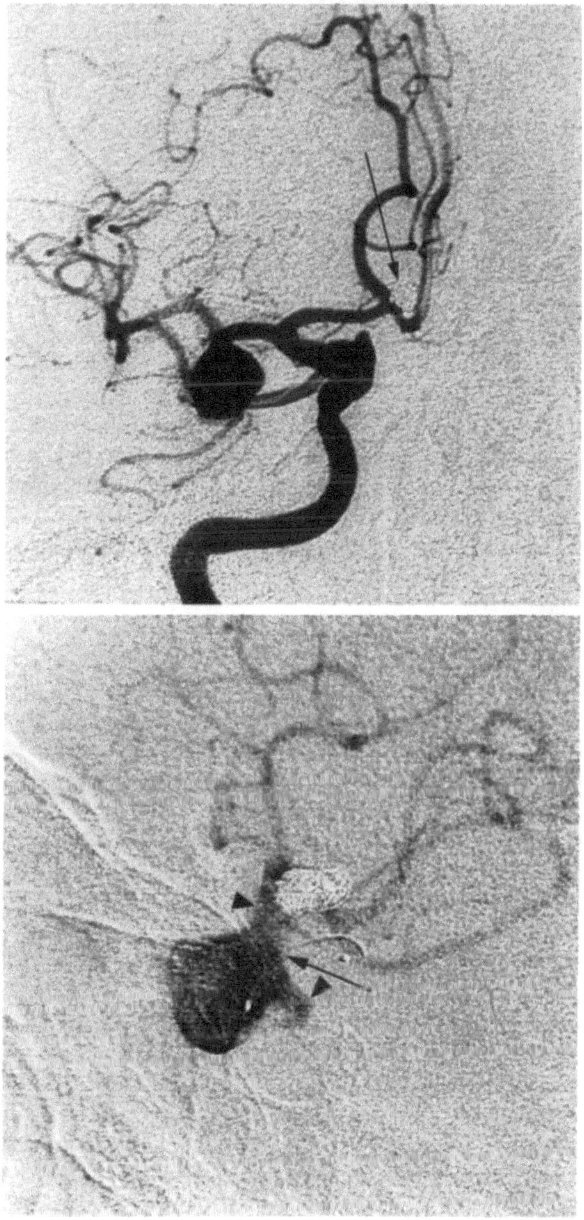

c

d

Fig. 5.8

reasonable to believe that, in vivo, the orifice is oval in shape. The orifice size is generally proportional to sac size, thus small aneurysms often have small orifices, and large and giant aneurysms large orifices that may incorporate part of the origins of adjacent arteries (Fig. 5.8).

From the endovascular perspective; (a) the size of the aneurysm neck, (b) the shape of the aneurysm, (c) the dimension of the neck compared to the size and shape of the aneurysm, and (d) the dimension of the aneurysm neck compared to the size of the parent vessel are important in predicting angiographic results of endosaccular packing.

Manuals of operative neurosurgery are available which describe the manipulation of cranial tissues and the dissection needed to expose intracranial aneurysms at different lesion locations. Pre-operative planning requires an accurate assessment of the aneurysm location. The endovascular perspective is different since the aneurysm is visible on angiography and real-time fluoroscopy. The endovascular therapist needs to determine the size and angle of origin of the aneurysm from the parent artery and use these data to determine the optimum angiographic ("working") projection to use during coil deployment, as well as the best shape (formed by steaming) for the distal portion of the microcatheter and size and type of GDC to use for endosaccular packing. The process of femoral puncture, carotid or vertebral artery negotiation, and aneurysm catheterisation, is analogous to neurosurgery which involves craniotomy, brain retraction and careful dissection to expose the aneurysm neck. Similarly, the relationship of the aneurysm neck to surrounding arterial branches must therefore be carefully imaged and analysed in order to plan safe endovascular treatment (Fig. 5.8).

5.4.2
Principles of Endosaccular Packing with GDC

The GDC technique includes various steps. The tip of a microcatheter is positioned in the aneurysm with the aid of a microguide wire (Fig. 5.9). Through the microcatheter, the platinum portion of a GDC is introduced into the aneurysm while still soldered to the stainless steel delivery wire. In the microcatheter the coil assumes a straight configuration. As soon as it exits the tip of the microcatheter the coil folds on itself with a predetermined circular memory. The platinum portion of the GDC is radiopaque and this allows fluoroscopic visualisation while it is being positioned within the aneurysm. If the correct size has been deployed, the platinum coil will adapt to the shape of the aneurysm sac. If the coil is inappropriate in size or loops extrude into the parent vessel, it can be withdrawn and repositioned. When the operator is satisfied that the coil is properly positioned inside the aneurysm, a 1 mA direct electric current is applied to the proximal end of the delivery wire. To do this, a negative ground electrode is connected to the patient by placing a hypodermic needle or a conductive pad in/on the groin or shoulder. A positive electrode is connected to the external end of the delivery wire, which causes the positively charged intra-aneurysmal platinum to attract negatively charged blood elements. At the same time the electric current dissolves the stainless steel of the delivery wire, immediately proximal to the solder between platinum and stainless steel, by electrolysis. Electrolytic detachment typically occurs in 1–3 min and the steel delivery wire is withdrawn, leaving the platinum coil inside the aneurysm. The platinum coil(s) packed in the aneurysm sac acts as a dense mesh that holds throm-

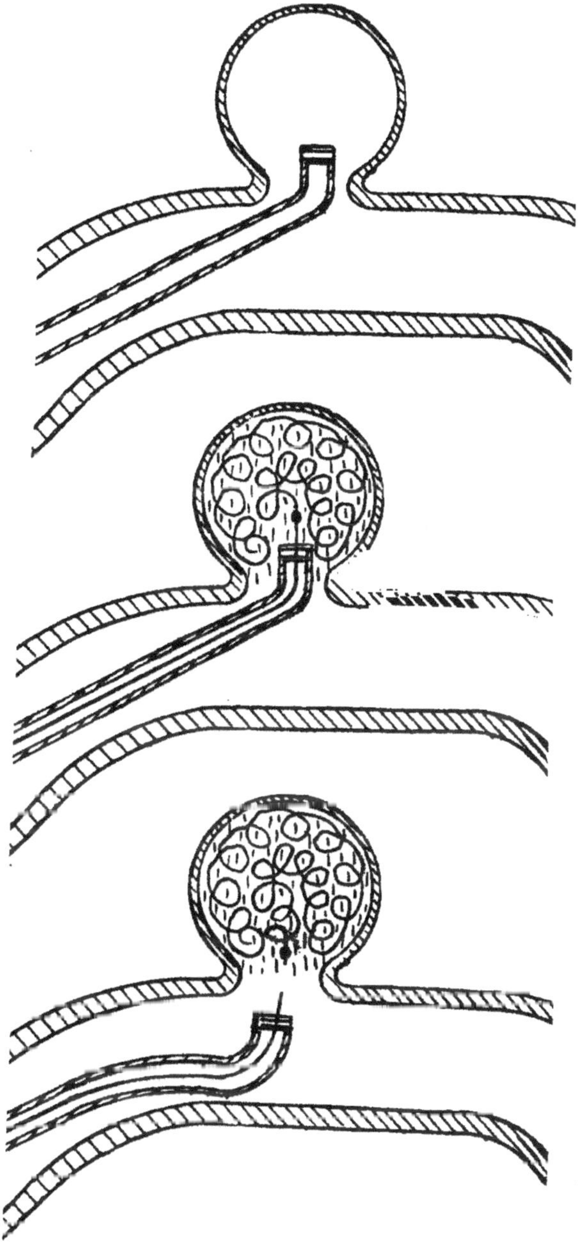

a

b

c

Fig. 5.9 a-c. A representation of the Guglielmi detachable coil (GDC) technique. **a** The tip of a microcatheter is positioned inside the aneurysm. **b** The platinum portion of the GDC is delivered into the aneurysm and a positive direct electric current is applied to the stainless steel delivery wire so that the positively charged platinum attracts the negatively charged blood components. **c** Within 1–3 min the junction between coil and delivery wire is dissolved by electrolysis, detaching the platinum coil within the aneurysm

bus, thus preventing thromboembolism into the parent artery and distal vascular tree. Additional GDCs are placed and detached in the aneurysm to completely, and densely, fill its sac and neck (Fig. 5.10).

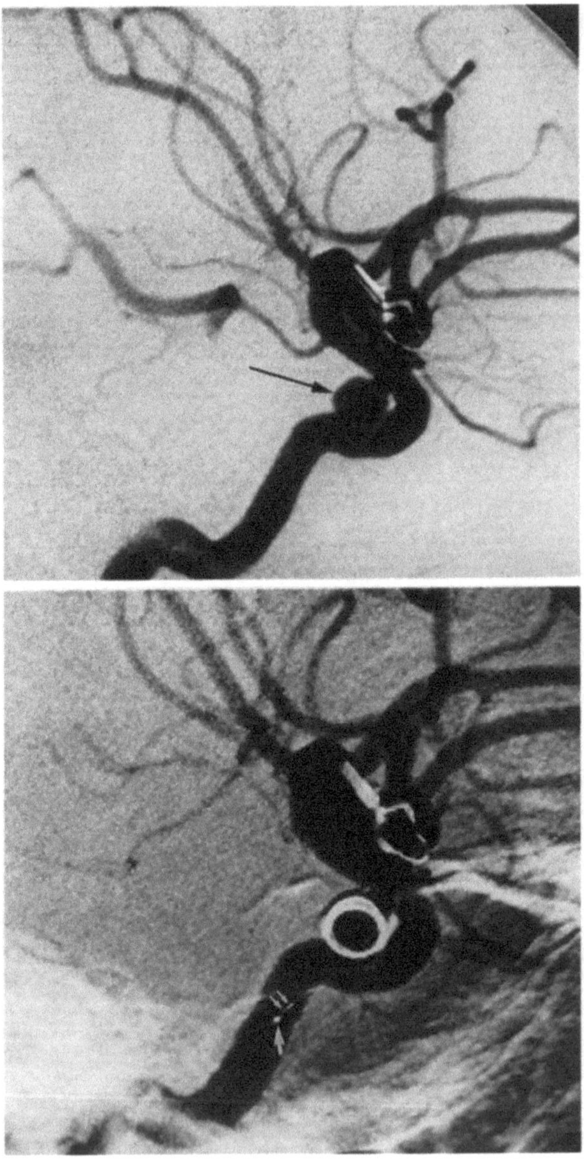

a

b

Fig. 5.10.
a Patient with a small-necked, superior hypophyseal aneurysm (*arrow*) found co-incidentally. b After aneurysm catheterisation with a Tracker-10, the first Guglielmi detachable coil (GDC) is delivered. Several loops of the first coil cross the aneurysm neck; this constitutes the ideal positioning of the first coil. The radiopaque markers – one on the GDC delivery wire (*twin arrows*) and one on the microcatheter (*single arrow*) – are in the correct pre-detachment position for electrolytic detachment of the coil. c Additional, smaller GDCs are then delivered and detached within the frame formed by the first coil to densely fill the aneurysm (c see p. 149)

5.4.3 Aneurysm Catheterisation and Coil Delivery

The usual procedure practiced by one of the authors (GG) to perform endosaccular packing will be described in detail. A 6-F femoral artery sheath is placed following percutaneous puncture with the patient under general anaesthesia. A continuous infusion of heparinised saline is maintained to pre-

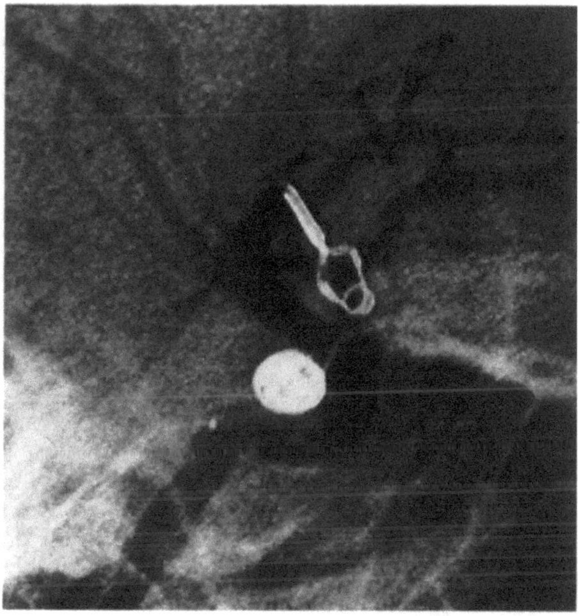

Fig. 5.10 c

vent thrombosis. The appropriate carotid or vertebral artery is catheterised with a 6-F, thin walled, soft tip, non-tapered guiding catheter. For small posterior circulation aneurysms, a 5-F guiding catheter may be utilised with a Tracker 10 microcatheter. The 6 F catheter should be used with the Tracker 18 microcatheter to obtain an adequate flow of contrast for angiography. The guiding catheter must be continuously flushed with heparinised and pressurised saline via a side-arm adapter. Guidewires and the microcatheter are then introduced through the valve of the side-arm adapter in order to maintain a continuous flow of heparinised saline and prevent thromboembolic complications. Angiography is performed by gentle hand-injection of radiographic contrast media. A mechanical pump injection should not be used when performing angiograms in patients harbouring intracranial aneurysms, in case the greater intra-arterial pressures generated cause aneurysm rupture.

Diagnostic angiography is performed through the guiding catheter, in multiple projections if necessary, in order to obtain the best view of the aneurysm sac and neck. The best view is the projection which clearly separates aneurysm (sac and neck) from parent artery. It is selected and used to monitor coil delivery (see Fig. 5.8). The ability to obtain a clear visualisation of the aneurysm neck is crucial and if this "working projection" cannot be identified, the procedure should be aborted. There are no standard projections that can be suggested for aneurysms at different sites, since every aneurysm is different and the correct projection, has to be "discovered" for each particular aneurysm. In this respect, the experience of the operator is important. There are, however, some general principles that can be applied. Working projections for anterior communicating artery (ACoA) and basilar termi-

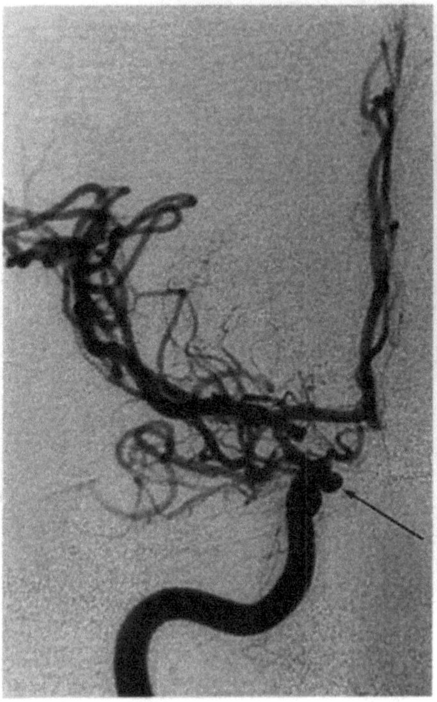

a

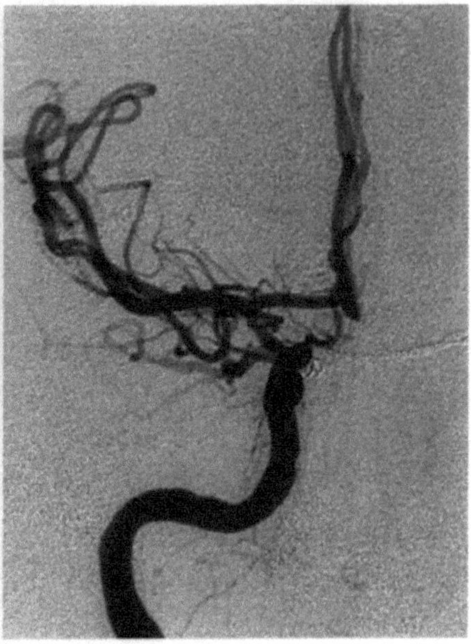

b

Fig. 5.11. a This slightly oblique antero-posterior view demonstrated the neck of a small paraophthalmic aneurysm (*arrow*). **b** Utilising one Guglielmi detachable coil the aneurysm was excluded from the circulation

nation aneurysms should be in the antero-posterior (AP) view, with the correct cranio-caudal incidence of the AP X-ray tube determined from an evaluation of the lateral view. The projection needs to be angled perpendicular to the longest axis of the aneurysm. Carotid-ophthalmic, para-ophthalmic and middle cerebral artery (MCA) aneurysms often require complex oblique views using either the lateral or the AP X-ray tube (Fig. 5.11).

Once the operator has determined the optimum angiographic projection and has made an angiographic analysis of the aneurysm and the rest of the intracranial vasculature, the aneurysm is catheterised. This is done with road-map fluoroscopic control, which is also used to deliver the first coil. Road-map fluoroscopy is performed in order to ensure that the coil is deployed in the aneurysm lumen without herniating into the parent artery. Subsequent coils may be better delivered using regular fluoroscopy since the first coil acts as a reference point for the aneurysm neck, i.e. the boundary between aneurysm and parent artery. The aneurysm is catheterised with either a Tracker 10-GDC or a Tracker 18-GDC microcatheter with two markers. The criteria for choosing which catheter to employ depends on the size of the aneurysm and of the coils to be introduced, as well as the clinical circumstances. Thus the Tracker 10 is used in small, recently ruptured aneurysms, whilst the Tracker 18 is used for unruptured or large or giant aneurysms.

The tip of the microcatheter should be steam-shaped to conform to the anatomical configuration of the aneurysm–parent vessel complex. This step is very important and, if correctly performed, makes catheterisation faster and easier. It prevents microcatheter kinking and helps to maintain a stable catheter position within the aneurysm. Again, operator experience is important in achieving the optimum shape. Some aneurysms, such as smaller carotid-ophthalmic aneurysms, require complex shapes to obtain a stable position of the catheter tip within the aneurysm. However, for others, e.g. basilar termination or internal carotid artery (ICA) bifurcation aneurysms where the aneurysm generally points in the same direction (axis) as the parent artery, little or no shaping is required.

A guidewire, such as the Seeker 10 or Dasher 14 (Target Therapeutics, Fremont, California), is used in combination with the microcatheter during aneurysm catheterisation. The tip of the microcatheter and the guidewire should not touch the wall of the aneurysm. When the guidewire is withdrawn, forward movement of the microcatheter tip can be anticipated and prevented by retrieving any slack in the body of the microcatheter. In patients with tortuous vasculature, in particular elderly patients, the Fastracker 10-GDC or 18-GDC microcatheters with two markers are now available. The outer hydrophilic layer reduces friction between the catheter and the inner arterial wall, facilitating distal catheterisation. Sudden forward movements of these hydrophilic coated microcatheters can occur and therefore great care should be taken when manoeuvering them in close proximity to the aneurysm. They also have a greater tendency than standard microcatheters for the tip to recoil when coils are being delivered into the aneurysm. We generally prefer to use uncoated catheters if access to the aneurysm permits. Once the tip of the microcatheter is positioned inside the aneurysm, a controlled infusion (one drop every 5 s) of heparinised saline is connected to its hub via a side-arm adapter in order to prevent back flow of blood. Flushing the microcatheter reduces friction between the catheter and coils since blood is more viscous than saline. Intra-aneurysmal angiograms should be avoided, except in unusual cases such as uncertainty as to whether an aneurysm is saccular or fusiform in nature (see Fig. 5.8).

The first coil is then chosen and introduced. This first GDC should have the largest possible circular memory that can be contained by the aneurysm lumen, in order to cross the neck area with several loops and to form an intra-aneurysmal "basket" (Fig. 5.12; see also Chap. 7, Fig. 7.6). Then, progressively smaller coils are delivered to fill the centre of the aneurysmal sac within the basket formed by the first coil (see Fig. 5.10). As already mentioned, there are two main versions of GDCs, the GDC-10 and the GDC-18. Both kinds can be delivered through the Tracker 18 microcatheter but only short GDC-10s should be used with the Tracker 18 since mismatching the size of catheter and coil, increases friction due to "snaking" of the coil within the catheter and causes stretching or breakage of coils during retrieval (Fig. 5.13). The standard GDC-18 is heavier and less malleable than the GDC-10, but "soft" versions of both are now available (Fig. 5.14). These are constructed of thinner platinum core wire, making them softer and more suitable for use in recently ruptured aneurysms.

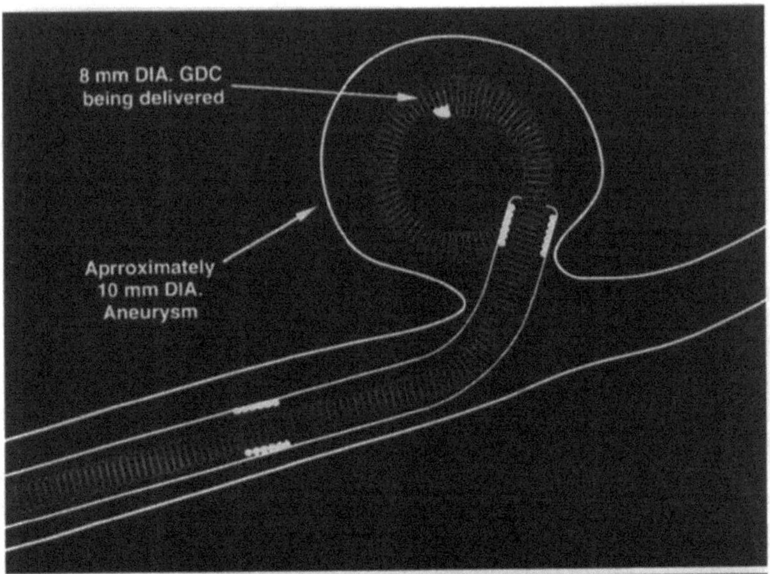

a

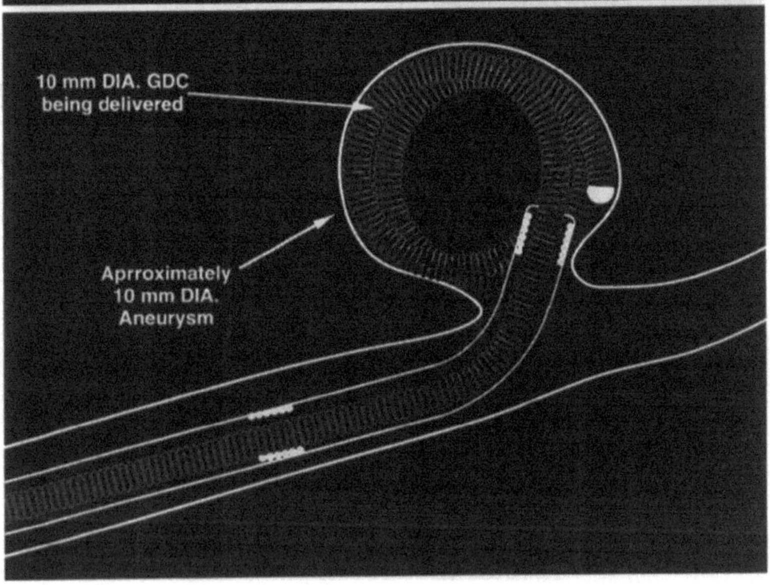

b

Fig. 5.12. a An incorrectly sized first coil. The circular memory is too small which may allow coil migration into the parent artery or cause subtotal aneurysm occlusion. **b** The correct size of coil has been selected. Several loops cross the aneurysm neck area. This allows complete aneurysm occlusion after smaller coils are placed within the basket formed by the first coil. *GDC*, Guglielmi detachable coil

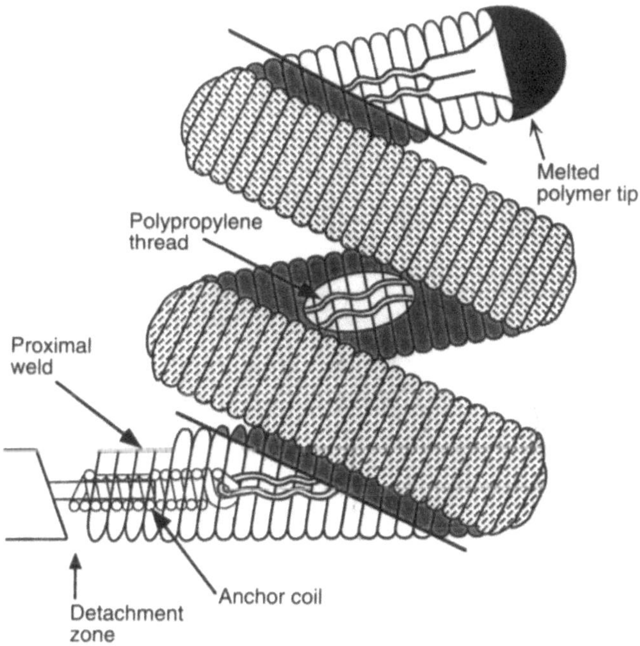

Fig. 5.13. Diagram of a stretch resistant Guglielmi detachable coil (GDC) which is manufactured with a polypropylene thread within the distal platinum section. The addition of the thread is intended to strengthen this section and reduce the risk of the coil stretching and/or breaking during retrieval. This new design is currently undergoing clinical evaluation. (Courtesy of J. Eder, Target Therapeutics)

If the chosen first coil is too large it will herniate into the parent vessel or cause excessive pressure on the sac wall and risk perforation. If it is too small it will not stabilise in the sac and may also herniate into the parent artery. In either case, it has to be partially withdrawn and repositioned or exchanged for one of a different size. Shaped coils are now available to reduce the tendency of the initial loops of the first coils to herniate into the parent artery. These 2D coils are manufactured so that the first one and a half loops of coil have a diameter 25% smaller than the rest. The manoeuvre for withdrawing the coil is a delicate one and should be avoided if possible, since the coil may become stretched and break. This complication is more likely to occur with the lighter and more delicate GDC-10 and particularly when deploying them in the larger Tracker 18 microcatheter. It is recommended to ensure that there are no kinks in the microcatheter (by gently retrieving it into the aneurysm neck area) before coil withdrawal to reduce friction between coil and microcatheter. Coil withdrawal is performed slowly and intermittently, to allow the axial pulling force to be transmitted to the entire coil and so avoid stretching.

Once the coil is positioned, angiography, via the guiding catheter, should be performed in two planes before GDC detachment to ensure that the parent and adjacent arteries are not compromised. The GDC is detached by applying a 1-mA direct electric current. The correct pre-detachment position of

GDC®-10
Guglielmi Detachable Coil

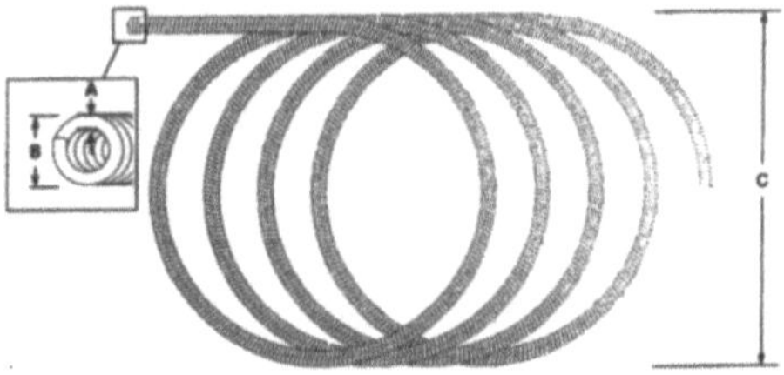

Sizing Chart

GDC-10 Part Number	Platinum Core Wire Diameter (A)	GDC Primary Coil Diameter (B)	GDC Helical Diameter (C)	Overall Length
341202 *soft*	0.00175"	0.0095"	2mm	2cm
341203 *soft*	0.00175"	0.0095"	2mm	3cm
341204 *soft*	0.00175"	0.0095"	2mm	4cm
341206 *soft*	0.00175"	0.0095"	2mm	6cm
341208 *soft*	0.00175"	0.0095"	2mm	8cm
341303 *soft*	0.00175"	0.0095"	3mm	3cm
341304 *soft*	0.00175"	0.0095"	3mm	4cm
341306 *soft*	0.00175"	0.0095"	3mm	6cm
341308 *soft*	0.00175"	0.0095"	3mm	8cm
341310 *soft*	0.00175"	0.0095"	3mm	10cm
340204	0.002"	0.010"	2mm	4cm
340208	0.002"	0.010"	2mm	8cm
340304	0.002"	0.010"	3mm	4cm
340306	0.002"	0.010"	3mm	6cm
340308	0.002"	0.010"	3mm	8cm
340312	0.002"	0.010"	3mm	12cm
340406	0.002"	0.010"	4mm	6cm
340410	0.002"	0.010"	4mm	10cm
340510	0.002"	0.010"	5mm	10cm
340515	0.002"	0.010"	5mm	15cm
340610	0.002"	0.010"	6mm	10cm
340620	0.002"	0.010"	6mm	20cm
340710	0.002"	0.010"	7mm	10cm
340730	0.002"	0.010"	7mm	30cm
340810	0.002"	0.010"	8mm	10cm
340820	0.002"	0.010"	8mm	20cm
340830	0.002"	0.010"	8mm	30cm
340915	0.002"	0.010"	9mm	15cm
340930	0.002"	0.010"	9mm	30cm
340103	0.002"	0.010"	10mm	30cm

a

Fig. 5.14 a, b. Lists of the (**a**) Guglielmi detachable coil (GDC)-10 and (**b**) GDC-18 currently available (as of November 1996) (see p. 155)

GDC®-18

Guglielmi Detachable Coil

Sizing Chart

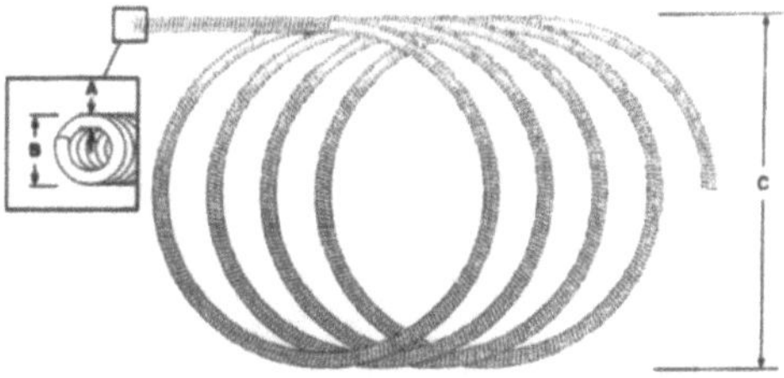

GDC-18 Part Number	Platinum Core Wire Diameter (A)	GDC Primary Coil Diameter (B)	GDC Helical Diameter (C)	Overall Length
351204 *soft*	0.00225"	0.0135"	2mm	4cm
351208 *soft*	0.00225"	0.0135"	2mm	8cm
351304 *soft*	0.00225"	0.0135"	3mm	4cm
351308 *soft*	0.00225"	0.0135"	3mm	8cm
351406 *soft*	0.00225"	0.0135"	4mm	6cm
351410 *soft*	0.00225"	0.0135"	4mm	10cm
350515	0.003"	0.015"	5mm	15cm
350520	0.003"	0.015"	5mm	20cm
350620	0.003"	0.015"	6mm	20cm
350730	0.003"	0.015"	7mm	30cm
350820	0.003"	0.015"	8mm	20cm
350830	0.003"	0.015"	8mm	30cm
350915	0.003"	0.015"	9mm	15cm
350930	0.003"	0.015"	9mm	30cm
350103	0.003"	0.015"	10mm	30cm
350123	0.003"	0.015"	12mm	30cm
350143	0.003"	0.015"	14mm	30cm
350163	0.004"	0.015"	16mm	30cm
350183	0.004"	0.015"	18mm	30cm
350203	0.004"	0.015"	20mm	30cm

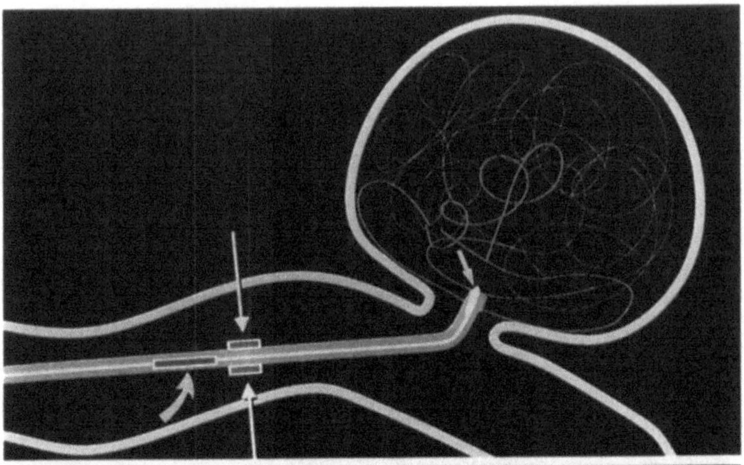
a

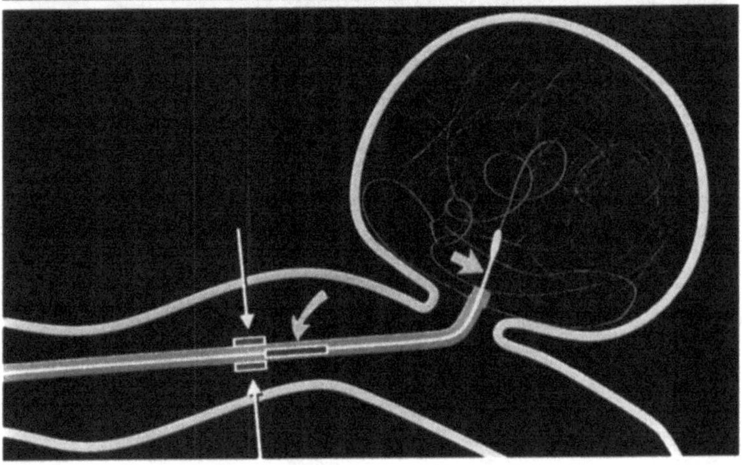
b

Fig. 5.15 a, b. The rationale for the double markers in the Guglielmi detachable coil (GDC) system. **a** The marker on the GDC delivery wire (*curved arrow*) is proximal to the proximal marker (between *two arrows*) on the microcatheter. The junction of platinum-stainless steel (*short single arrow*) is still inside the microcatheter which acts as an electric insulator and prevents detachment of the coil. **b** After gentle advancement of the delivery wire the junction (*short single arrow*) is exposed. The marker on the delivery wire (*curved arrow*) is now just distal to the marker on the microcatheter (between *two arrows*)

the coil is insured by two markers (Fig. 5.15). The GDC coil has a 0.5-cm long radiopaque (platinum) marker positioned in the stainless steel delivery wire 3 cm proximal to the platinum-stainless steel junction or detachment zone and the microcatheter has a short radiopaque marker 3 cm proximal to its tip. These radiopaque marks have been engineered to increase the safety of the procedure since, after detachment of the first coil, it is difficult to visualise the platinum-stainless steel junction of subsequent coils within the intra-aneurysmal coil mesh. Alignment of the two radiopaque markers (3 cm proximal to the catheter tip and, therefore, in the parent vessel and outside

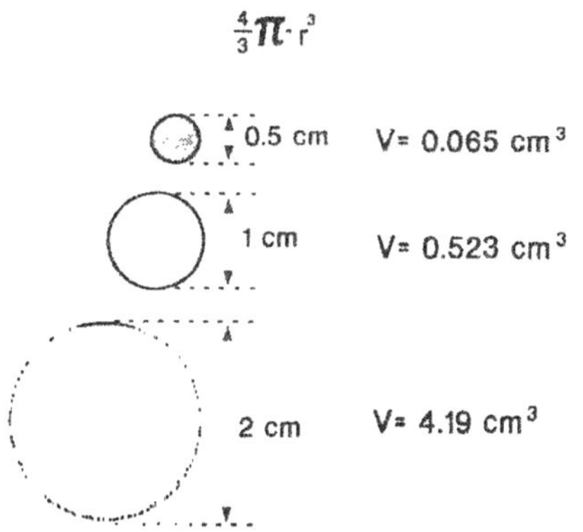

Fig. 5.16. The non-linear relationship between aneurysm volume and aneurysm diameter. The volume (V) is calcalated from the formula $3/4\,\pi r^3$ (r = radius of the sac)

the aneurysm) allows precise placement of the junction within the aneurysm, even if the actual junction cannot be visualised. It is imperative that the platinum–stainless steel junction is no more that 2 mm beyond the microcatheter tip because of its relative stiffness, which could perforate the aneurysm if advanced too far. Alignment of the proximal radiopaque markers on the microcatheter and GDC ensures that the junction is no more than 2 mm beyond the microcatheter tip.

Subsequent, progressively smaller GDCs are delivered and detached to fill the centre of the aneurysm, within the basket formed by the first coil [17]. In order to achieve dense packing, it is important to appreciate the non-linear relationship between aneurysm diameter and volume. The volume of a 10-mm aneurysm, for instance, is eight times larger than the volume of a 5-mm aneurysm (Fig. 5.16). Once dense aneurysm packing is achieved, the procedure is terminated (Fig. 5.17). The microcatheter is slowly removed from the aneurysm and a post-treatment angiogram is performed to assess the degree of aneurysm occlusion and the patency of the distal vascular tree.

A strict protocol of follow-up angiograms should be implemented. Follow-up angiograms are usually performed in our institution at 3 months, 12 months, 2 years, and 4–6 years (Figs. 5.18, 5.19).

5.4.4 Patient Management During Embolisation

General anaesthesia with intubation should be utilised for patients that are uncooperative or those with small aneurysms so that high quality motionless road-mapping can be obtained for precise aneurysm catheterisation without touching the aneurysmal wall. General anaesthesia must be utilised in the treatment of ruptured aneurysms treated in the acute phase following subarachnoid haemorrhage (SAH) in order to better manage possible intraprocedural complications. Neuroleptic analgesia may be used for the treatment of cooperative patients with large or giant unruptured aneurysms.

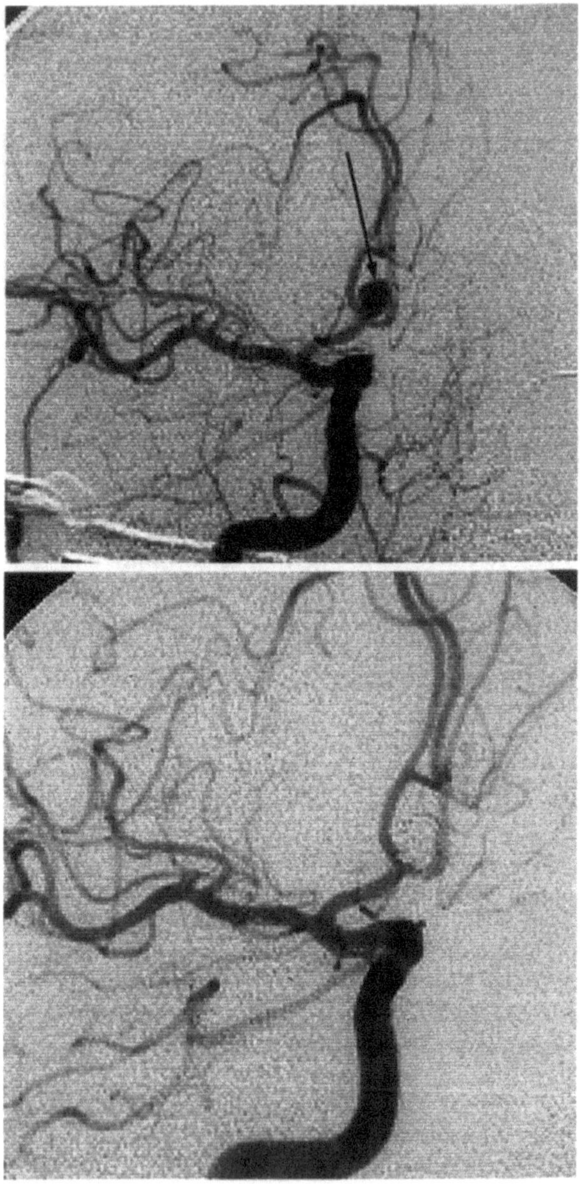

Fig. 5.17.
a Patient with a small, ruptured anterior communicating artery aneurysm (*arrow*) which was treated with one 6×20, one 4×10, two 3×6, one 2×8-soft, and two 2×4-soft Guglielmi detachable coil (GDC)-10 coils.
b The aneurysm is densely packed and completely occluded

To prevent thromboembolic complications, patients are anticoagulated during coil embolisation. For procedures performed in the subacute-chronic phase post-SAH, or for unruptured aneurysms, a bolus of 3000 IU of heparin is administered at the beginning of the procedure, i.e. as soon as a sheath has been placed in the femoral artery. This is followed by hourly intravenous injections of 1000 IU of heparin. Heparin (5000 IU/l) is always added to the saline that is used to continuously flush the catheters. For pa-

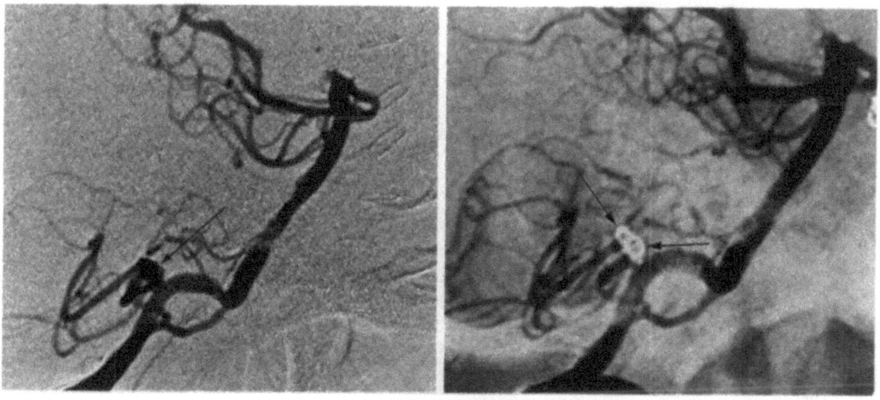

a b

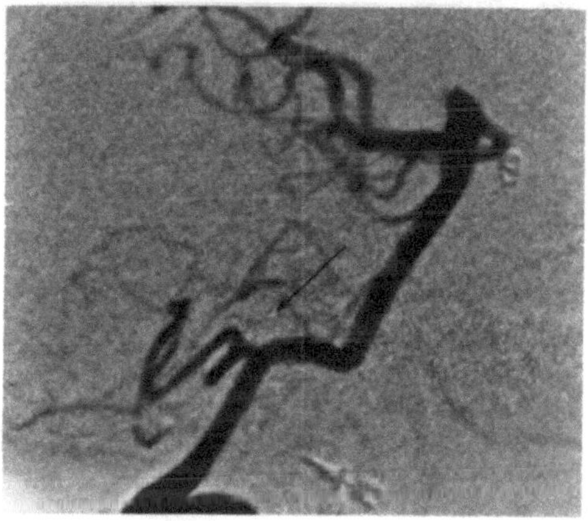

c

Fig. 5.18.
a Patient with a small, ruptured posterior inferior cerebellar artery aneurysm, who had undergone unsuccessful surgical clipping. Guglielmi detachable coil treatment was then performed. The aneurysm re-ruptured during the deposition of the second and last coil. Continuous coil delivery into the aneurysm and immediate reversal of systemic heparinisation halted the bleeding.
b, c The post-treatment (b) and 18-month follow-up angiograms (c) show complete occlusion of the aneurysm (*arrows*)

tients treated soon after aneurysm rupture, heparin is only used in the flushing solutions. During treatment in this acute phase, systemic heparinisation may be instituted, after the detachment of initial coils or once the fundus or putative bleeding site of the aneurysm no longer fills with radiographic contrast. Anticoagulation is monitored by estimation of the activated clotting time (ACT) during the procedure. The amount of heparin given is adjusted to ensure that clotting times are maintained at between two and three times baseline values.

Following embolisation, the anticoagulant effect of heparin may be reversed by administration of protamine sulphate. In wide-necked aneurysms, and if there is some coil impingement upon the parent vessel, heparin is not reversed and aspirin (325 mg/day) is administered to reduce the risk of distal embolisation. Patients treated for recently ruptured aneurysms may be given heparin intravenously by continuous pump infusion for the same indications as after elective procedures, but antiplatelet medication (i.e. aspirin) is not given because its effect is longer-lasting and can not be easily reversed should a surgical procedure, such as CSF drainage for hydrocephalus, be required.

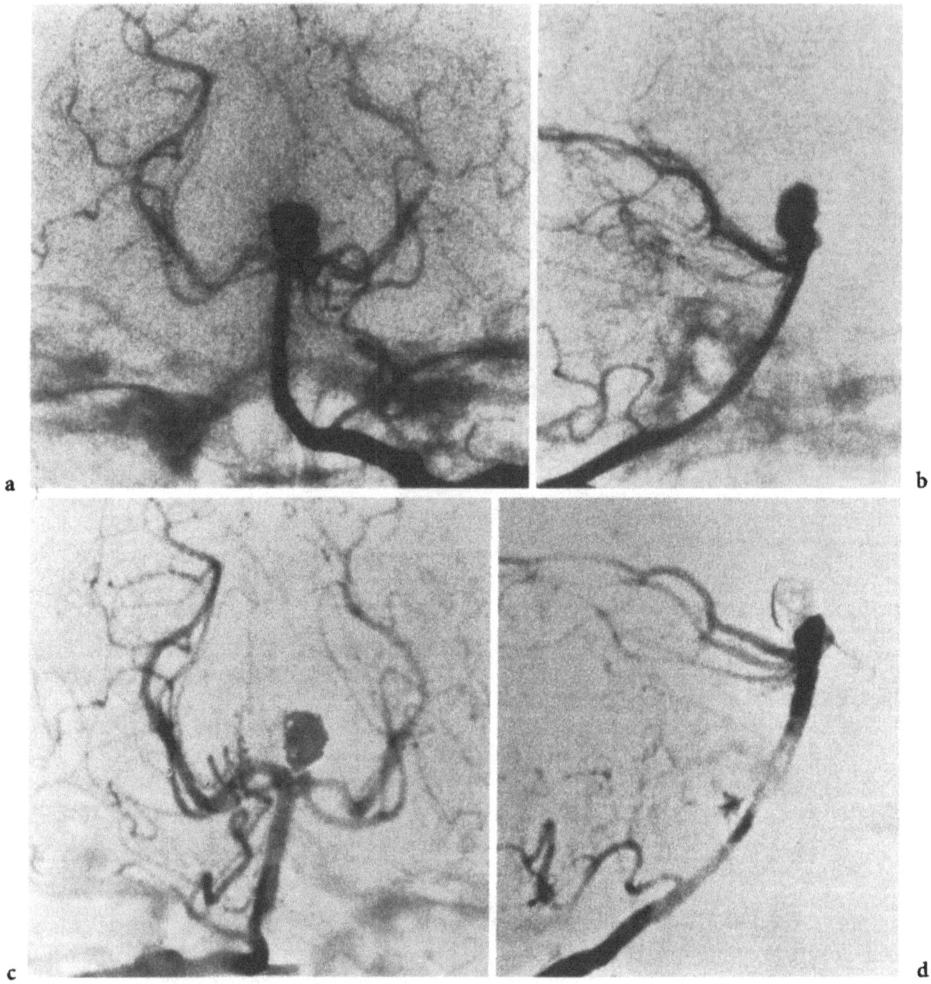

Fig. 5.19. a, b Patient with a ruptured aneurysm of the basilar artery termination; anteroposterior (**a**) and lateral (**b**) views. A surgical attempt to clip this aneurysm was unsuccessful. The aneurysm was treated with two Guglielmi detachable coil (GDC)-10 coils (one 8×40 and one 5×15). **c, d** Follow-up angiograms after 6 years show persistent complete aneurysm occlusion

5.4.5 Periprocedural Complications and Their Management

Although coil embolisation is less invasive than extravascular treatment, it does not warrant the label "minimally invasive", which is sometimes used to describe this endovascular technique. Even in experienced hands, complications may occur and their consequences may be serious and even fatal.

5.4.5.1
Aneurysm Rupture

The incidence of peri-operative aneurysm rupture during extravascular neurosurgery is 15%–20% [11]. Aneurysm rupture also occurs during endovascular treatment but the incidence is lower [18, 8]. In a series of 150 aneurysms [18] treated with GDCs, there were six cases (4%) of aneurysm rupture during the procedure. One rupture occurred during aneurysm catheterisation, one during the detachment of the sixth (and final) coil, and the remaining four ruptures occurred while delivering the final coil into the aneurysm.

All ruptures occurred in small aneurysms; five aneurysms were treated soon after SAH and one had never previously ruptured. Four of these six patients were in good Hunt and Hess grading (0–III) on admission, while two were in grades IV and V. In all six cases it was possible to quickly stop the haemorrhage (vide infra). One of these patients required subsequent aneurysm clipping, while in the remaining five cases the aneurysm was completely occluded with coils (see Fig. 5.18). The four patients that were originally in grades 0–III made an excellent recovery, while the two patients in grades IV and V eventually died.

To summarise, the final outcome, despite periprocedural aneurysm rupture, can be good and seems related to the patients condition (grade) prior to treatment. To prevent the frightening occurrence of intraprocedural aneurysm rupture, some criteria need to be adopted, particularly in small aneurysms. We suggest the following precautions:

- General anaesthesia should be utilised
- Catheterisation of the aneurysm should be performed cautiously and care taken to remove any "slack" from the microcatheter
- The microcatheter should be steam-shaped with an appropriate distal curve in order to maintain a central position in the sac and not to touch the aneurysm walls
- It is preferable to position the microcatheter tip near the neck of the aneurysm rather than near the fundus
- Only GDC-10 "soft" should be utilised in lesions of 4 mm or smaller and they should also be used to fill the centre of small aneurysms after the delivery of larger coils
- All the above-mentioned steps should be followed when treating small and recently ruptured aneurysms.

If, in spite of such precautions, an aneurysm ruptures during the procedure, we recommend the following management:

- Anticoagulants should be reversed with protamine sulphate
- The aneurysm must be completely occluded by expeditiously adding more coils
- Upon completion of the procedure, a computed tomograph should be performed and, if appropriate, ventricular CSF drainage performed
- If the aneurysm is not completely occluded, emergency surgery should be considered [26].

5.4.5.2
Thromboembolic Events

In a series of 200 patients [18] treated with GDCs, transient, mild clinical worsening (mono-hemiparesis, hemianopsia, dysphasia, sensory deficit) was observed following endosaccular packing with GDCs in 4% of patients. These symptoms and signs resolved within 24–48 h of onset and were probably due to micro-thromboembolic events. Permanent neurological deficit due to periprocedural thromboembolism occurred in 2% of the same series of patients (two cases of hemianopsia, one case of mild hemiparesis, and one case of severe hemiparesis). In two of these four patients, the source of the embolus was the guiding catheter.

Our current protocol includes the use of heparin during the procedure in order to prevent such complications. The use of systemic heparinisation when embolisation is performed soon after spontaneous aneurysm rupture is controversial. The potential risk of exacerbating bleeding should periprocedural rupture occur, has to be balanced against the risk of thromboembolic events. One of the authors (GG) uses heparin only in the flushing solutions when treating patients acutely after SAH. Aspirin is administered after embolisation if there is contrast stagnation in the network of coils within the neck area, or if there is some degree of coil impingment upon the parent vessel. Aspirin is also prescribed, for longer (1 year or more), if there is any extension of coils into the parent artery.

5.5
Delayed Complications and Their Management

5.5.1
Aneurysm Rebleeding

Coil embolisation has been shown to protect patients presenting with aneurysmal SAH in the short-term [8, 13] but delayed rebleeding may occur (see also Chap. 7, Sect. 7.3.5). In a series of 200 patients [18] treated with GDCs, there were two cases of aneurysm rebleeding. The first occured in a patient with a giant right posterior communicating artery (PCoA) aneurysm that had bled twice before treatment with GDC. Fifty days after treatment the patient re-haemorrhaged. An emergency angiogram showed that the coils had compacted, re-exposing the neck and a small part of the body of the aneurysm to the parent artery blood flow. In this case, as rarely occurs, the original rupture was near the neck of the aneurysm. The residual portion was retreated with GDC and complete occlusion of the aneurysm was achieved in two sessions. Angiography performed 6 months, 16 months, and 3 years later confirmed stable aneurysm occlusion and physical examination at 3 years revealed a mild left upper extremity weakness only. The second instance of rebleeding occurred in a patient with severe diffuse intracranial atherosclerosis and a large PCoA aneurysm that, after SAH, underwent an unsuccessful attempt at surgical clipping. Endovascularly, it was possible to achieve subtotal occlusion of this wide-necked aneurysm in two sessions. Two years later the aneurysm rebled and the patient is now in poor neurological status. Byrne et al. [6] reported a similar incidence of late bleeding after coil embolisation in a series of 199 patients, followed for up to 3.5 years. Rebleeding occurred in three patients, and one further patient experienced SAH due to rupture of a co-incidental aneurysm.

5.5.2 Rupture of Previously Unruptured Aneurysms

Rupture of previously unruptured aneurysms may occur. In the same series of 200 patients [18] treated with GDCs, rupture occurred for the first time 1–2 years after partial GDC treatment of four giant aneurysms. Three of these lesions were judged inoperable and one had previously undergone unsuccessful surgical exploration. The haemorrhages were fatal in all four patients. These cases and the reported experience of others [7, 9] suggest that partial endosaccular packing does not ensure protection against future rupture, even in previously unruptured aneurysms and highlight the need for careful angiographic follow-up.

References

1. ApSimon T, Khangure M, Ives J et al (1995) The Guglielmi coil for transarterial occlusion of intracranial aneurysm: preliminary Western Australian experience. J Clin Neurosci 2:26–35
2. Araki C, Handa H, Yoshida K et al (1995) Electrically induced thrombosis for the treatment of intracranial aneurysms and angiomas. In: de Vet AC (ed) Proc 3rd Int Congr Neurological Surgery, Copenhagen, vol 110. Excerpta Medica, Amsterdam 1966, pp 651–654
3. Bigelow FS, De Foyes JF (1953) Cited by Sawyer P, Pate J. Am J Physiol 175:103–107
4. Black SPW, Leo HL, Carson WL (1988) Recording and measuring the interior features of intracranial aneurysms removed at autopsy: method and initial findings. Neurosurgery 22:40–43
5. Bradac GB, Riva M, Bergui M (1995) Endovascular coil embolisation of cerebral aneurysms. Riv Neuroradiol 8:637–644
6. Byrne J, Bacon F, Higgins N et al. (1996) Coil embolisation of intracranial aneurysms: follow-up results. Proceeding of 34th annual meeting of the American Society of Neuroradiology, Seattle 23–27 June, p138
7. Byrne JV, Hubbard N, Morris JH (1994) Endovascular coil occlusion of experimental aneurysms: partial treatment does not prevent subsequent rupture. Neurol Res 16:425–427
8. Byrne JV, Molyneux AJ, Brennan RP, Renowden SA (1995) Embolisation of recently ruptured intracranial aneurysms. J Neurol Neurosurg Psychiatry. 59:616–620
9. Casasco AE, Aymard A, Gobin P et al (1993) Selective endovascular treatment of 71 intracranial aneurysms with platinum coils. J Neurosurg 73:3–10
10. Civit T, Auque J, Marchal JC et al (1996) Aneurysm clipping after endovascular treatment with coils: a report of eight patients. Neurosurgery 38:955–961
11. Giannotta SL, Oppenheimer JH, Levy ML et al (1991) Management of intraoperative rupture of aneurysms without hypotension. Neurosurgery 28:531–535
12. Gobin P, Viñuela F, Gurian J et al (1996) Treatment of large and giant fusiform intracranial aneurysms with Guglielmi detachable coils. J Neurosurg 84:55–62
13. Graves V, Strother C, Duff T et al (1995) Early treatment of ruptured aneurysms with Guglielmi Detachable Coils: effect on subsequent bleeding. Neurosurgery 37:640–648
14. Guglielmi G (1992) Embolization of intracranial aneurysms with detachable coils and electrothrombosis. In: Viñuela F, Halbach F, Dion J (eds) Interventional neuroradiology. Raven Press, New York, pp 63–75

15. Guglielmi G (1992) Endovascular treatment of intracranial aneurysms. In: Viñuela F, Dion J, Duckwiler G (eds) Neuroimaging clinics of North America. Saunders, Philadelphia, pp 269–278
16. Guglielmi G (1993) Endovascular treatment of intracranial aneurysm with detachable coils and electrothrombosis. In: Valavanis A (ed) Interventional neuroradiology. Springer, Berlin Heidelberg New York, pp 111–122
17. Scotti G, Righi C (1994) The "hypoteloric happy face" sign: a misleading indicator of complete aneurysm closure with GDC coils. Am J Neuroradiol 15:796–797
18. Guglielmi G (to be published) The interventional neuroradiological treatment of intracranial aneurysms. In: Cohadon F (ed) Advances and technical standards in neurosurgery. Springer, Berlin Heidelberg New York
19. Guglielmi G, Viñuela F (1994) Endosaccular treatment of intracranial saccular aneurysms with GDC platinum detachable coils: small-necked aneurysms. In: Pasqualin A, Da Pian R (eds) New trends in management of cerebro-vascular malformations. Proc Int Conf Verona, Italy, 8–12 June, 1992. Springer, Berlin Heidelberg New York, pp 269–271
20. Guglielmi G, Viñuela F (1994) Intracranial aneurysms: Guglielmi electrothrombotic coils. In: Hopkins LN (ed) Neurosurgery clinics of North America, vol 5, no 3. Saunders, Philadelphia, pp 427–436
21. Guglielmi G, Viñuela F, Sepetka I et al (1991) Electrothrombosis of saccular aneurysms via endovascular approach. Part 1. Electro-chemical basis, technique, and experimental results. J Neurosurg 75:1–7
22. Guglielmi G, Viñuela F, Dion J et al (1991) Electrothrombosis of saccular aneurysms via endovascular approach. Part 2. Preliminary clinical experience. J Neurosurg 75:8–14
23. Guglielmi G, Viñuela F, Briganti F et al (1992) Carotid-cavernous fistula due to a ruptured intracavernous aneurysm: endovascular treatment by electrothrombosis with detachable coils. Neurosurgery 31:591–597
24. Guglielmi G, Viñuela F, Duckwiler G et al (1992) Endovascular treatment of posterior circulation aneurysms by electrothrombosis using electrically detachable coils. J Neurosurg 77:515–524
25. Guglielmi G, Viñuela F, Duckwiler G et al (1995) High-flow, small hole arteriovenous fistulae: treatment with electrodetachable (GDC) coils. Am J Neuroradiol 16:325–328
26. Gurian J, Martin N, King W et al (1995) Neurosurgical management of cerebral aneurysms following unsuccessful or incomplete endovascular embolization. J Neurosurg 83:843–853
27. Gurian J, Viñuela F, Gobin P et al (1995) Aneurysm rupture after parent vessel sacrifice: treatment with Guglielmi detachable coil embolization via retrograde catheterization: case report. Neurosurgery 37:1216–1221
28. Lylyk P, Viñuela F, Dion J et al (1993) Therapeutic alternatives for vein of Galen vascular malformations. J Neurosurg 78:438–445
29. Massoud T, Guglielmi G, Viñuela F et al (1994) Saccular aneurysms in Moya Moya disease. Endovascular treatment using electrically detachable coils. Surg Neurol 41:462–467
30. Massoud T, Guglielmi G, Viñuela F et al (1996) Multiple intracranial aneurysms involving the posterior circulation: endovascular treatment with electrolytically detachable coils. Am J Neuroradiol 17:549–554
31. McDougall C, Halbach V, Dowd C et al (1996) Endovascular treatment of basilar tip aneurysms using electrolytically detachable coils. J Neurosurg 84:393–399
32. Miller MD, Johnsrude IS, Limberakis AJ et al (1978) Clinical use of transcatheter electrocoagulation. Radiology 129:211–214
33. Molyneux A, Ellison D, Morris J, Byrne JV et al (1995) Histological findings in giant aneurysms treated with Guglielmi detachable coils. J Neurosurg 83:129–132
34. Nichols D (1993) Endovascular treatment of the acutely ruptured intracranial aneurysm. J Neurosurg 79:1–2 (commentary)
35. Pierot L, Boulin A, Castaings L et al (1966) Selective occlusion of basilar artery aneurysms using controlled detachable coils. Report of 35 cases. Neurosurgery 38:948–954
36. Piton J, Billerey J, Constant P et al (1996) Selective vascular thrombosis induced by a direct electrical current: animal experiments. J Neuroradiol 5:139–152
37. Salazar A (1961) Experimental myocardial infarction. Induction of coronary thrombosis in the intact closed chest dog. Circ Res 9:1351–1356
38. Sawyer P, Pate J (1953) Bio-electric phenomena as an etiologic factor in intravascular thrombosis. Am J Physiol 175:103–107
39. Sawyer P, Pate J (1953) Electric potential differences across the normal aorta and aortic grafts of dogs. Am J Physiol 175:113–117

40. Sawyer P, Pate J, Weldon C (1953) Relations of abnormal and injury electric potential differences to intravascular thrombosis. Am J Physiol 175:108–112
41. Scotti G, Righi C, Simionato F et al (1994) Endovascular therapy of intracranial aneurysms with Guglielmi detachable coils (GDC). Riv Neuroradiol 7:723–733
42. Standard S, Chavis T, Wakhloo A et al (1994) Retrieval of a Guglielmi detachable coil after unraveling and fracture: case report and experimental results. Neurosurgery 35:994–999
43. Tenjin H, Fushiki S, Nakahara Y et al (1995) Effect of Guglielmi detachable coils on experimental carotid artery aneurysms in primates. Stroke 26:2075–2080
44. Thompson W, Pizzo S, Jackson D et al (1977) Transcatheter electrocoagulation: a therapeutic angiographic technique for vessel occlusion. Invest Radiol 12:146–153
45. Turjman F, Massoud T, Ji C et al (1994) Combined stent implantation and endosaccular coil placement for treatment of experimental wide-necked aneurysms: a feasibility study in swine. Am J Neuroradiol 15:1087–1090
46. Yasargil MG (1984) Pathological considerations. In: Yasargil MG (ed) Microneurosurgery. Thieme, Stuttgart, pp 280–281
47. Zubillaga A, Guglielmi G, Viñuela F et al (1994) Endovascular occlusion of intracranial aneurysms with electrically detachable coils: correlation of aneurysm neck size and treatment results. Am J Neuroradiol 15:815–820

CHAPTER 6

Coil Embolisation of Saccular Aneurysms at Specific Sites

6.1 Introduction

The site of an intracranial aneurysm has a profound effect on how the patient presents and is treated. The clinical syndromes caused by ruptured or unruptured aneurysms at various sites have been considered in Chap. 2. In the present chapter the vascular anatomy of common aneurysm sites will be described and local factors relevant to endovascular treatment emphasised. The dissection needed to clip aneurysms of the posterior fossa is generally more difficult than for aneurysms of the anterior circulation. The endovascular route, though it allows easier access to some aneurysm locations, is not immune to constraints of local anatomy. The aneurysm site thus determines surgical difficulty, both endovascular and extravascular which is reflected in treatment results and procedural morbidity figures.

There is a considerable literature of operative techniques and microvascular anatomy for the exposure and clipping of intracranial aneurysms. The surgeon, in undertaking the treatment of a particular aneurysm, must be aware of the anatomical route to reach the aneurysm and needs to know the relative priority of structures that may be vulnerable during the procedure. Applying this principle of operative surgery to endovascular techniques means that the endovascular therapist needs the optimum pre-operative anatomical display of the aneurysm and relevant cerebral vasculature. He or she needs to be aware of the position of parent and adjacent arteries, as well as the likely consequences of their intentional or inadvertent occlusion.

Before describing individual aneurysm locations it is worth considering their relative incidences. As has been previously discussed, reported incidences vary depending on sampling criteria. The frequencies quoted in previous chapters are largely derived from autopsy or multicentre studies of treated patients. The international cooperative study on the timing of aneurysm surgery recruited 3521 patients, presenting within 3 days of aneurysmal subarachnoid haemorrhage (SAH) and reported aneurysms of the anterior circulation in 92% [internal carotid artery (ICA), 29.8%; middle cerebral

Table 6.1. Sites of intracranial aneurysms (% of total at each location)

Site	Treated and untreated (Ferguson[a] [43]) n=5808	Coil embolisation (Oxford Series) n=473	Operated patients (Newcastle Series [47]) n=500
ICA			
Cavernous	3.7	2.1	0.6
COA	4.8	7.2	4.8
PCoA	19.3	14.4	23.2
AChA	1.9	1.8	2.0
Bifurcation	7.3	4.5	6.4
Unspecified	-	-	2.4
Total	37.0	30.0	39.4
ACA			
A1	0.9	0.4	0.8
ACoA	25.0	17.9	32.0
DACA	4.8	2.0	2.0
Total	30.7	20.3	34.8
MCA			
M1	-	2.3	-
Bifurcation	-	13.3	-
DMCA	-	1.1	-
Total	13.4	16.7	19.8
Posterior circulation			
PCA	0.9	1.2	0.4
BA Termination	7.0	22.0	2.8
SCA	2.0	2.3	0.4
AICA/Trunk	0.9	2.3	0
VB Junction	0.9	2.7	0.4
PICA	1.8	2.5	2.8
Total	13.5	33.0	6.0

[a]Ferguson's figures derived from Fox [15] and Drake [8] for anterior and posterior circulations, repectively. An additional 5.4% of aneurysms were sited on minor arteries and are not included.

artery (MCA), 22.3%; anterior cerebral artery (ACA), 39%] and of the posterior circulation in 8% of patients [23]. However, Fox [15], who conducted a literature review of over 4000 reports and in 1983 published data on 4957 patients with 5808 intracranial aneurysms, found that 86.5% occurred in the anterior circulation and that 95% of aneurysms arose from five arteries [ICA, ACA, MCA, basilar artery (BA) and vertebral artery (VA) in descending order of frequency] with the remaining 5% from 15 other arteries [43]. His data were used by Redekop and Ferguson [43] to compile a frequency list (Table 1). For comparison the relative percentage of aneurysm locations in patients treated consecutively by coil embolisation in Oxford between 1992 and 1996 and by extravascular surgery in Newcastle between 1969 and 1980 are also presented in Table 1. The Oxford series comprises 400 patients in whom 473 aneurysms were treated. The Newcastle series was selected for comparison since it is the most recent and largest single-centre surgical series published in the United Kingdom. The former contains over twice as many posterior circulation aneurysms as the pooled data of Redekop and Ferguson and five times the number in the surgical series. The demographics of patients in these series must reflect different treatment selection criteria and the relative ease and safety of endovascular treatment in the posterior circulation. The reader should also be aware that the role of embolisation in the management of surgically accessible aneurysms, such as those at the anterior communicating artery (ACoA) or MCA bifurcation, is controversial and universally accepted selection criteria have yet to be determined.

6.2 Internal Carotid Artery Aneurysms

Internal carotid artery (ICA) aneurysms account for 30–40% of all intracranial saccular aneurysms [11, 15, 43]; the ICA, therefore, represents the commonest aneurysm bearing intracranial artery. Saccular aneurysms usually occur at the site of side branches and aneurysms are described according to the nearest branches of ICA. The posterior communicating artery (PCoA) origin is the single commonest site on the ICA. The sites and relative incidences of saccular ICA aneurysms are as follows:

- Cavernous ICA (10%)
- Origin of ophthalmic artery (13%)
- Origin of PCoA (52%)
- Origin of AChA (anterior choroidal artery) (5%)
- Termination of ICA (20%).

(Modified from Ferguson [11].)

6.2.1 Vascular Anatomy

The ICA can be divided for description into four parts: cervical, petrous, cavernous and supraclinoid. The cervical portion has no branches and is rarely the site of aneurysms. The aetiology of such aneurysms is usually traumatic dissection. They may be fusiform or saccular and, although the latter have been treated by endosaccular packing, they are so uncommon that they will not be considered further here.

The petrous ICA tranverses the temporal bone in the carotid canal to emerge from the foramen lacerum to lie lateral to the sphenoid sinus and anteromedial to the Gasserian ganglion. In its petrous portion it gives the caroticotympanic artery which arises at the point where the proximal vertical part turns horizontal to run anteromedially and an inconstant artery of the pterygoid canal (Vidian artery). This section is again an unusual site for aneurysms (see Chap. 2, Sect. 2.5.1).

The cavernous artery initially runs vertically and then turns forwards and slightly inferiorly, within the cavernous sinus, before turning superiorly to penetrate the dura forming the roof of the sinus and emerge as the supraclinoid artery. It therefore makes two loops: a posterior loop between the proximal vertical and the horizontal sections, and an anterior loop between the horizontal and the distal vertical sections. The ICA gives several small branches within the sinus; these are the meningohypophyseal trunk, the inferior cavernous artery and the capsular artery using the nomenculature of Parkinson [39]. The meningohypophyseal trunk is the origin of arteries that supply the meninges, hypophysis and nerves of the regions, i.e. the artery of the tentorium (artery of Bernasconi and Casinari [4]), the dorsal meningeal artery and the inferior hypophyseal artery, all of which may arise separately. Lasjaunias and Berenstein [32] describe this vessel as the primitive maxillary artery which may have a common origin with the trigeminal artery and the posterior inferior hypophyseal artery [32]. The older descriptions of Parkinson [39] and McConnell [34] can be further confusing since the inferior cavernous artery is now generally known as the inferolateral trunk and the capsular artery (of McConnell) usually arises as two branches [32]. Because the intracavernous ICA is relatively fixed as it traverses the dura in the region of the anterior clinoid process, its anterior portion is the most common site of traumatic aneurysms, whereas saccular aneurysms, which are usually idiopathic or due to atherosclerosis are sited in the horizontal section where branch vessels arise. These small arteries are generally difficult to image in the presence of an aneurysm.

Once intradural the supraclinoid ICA passes below the optic nerve and turns posteriorly below the anterior perforating substance to its terminal bifurcation. This section gives the ophthalmic artery (OphA), superior hypophyseal artery, PCoA and AChA.

6.2.2
Anatomical Variations of the Internal Carotid Artery

Agenesis and hypoplasia. Complete or sequential underdevelopment of the ICA may result in compensatory hypertrophy of the circle of Willis and aneurysm formation [52]. For example, in a series of 24 cases of agenesis of ICA reported by Turnball [53] aneurysms of the ACoA were present in four patients.

Variants of the intrapetrous and intracavernous ICA. Intratympanic and trans-sellar variations in the course of the extradural ICA are well described. Extension of the intrapetrous artery into the middle ear cavity due to an incomplete bony carotid canal may simulate an intrapetrous aneurysm by causing pulsatile tinnitus and a mass deep to the tympanic membrane [30].

Persistent embryological caroticovertebral and caroticobasilar communications. The persistent primitive trigeminal artery (PPTA) is the most frequently encountered persistent segmental artery. Three types are described:

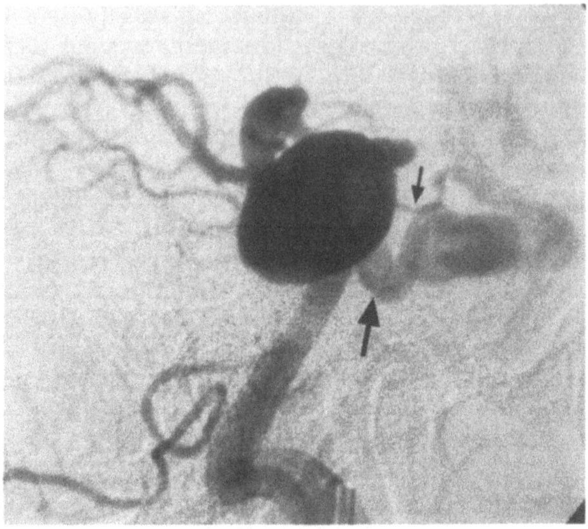

Fig. 6.1.
Lateral vertebral intra-arterial digital subtraction angiogram showing a large aneurysm arising at the junction of the basilar artery (BA) trunk and a persistent primitive trigeminal artery (*large arrow*). The latter is ectatic, as is the BA termination and posterior cerebral artery. The ipsilateral posterior communicating artery is patent (*small arrow*). (Courtesy of Dr A.J. Molyneux)

in type 1, the PPTA supplies bilateral posterior cerebellar arteries (PCAs) and superior cerebellar arteries (SCAs); in type 2, it supplies one PCA (usually the contralateral) and both SCAs; and in type 3 both PCAs are supplied by PCoAs and the PPTA supplies both SCAs [46] only. The PPTA connects BA [between SCA and the anterior inferior cerebellar artery (AICA)] with the ICA at the junction of its intrapetrous and intracavernous portions (Fig. 6.1). Other persistent segmental arteries of the ICA theoretically occur proximal to PPTA; namely the otic artery, hypoglossal artery and proatlantic artery type 1. All are extremely rare in comparison with PPTA. The hypoglossal artery, if present, arises from the cervical ICA and enters the cranium via the hypoglossal canal to join the centrolateral VA and form the BA. This vessel is associated with hypoplasia of the ipsilateral VA. The proatlantic artery type 1 arises from the cervical ICA at the C2 vertebral level and joins the contralateral VA [31].

6.2.3 Intracavernous Aneurysms

The mid-section, i.e. between the two loops, is the most common site of aneurysms. They may, less frequently, arise from the anterior loop or the posterior vertical section (Fig. 6.2). It may be difficult to determine whether an anterior aneurysm is intracavernous or intradural or both. They are caused by incomplete rupture or degeneration of the vessel wall and the defect forming the neck tends to be wide. Larger aneurysms, in which the exact site of the defect is difficult to define, develop in the horizontal or vertical portions because the vessel is less constrained by bone. They usually project laterally but may point dorsally and less often medially or anteriorly.

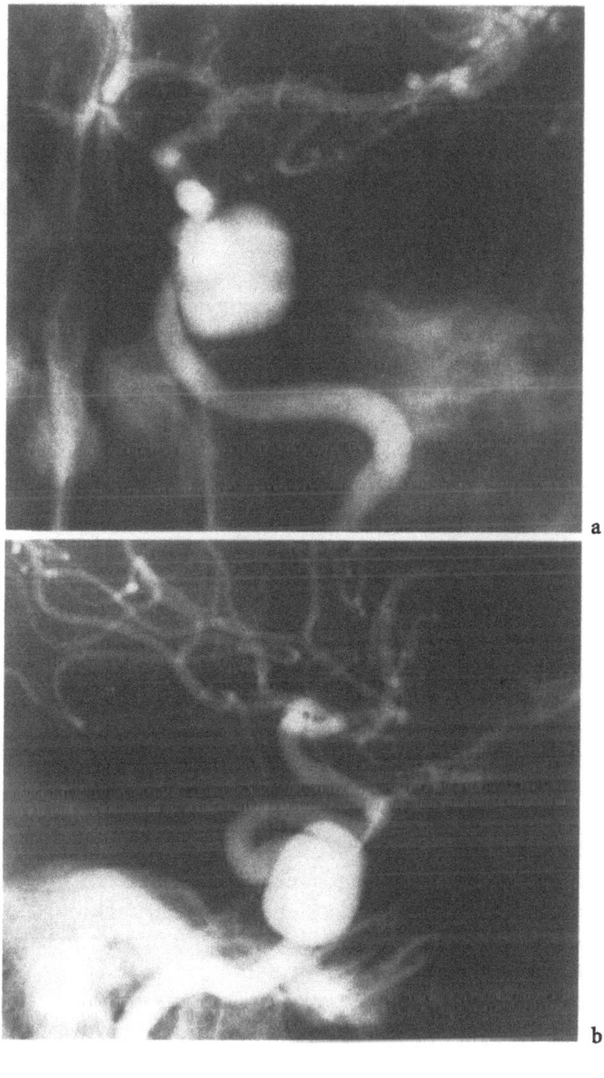

Fig. 6.2 a, b.
Unsubtracted internal carotid artery (ICA) angiograms in lateral (**a**) and frontal (**b**) projections. There is an intracavernous carotid aneurysm arising from the proximal portion of the ectatic intracavernous ICA. The neck of the aneurysm is difficult to define. Aneurysms at this site project laterally but are confined by the dura of the cavernous sinus wall

The surgical management of these aneurysms remains controversial; there are advocates of a direct surgical approach but this is technically demanding. Results of endosaccular packing with coils in order to avoid ICA occlusion have been disappointing, principally because larger aneurysms have wide necks. Furthermore, deploying coils is difficult in small or large aneurysms because the relatively rigid dural walls of the sinus tend to distort the coil ball and frustrate tight packing. Endovascular treatment, therefore, usually requires ICA occlusion.

6.2.4 Carotid-ophthalmic Aneurysms

The carotid-ophthalmic aneurysm (COA) was defined by Drake et al. [9] as an ICA aneurysm arising at the level of the ophthalmic artery (OphA). Some authors have considered the section of ICA from which COA may originate to extend from the OphA origin to PCoA, or even the ICA termination, so long as the sac points medially. This is confusing since it includes aneurysms developing at the superior hypophyseal artery origin. Furthermore, Drake's definition included those aneurysms that project inferiorly or laterally, but some authors describe aneurysms that are directed inferiorly as paraclinoid aneurysms [9, 16] or even carotid cave aneurysms [25]. There is no doubt that most arise from the superomedial or superior wall of the proximal supracliniod ICA and only rarely from its inferomedial or lateral wall.

There is a general consensus that the medially directed COA grows either above or below the anterior optic pathway (i.e. intracranial optic nerve and chiasm); the direction influences the mode of presentation of unruptured aneurysms (see Chap. 2, Sect. 2.5.2). Size is important to the angiogram analysis since small aneurysms remain lateral to the optic pathway, whilst larger ones extend horizontally under the nerve or superiorly above it to elevate the anterior circle of Willis (COW) and roof of the chiasmatic cistern. The rare aneurysm which arises from the inferior wall may be confused with a PCoA origin. The angiogram in the frontal projection is useful in making the distinction since the PCoA aneurysm usually extends lateral to the ICA whereas the COA medially. This location is, like the MCA bifurcation, a common site for bilateral aneurysms.

The position of the neck relative to the anterior clinoid process is important for surgical exposure but is less relevant to the endovascular therapist. Since most unruptured aneurysms are large or giant in size at presentation, an excessively wide neck may prevent packing. Ferguson [10] found that patients presented with relatively large unruptured aneurysm; in a series of 100 COAs 32 were giant at presentation and 61 unruptured. Kothandaram et al. termed very large ICA aneurysms global aneurysms since the position of the neck may be indeterminant [26]. The OphA origin may become incorporated in the aneurysm wall which may extend below the dural ring into the cavernous sinus.

Catheterisation of larger aneurysms is generally straightforward but coil transfers may be difficult because of the microcatheter kinking in the loops of the cavernous and petrous ICA. This tendency may be due to the slightly stiffer terminal section of the two tip-maker microcatheter combined with the proximity of the aneurysm neck to the fixed anterior loop of the cavernous ICA. In large or giant aneurysms a large part of the circumference of the ICA is involved in the neck; attempts to embolise the aneurysm sac and refashion the ICA lumen may prove fruitless and parent occlusion after remains the better option (Fig. 6.3).

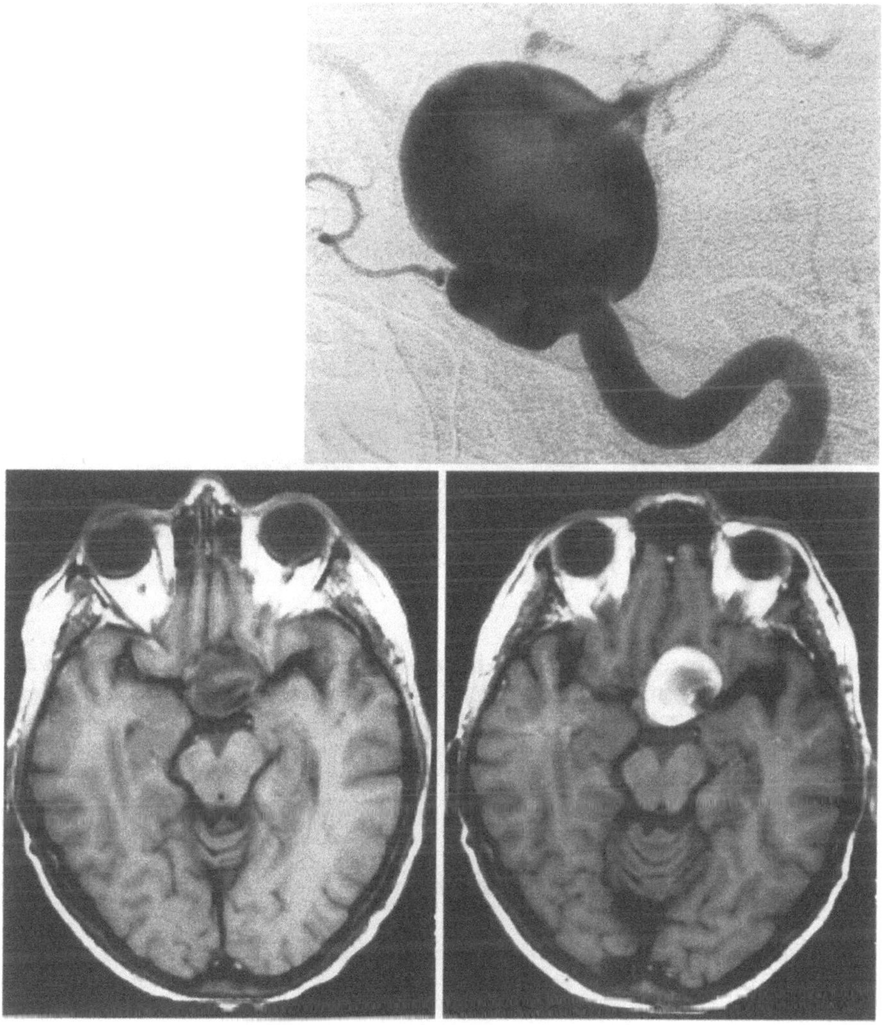

a

b

c

Fig. 6.3 a. A very large aneurysm arising from the internal carotid artery (ICA) distal to the ophthalmic artery origin, pointing upwards and medially. Aneurysms at this site are variously described as carotid-ophthalmic, paraclinoid or global ICA aneurysms. The neck is very wide and this lesion was treated by parent artery occlusion. **b** T1-weighted axial magnetic resonance imaging (MRI) showing the aneurysm filling the chiasmatic cistern with the chiasm displaced to the right. **c** T1-weighted axial MRI shortly after left ICA balloon occlusion. The aneurysm sac is substantially thrombosed

6.2.5
Superior Hypophyseal Artery Aneurysms

The superior hypophyseal artery (SHA) arises distal to the OphA and runs medially and ventrally beneath the optic nerve to supply the optic nerve, chiasm, pituitary stalk, pituitary gland and the floor of the third ventricle.

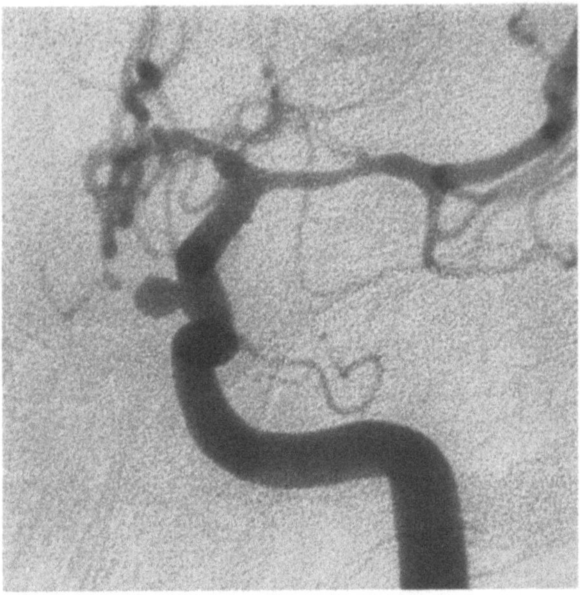

Fig. 6.4.
Internal carotid intra-arterial digital subtraction angiogram showing a small superior hypophyseal aneurysm arising from the supraclinoid artery and pointing medially. The aneurysm arises at the level of the superior hypophyseal artery, but this vessel is rarely visible on angiography

Aneurysms point either medially below the anterior optic pathway or ventrally beneath the anterior clinoid process [7]. They are therefore easily confused with COA and similarly may be bilateral. The principles of their endovascular management are the same (Fig. 6.4).

6.2.6 Posterior Communicating Artery Aneurysms

The majority of PCoA aneurysms arise from the ICA in the region of the PCoA origin. True PCoA aneurysms may occur and are associated with a "fetal" PCA [i.e. ICA origin of the posterior cerebral artery (PCA) with small or absent P1 segment of PCA]. The PCoA runs posteromedially below the tuber cinereum and above the sella turcica and oculomotor nerve to join the PCA at the P1/P2 junction. It gives small branches to supply the pituitary stalk, optic tract, chiasm, the floor of the third ventricle and perforating arteries to the medial surface of the thalamus. The anterior thalamoperforating artery arises from its superior surface, often as two or more vessels, and supplies the anterior and lateral aspect of the thalamus.

The ICA turns ventrally at the level of the PCoA origin so that the geometry simulates a termination aneurysm and aneurysms at this site consistently point posteriorly and usually laterally or inferiorly (Fig. 6.5). This configuration makes catheterisation for endosaccular packing relatively simple but steam shaping of the microcatheter tip is often necessary to gain access and to help stabilise its position within small aneurysms during coil placement. Focal dilation of the ICA and proximal PCoA are relatively common and an

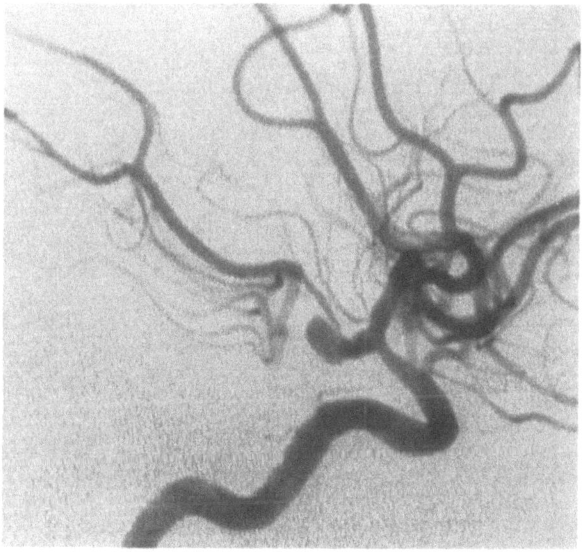

Fig. 6.5.
Oblique lateral intra-arterial digital subtraction angiogram following internal carotid artery (ICA) injection of contrast. There is a small aneurysm arising at the posterior communicating artery (PCoA) origin and pointing backwards and upwards. This appearance is unusual since most aneurysms at this location point downwards, backwards and laterally. Focal vasospasm of the adjacent ICA and PCoA is present

infundibulum can be distinguished from a saccular aneurysm because PCoA arises at the apex of the infundibulum [14].

Total or partial oculomotor palsies with or without SAH are present in 30–40% of patients at presentation and current surgical practice is for early craniotomy and clipping. Absence of the pupillary disturbance associated with third cranial nerve dysfunction usually implies a more laterally directed aneurysm (see Chap. 2, Sect. 2.5.4). Surgical clipping or coil embolisation are generally considered straightforward procedures but if the primitive PCoA/PCA variation is present, the associated procedural morbidity may be increased.

6.2.7 Anterior Choroidal Artery Aneurysms

The AChA arises from the posterolateral aspect of the ICA origin distal to PCoA; it runs posterosuperiorly below the optic tract and above PCoA to reach the medial temporal lobe where it enters the temporal horn through the choroidal fissure. It gives an uncal branch at or soon after its origin which, if it is very close to ICA, may simulate duplication of the origin [45]. It may also arise from the MCA or PCoA. Carpenter et al. found AChA origins from MCA in seven and PCoA in four of 60 dissections [5].

The structures potentially supplied by AChA are the optic tract, lateral geniculate body, cerebral peduncle, subthalamic region, optic radiation, uncus, hippocampus, ventrolateral thalamus, choriod plexus, posterior limb of internal capsule and parts of the caudate, amygdaloid nucleus and globus pallidus [45]. It principly supplies the choroid plexus, hippocampus and basal ganglia. Aneurysms are relatively rare; they develop just distal to AChA

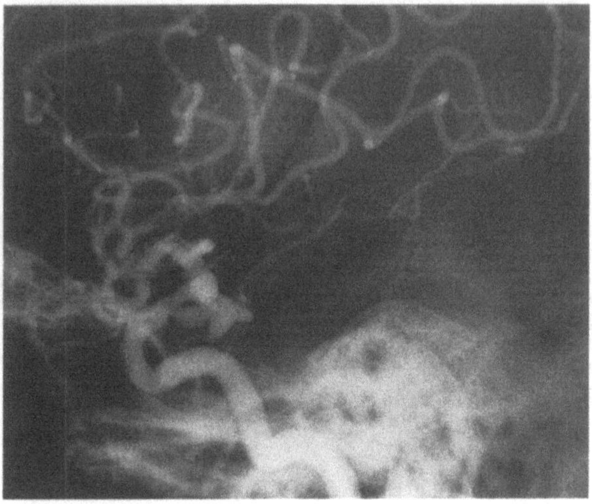

Fig. 6.6.
Carotid angiogram in the lateral projection showing small saccular aneurysms of the internal carotid artery (ICA) arising at the origin of the posterior communicating artery and the anterior choroidal artery (AChA). Both aneurysms point posteriorally and the AChA aneurysm is bilobed

origin and like PCoA aneurysms usually point posteriorly or posterolaterally. If the neck is wide it may be difficult to distinguish an AChA origin from PCoA. Their endovascular management is as for PCoA aneurysms (Fig. 6.6).

6.2.8
Carotid Termination Aneurysms

The termination of the ICA, from the perspective of the endovascular therapist, has many similarities to the BA termination. The geometry is similar and the aneurysmal sacs at both locations are intimately related to small perforating arteries arising from adjacent branch arteries. Carotid termination aneurysms generally point ventrally or ventrally and posteriorly (Fig. 6.7). Less often they project anteriorly or directly backwards. Rupture frequently causes intraventricular or intraparenchymal haemorrhage involving the internal capsule and/or thalamus.

The neck of larger aneurysms can be too wide for endosaccular packing but large and giant aneurysms may also be difficult to clip because of the proximity of perforators and the AChA. Tight packing of large ventrally directed aneurysms with coils both at this site and at the BA termination has been complicated by subsequent parent artery thrombosis - a complication that has been attributed to either distortion and/or compression of the terminal ICA and its branches by the mass of coils or more likely to thrombus forming on coils exposed by a wide aneurysm neck. Management of aneurysms with wide necks may therefore require additional proximal carotid artery occlusion. Neck remodeling techniques or combined treatment with partial microsurgical clipping of the neck and endosaccular packing have been advocated and no doubt, in the future, other technical solutions will emerge to reliably treat wide necked aneurysms at this location.

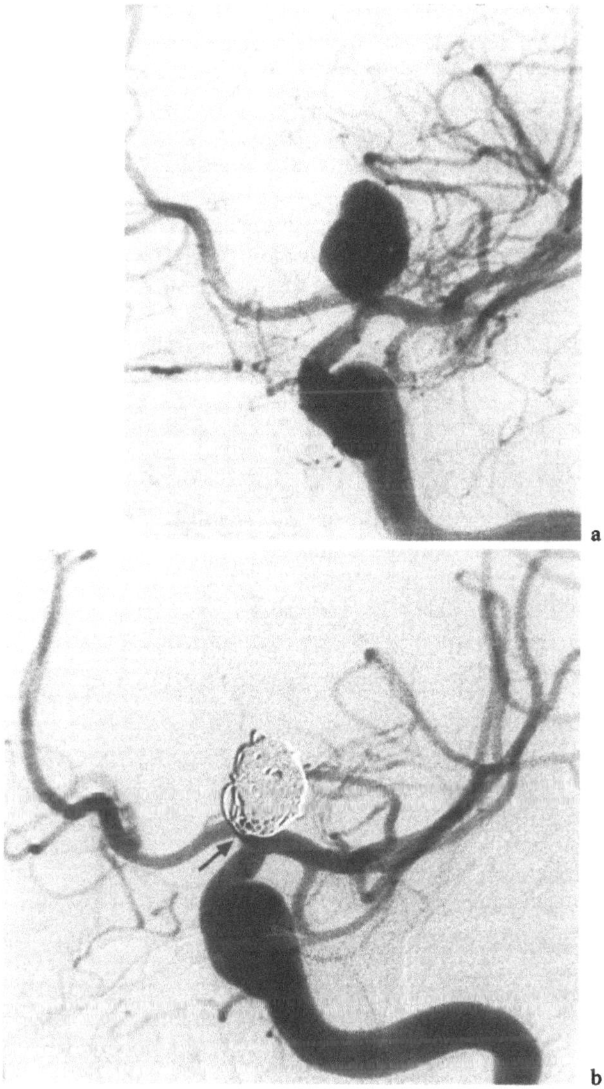

Fig. 6.7 a, b.
Oblique frontal angiograms of a large aneurysm of the terminal internal carotid artery (ICA). (**a**) before and (**b**) 6 months after coil embolisation. Aneurysms at this site often have wide necks which increases the risk of recurrence after coil embolisation. A microcatheter has been positioned in the central part of the aneurysm sac in (**a**). At follow-up (**b**) there is a small neck remnant (*arrow*) which will be monitored by further intra-arterial angiography

6.3 Aneurysms of the Anterior Cerebral Arteries

6.3.1 Vascular Anatomy

The anterior cerebral artery (ACA) arises as the medial terminal branch of the ICA and runs anteromedial crossing the optic nerve or chiasm to join the ACoA. This section, termed A1, gives multiple small branches from its superior surface which enter the anterior perforating substance. The recurrent artery of Heubner is a branch of the distal A1 or the proximal 0.5 mm of A2 in 88% of 50 brains examined [42]. It may be duplicated or triplicated [51]. The ACoA is usually smaller than the A1 but where significant asymmetry is evident between the A1 arteries it may be larger. Perforating arteries arise from its posterior and superior surfaces to supply the anterior chiasm and hypothalamus.

The ACA as the pericallosal artery is classically divided as follows [12]:

- A2: From ACoA to junction of rostrum and genu
- A3: Around genu to the point at which the artery turns sharply posteriorly
- A4: Horizontal portion anterior to the level of foramen of Monro
- A5: Horizontal portion posterior to foramen of Monro.

The perforating arteries of A1 and recurrent artery of Heubner supply the [51]:

- Head of caudate nucleus
- Anterior limb of internal capsule
- Anterior lentiform nucleus
- Anterior hypothalamus
- Olfactory trigone and tract
- Paraterminal gyrus and orbital frontal cortex.

Ischaemia and infarction in these territories are commonly manifest by contralateral facial and upper limb weakness and dysphasia if the dominant hemisphere is involved.

The perforating vessels arising from the A2 supply the:

- Gyrus rectus
- Inferior frontal lobe
- Anterior perforating substance
- Dorsal optic chiasm
- Suprachiasmatic hypothalamus.

Ischaemia and infarction may cause hypokinesia, visual field defects, affective and memory disorders and diabetes insipidus.

The cortical territory of ACA can be divided in areas supplied by one or two vessels. These, together with the supplying named artery in parentheses, are as follow [51]:

- Orbital surface of frontal lobe (orbitofrontal artery)
- Anterior aspect of frontal lobe (frontopolar artery)
- Medial surface of frontal lobe (callosomarginal arteries)
- Paracentral lobule (paracentral artery)
- Medial surface of parietal lobe (superior parietal artery)
- Corpus callosum and precuneus (pericallosal artery).

Neurological sequelae associated with ACA cortical territory infarctions are motor deficits of the lower limb with lesser involvement of the upper limb and sparing of the face. Weakness is typically more marked in the distal part of the lower limb due to involvement of the paracentral lobule [6].

Contralateral limb weakness is common as are hemisensory impairment, akinetic mutism and abulia, together with other psychomotor disorders and amnesia. Urinary incontinence may occur after unilateral or bilateral ACA occlusion [2].

6.3.2 Anatomic Variations

A1 and ACoA Variations. The literature concerning this subject is complicated by the difficulty in defining a normal COW. But there is consensus that relative hypoplasia of one A1 is associated with the presence of aneurysms [37]. Riggs and Rapp [44] found an incomplete or asymmetric COW in 79% of 992 routine autopsy specimens and reported asymmetry of the A1 arteries in 119 (9%), whilst in 40 patients with ACoA aneurysms Wilson et al. found A1 asymmetry in 85% [56]. Duplication of the A1 is a much rarer occurrence, reported in two of 50 autopsy specimens by Perlmutter and Rhoton [42], but duplications of the ACoA were present in 30% and triple ACoAs in 10% of their specimens. This variation is less commonly associated with aneurysms than A1 asymmetry [24].

A2 Variations. The paired A2 arteries and the distal pericallosal arteries contribute to the supply of the contralateral hemisphere in 64% of instances. In the classic description by Baptista [3], variations in ACA distal to ACoA were divided into three types (Fig. 6.8):

- Type 1: Single unpaired A2 or azygos ACA
- Type 2: Both A2 present but asymmetric with branches of the larger crossing the midline
- Type 3: Accessory A2 or median callosal artery.

The relative incidence of the type 1 configuration is 1–3% in autopsy studies but in patients harbouring aneurysm of the distal anterior cerebral arteries (DACA) the incidence reported by Ohno et al. [38] was 8–9%. The presence of this variation, i.e. azygos pericallosal artery, is obvious on diagnostic angiograms, but duplications of the ACoA and type 3 variations may not be as obvious and cause confusion when attempting catheterisation of ACoA aneurysms. Ogawa et al. [37] found the type 3 variation at operation in 27 of 206 patients with ACoA aneurysms, but only 11 of these could be identified easily on preoperative angiograms, and even after careful review eight (30%) were not identified on angiography (Fig. 6.9). Whether vessels that can only be identified at craniotomy through a microscope pose a problem to the endovascular therapist is doubtful but it should be remembered that the median callosal artery, if present, will supply the corpus callosum, septal nuclei, septum pellucidum, anterior fornix and a considerable part of the frontal lobes. A proximal origin of the callosomarginal artery, i.e. just beyond the level of ACoA, can also pose problems in defining the neck of aneurysms in this region because of overlap at angiography. They can usually be easily distinguished from frontopolar branches.

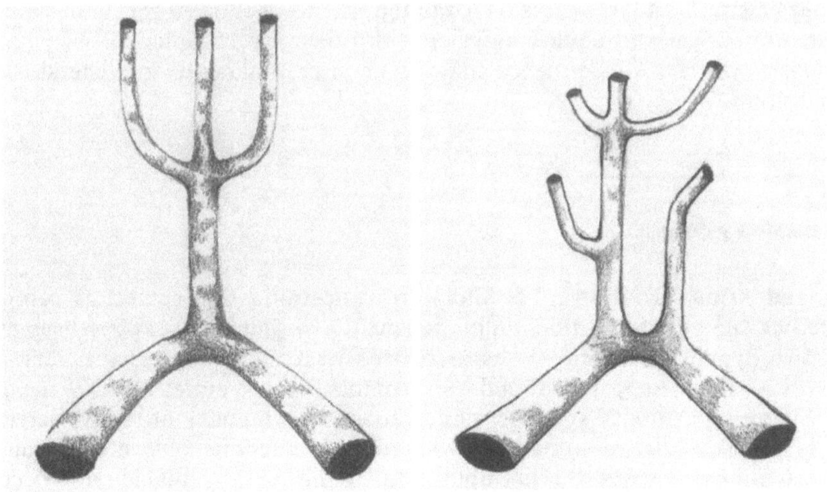

a

b

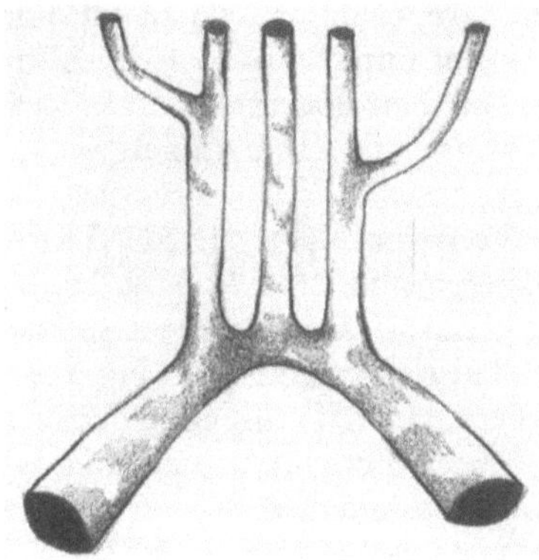

c

Fig. 6.8 a–c.
Variations of the anterior cerebral artery distal to the anterior communicating artery, according to Baptista [3]. **a** Type 1, **b** type 2, **c** type 3

6.3.3
Aneurysms of the Proximal ACA

Most aneurysms arise from the ACoA or its junction with A1 or A2, and only a minority arise from the proximal A1 section of the ACA (Table 1). Aneurysms of the A1 point upwards and forwards or backwards, and may arise at the origin of the recurrent artery of Heubner. Like aneurysms of the M1 section of the MCA, they are particularly suitable for treatment by endosaccular packing since small adjacent perforator arteries are unlikely to be compromised.

6.3.4
ACoA Aneurysms

ACoA aneurysms are distributed around the junction of the ACoA and the proximal and distal ACA in four regions (Fig. 6.10). If the median callosal ar-

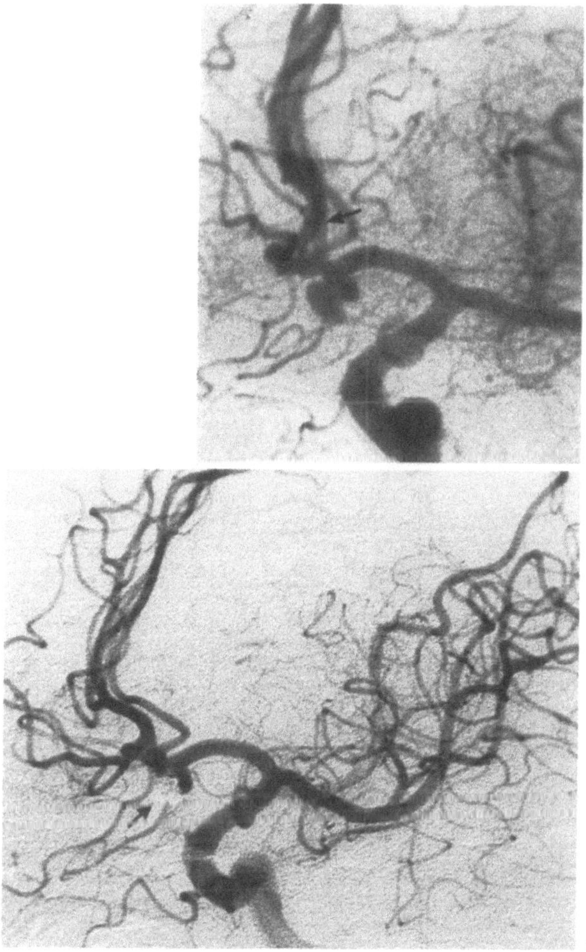

a

b

Fig. 6.9 a, b.
Oblique intra-arterial digital subtraction angiogram showing a small anterior communicating artery (ACoA) aneurysm arising from the junction of the left A1 and ACoA. **a** There is a median callosal artery (*arrow*) arising from ACoA, as well as small frontal branches arising from the pericallosal arteries and median callosal artery. **b** After endosaccular packing of the aneurysm (*arrow*) with detachable coils, the median callosal artery is difficult to identify because it is projected over the right A2

tery is present, 80% of aneurysms occur at the trifurcation between the ipsilateral A1, the median callosal artery and ACoA [37].

The majority of aneurysms at this location point forwards and laterally, either downwards or upwards. They may be directed backwards and if there is significant A1 asymmetry, they are directed away from the larger A1, i.e. the in-flow artery [59] (Fig. 6.11, Fig. 6.12 and Fig. 6.13). The direction in which they point is an important consideration in surgical planning. The aneurysm neck is usually approached from the non-dominant right side, but to expose the aneurysm neck with the minimum of disruption of the fundus, the side nearest the neck may be preferred [13]. In addition, surgical dissection may require resection of part of the gyrus rectus [59]. However, such considerations are not relevant to catheterisation, which is usually best performed via the larger A1. The theoretical advantages of endovascular treatments, which avoid craniotomy and resection of the gyrus rectus, are the

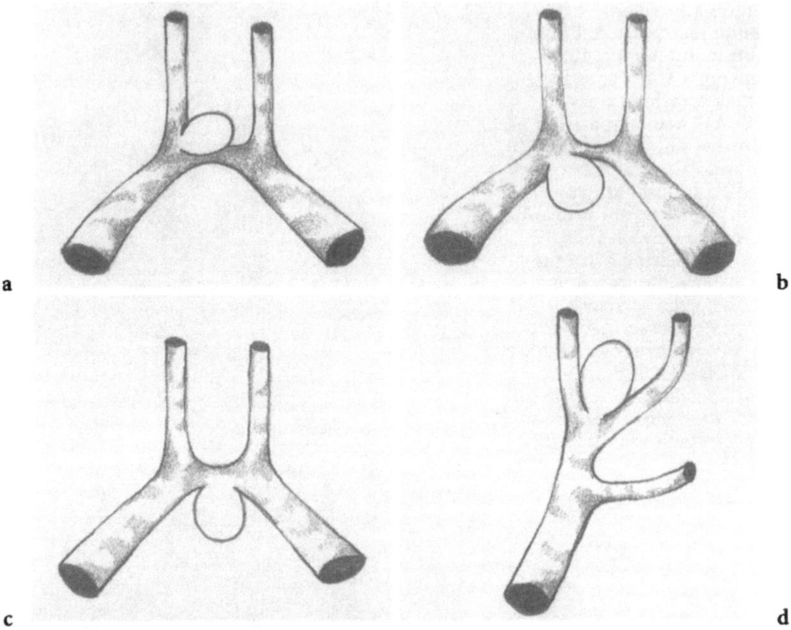

Fig. 6.10 a–d. Distribution of aneurysms around the anterior communicating artery (the relative frequency of aneurysms at these positions are given in parentheses). **a** Junction ACoA–A2 (40%), **b** junction A1–ACoA (20%), **c** ACoA (20%), **d** junction A2–A2 (20%). The most common configuration, representing 40% of the series of Ogawa et al. [37] is shown in Fig 2a; the aneurysm arising, and therefore the neck lying, between the origins of ACoA and the ipsilateral A_2. The other locations shown, occured equally frequently (20% each); Fig 1c represents a true ACoA origin. (From Ogawa et al. [37])

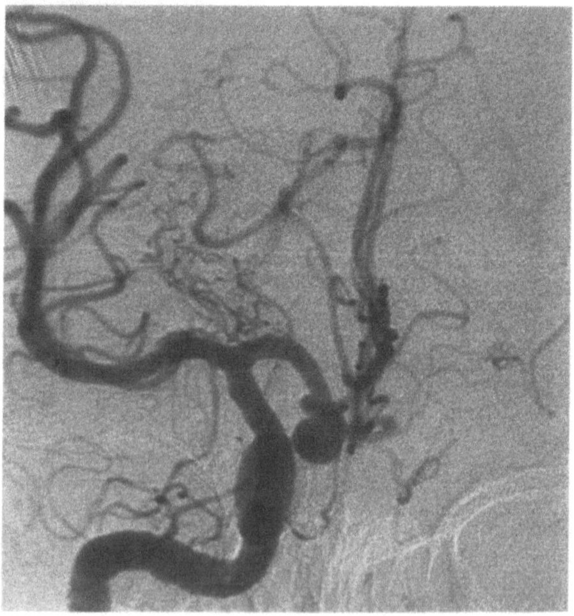

Fig. 6.11.
Frontal intra-arterial digital subtraction angiogram showing a small aneurysm arising at the junction of A1 and the anterior communicating artery (ACoA) and pointing downwards because of the direction of flow in an elongated right A1 artery. In this instance, the origins of A2 and ACoA are easily identified

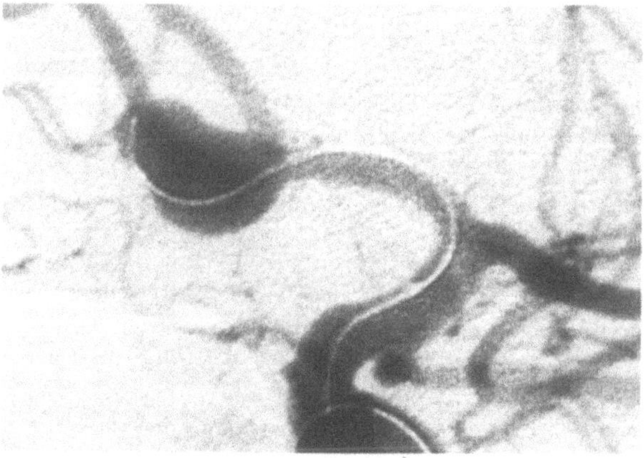

a

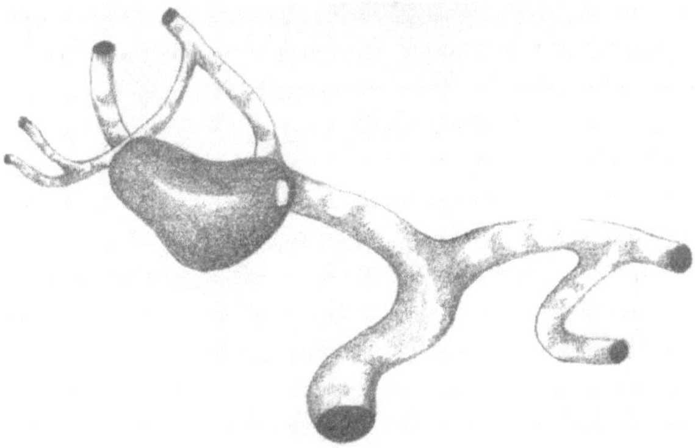

b

Fig. 6.12 a. Oblique frontal intra-arterial digital subtraction angiogram showing an aneurysm arising between the A2 branches of a dominant left A1 artery. The right A1 was hypoplastic. **b** Line drawing of the aneurysm sac which is obscuring the right A2 origin (see Fig. 6.10d)

subject of current research into long-term outcome in patients treated for ACoA aneurysms.

6.3.5 Distal ACA Aneurysms

Aneurysms of the ACA distal to the ACoA complex are generally termed pericallosal and occur at the origins of branch arteries. The commonest site in the distal ACA for aneurysms is at the branch artery at the level of the genu of the corpus callosum (i.e. anterior inferior frontal artery). The sites of aneurysms in the series of Ohno et al. [38] are shown in Fig. 6.14; 80% arose in the region of the genu of the corpus callosum. They are usually accessible to treatment by endosaccular packing and, given the eloquence of the distal ACA cortical territory, the parent artery should be preserved if possible.

Fig. 6.13 a–c.
Giant partially thrombosed anterior communicating artery aneurysm. The oblique frontal intra-arterial digital subtraction angiogram (**a**) and line drawing (**b**) show a relatively well defined neck with the aneurysm sac displacing the proximal A2 arteries. The contralateral (*left*) A2 runs inferior to the aneurysm sac and simulates a branch of the right A2. In the unsubtracted angiogram (**c**) the calcified walls of a similar aneurysm can be seen together with a displaced A2 artery and endosaccular platinum coils

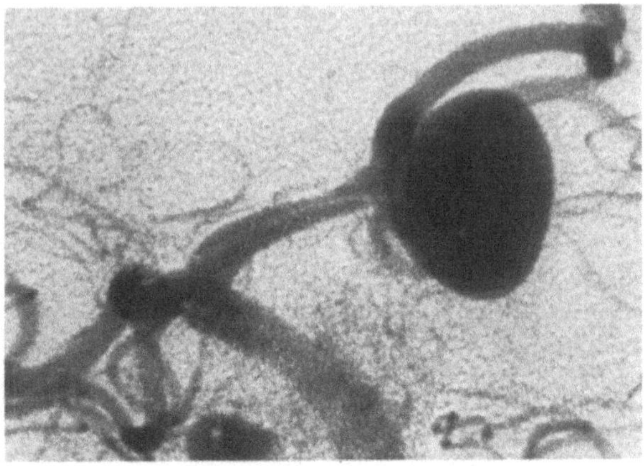

a

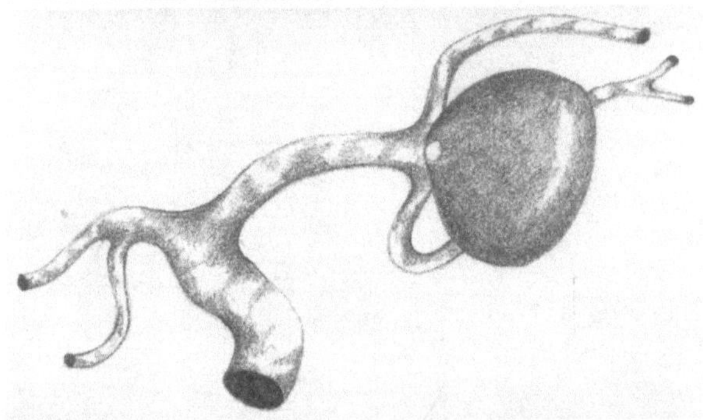

b

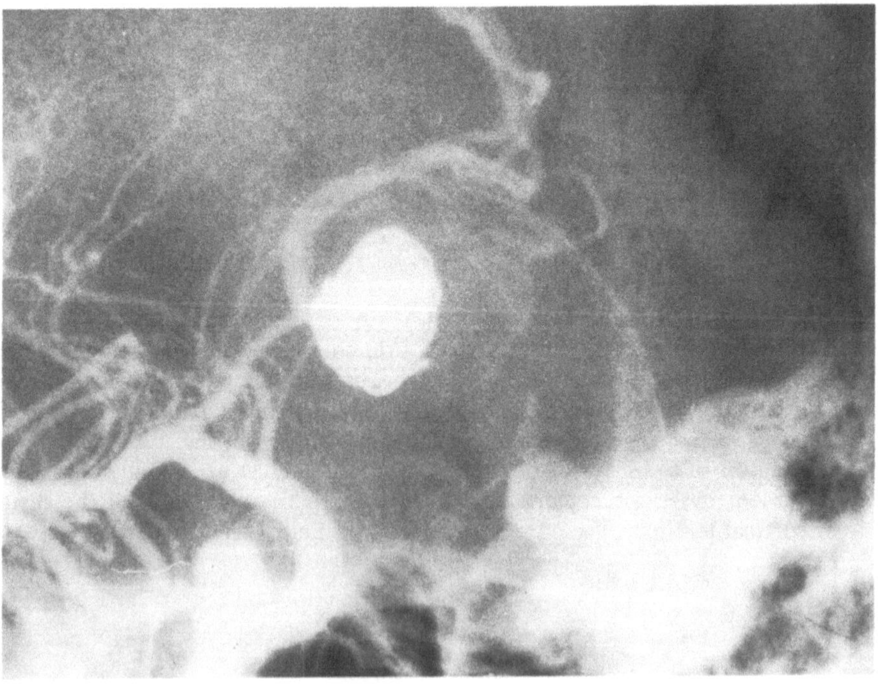

c

Fig. 6.14 a, b.
Aneurysms of the distal anterior cerebral artery (ACA) typically occur on the distal side of the pericallosal/callosal margin artery junction. They are most frequent in the region of the genu of the corpus callosum. The sites of 42 distal ACA aneurysms reported by Ohno et al. [38] are shown in (**a**). Lateral intra-arterial digital subtraction angiogram showing a small aneurysm at the origin of the anterior inferior frontal artery. The angiogram was performed soon after subarachnoid haemorrhage

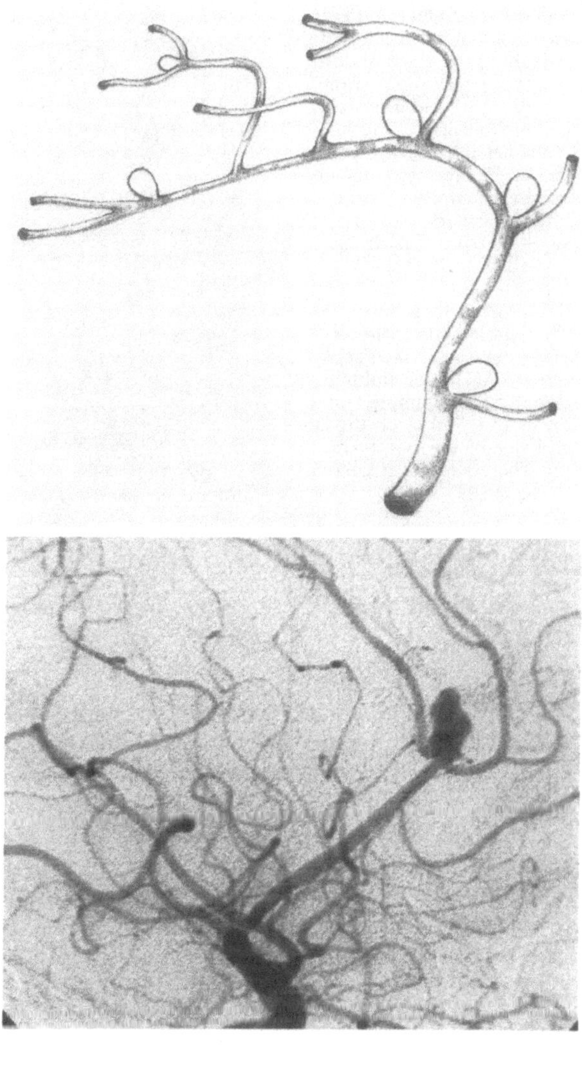

a

b

6.4 Aneurysms of the Middle Cerebral Arteries

6.4.1 Vascular Anatomy

The MCA is the continuation of the ICA distal to the ACA origin. It is up to 70% larger than the ACA and runs laterally within the Sylvian vallecula, parallel to the sphenoid ridge, before turning postero-superiorly at the limen insulae. This change of direction is described as the genu and usually corresponds to the point of bifurcation into superior and inferior trunks. It repre-

Fig. 6.15a–c. Oblique lateral views of a small saccular aneurysm at the right middle cerebral artery bifurcation before (**a**, **b**) and after (**c**) coil embolisation. The microcatheter tip seen on (**a**) lies in the aneurysm sac and not in the superior trunk branch, as shown in (**b**). The superior trunk has divided immediately after the M1 bifurcation and the aneurysm lies between these branches. The inferior trunk (*large arrow*) is clearly seen separately on (**c**) after embolisation. Note the pimple (*small arrow* in **a** and **c**) on the lateral side of the aneurysm sac where rupture occurred. (c see p. 189)

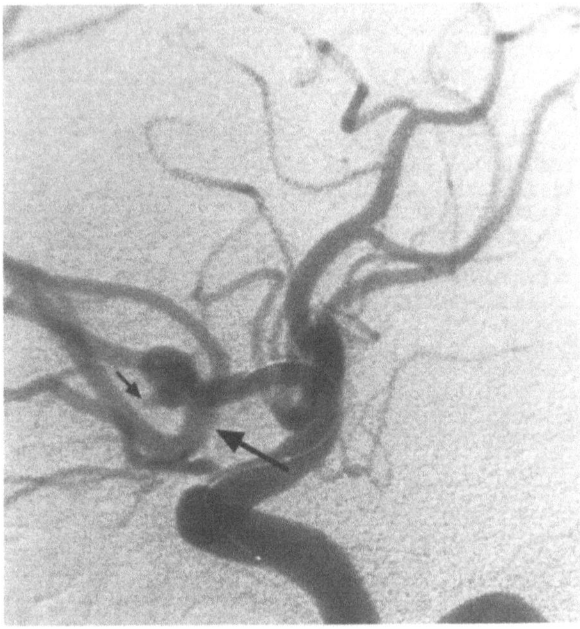
a

sents the junction of M1 and M2 segments. The traditional description of Fischer [12] divides the MCA into M1 (sphenoidal), M2 (insular), M3 (opercular) and M4 (cortical) segments. However, since the branching pattern beyond the M1 segment is so variable, the terms M2, M3 and M4 have little to recommend them in practice. Distal to the limen insulae, the branches lie on and supply the insula. It is in this portion of its course that most of the branching occurs. The distance travelled on the insular varies between anterior and posterior branches; the M3 segment begins once they reach the fronto-parietal and temporal opercular and ends on the surface of the Sylvian fissure. Terminal cortical branches then fan out over the hemisphere.

Since most aneurysms arise at the bifurcation, this is the area of most interest to the endovascular therapist. Branches of the superior or inferior trunks may arise just after the bifurcation, giving the impression of three or more trunks forming the termination of the M1 (Fig. 6.15). Similarly, frontal or temporal branches may arise from the main trunk, simulating a proximal bifurcation. Confusion over the nomenclature of the M1 termination is reflected in the literature. Gibo et al. [17] reported a bifurcation in 78%, a trifurcation in 12% and four or more trunks in 10% of 50 post mortem dissections, while Jain [22] recorded bifurcations in 90% and Lang [29] in only 20%. The inferior trunk was larger than the superior trunk in 42%, smaller in 36% and of equal size in 23% of specimens that bifurcated in Gibo et al.'s material [17].

Small perforating vessels arising from the M1 supply the head and body of caudate nucleus, putamen, anterior limb and genu of the internal capsule, the last being supplied by the most lateral vessels. These perforating arteries,

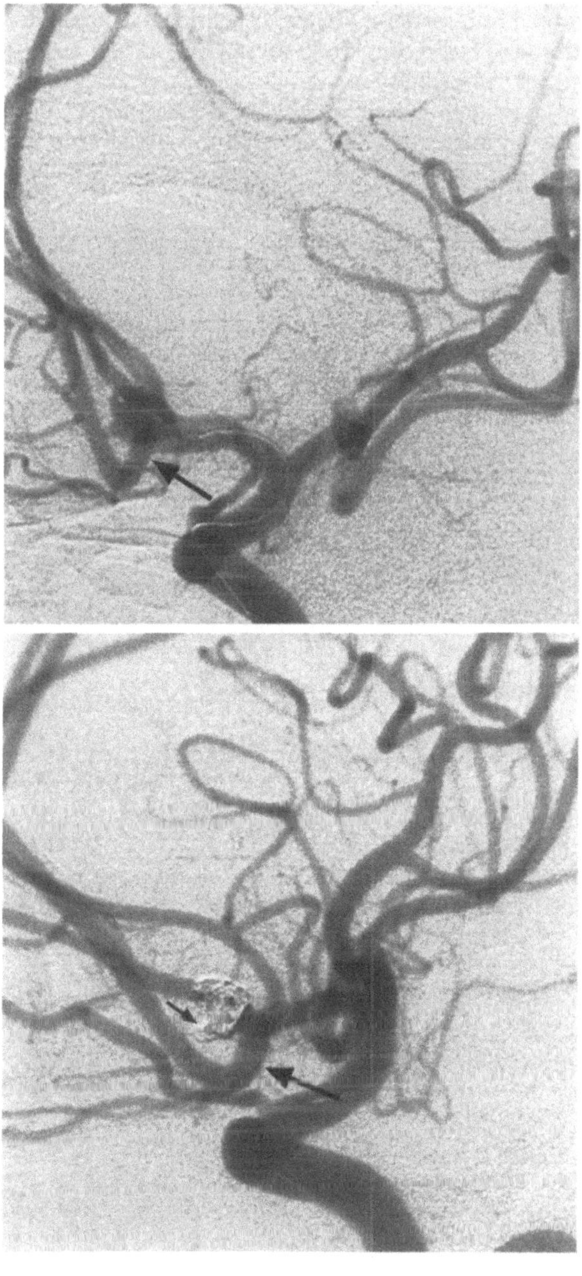

b

c

Fig. 6.15

termed anterolateral striate or lenticulostriate arteries, are arranged in medial and lateral groups of between six and 20 vessels in all, though only about a third are visible on angiography. They are generally about 100 µm in external diameter, and some may arise distal to the bifurcation. Jain [22] reported 79% arising from the main trunk or divisions and the rest from distal branches.

The cortical branches of the MCA are arranged as follows:

- Orbitofrontal artery — frontal lobe
- Prefrontal artery — frontal lobe
- Precentral artery — frontal lobe
- Central artery — frontal lobe
- Anterior parietal artery — parietal lobe
- Posterior parietal artery — parietal lobe
- Angular artery — parietal lobe
- Temporo-occipital artery — temporal lobe
- Posterior temporal artery — temporal lobe
- Middle temporal artery — temporal lobe
- Anterior temporal artery — temporal lobe
- Temporal polar artery — temporal lobe.

6.4.2 Anatomic Variations

Duplications and Accessory MCA. The incidence of this variation has been estimated as 0.3%. The accessory vessel may arise from the ICA trunk, the proximal ACA or distal ACA. In the last situation it represents a recurrent artery of Heubner with cortical supply. Gibo [17] puts it simply: a duplication of the MCA arises from the ICA and an accessory MCA from the ACA. In most instances perforating arteries arise from the superior vessel, according to Abanou et al. [1].

Fenestrations. The incidence has also been reported as 0.3%. Ueda et al. collected 13 cases and reported an association with the formation of aneurysms [54]. Differentiation of this variation from duplications or an accessory MCA depends on recognition of a single origin of the artery.

Anterior Choroidal Artery Origin from MCA. Incidences as high as 11% have been reported [32] but this variant is not specifically associated with aneurysm formation. Its recognition may require careful interpretation and high quality imaging if the AChA is small.

6.4.3 Aneurysms of the Proximal MCA

Proximal aneurysms arising from M1 point upwards if associated with the origin of a perforator artery. More distal M1 aneurysms are often associated

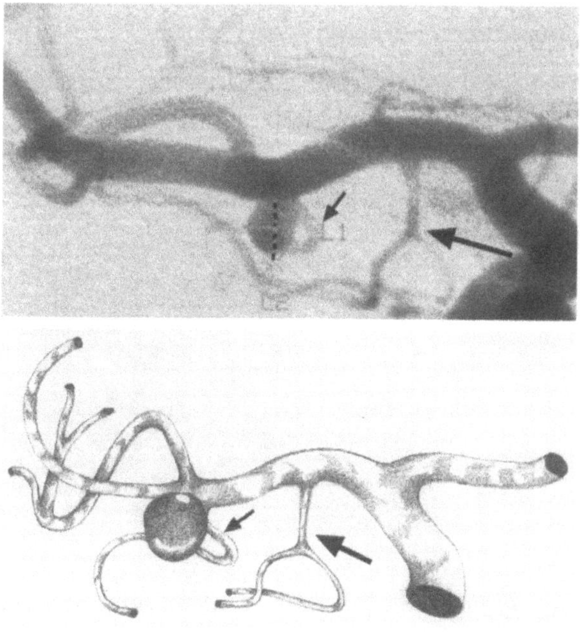

a

b

Fig. 6.16 a, b. Frontal oblique intra-arterial digital subtraction angiogram (a) and line drawing (b) showing a right middle cerebral artery (MCA) aneurysm arising at a proximal division of the MCA into superior and inferior trunks. There is an unusually proximal cortical branch arising from the M1 section (*large arrow*) medial to the aneurysm. The aneurysm is associated with the origin of an additional cortical branch (orbitofrontal) which is seen on the medial side of the sac (*small arrow*). The aneurysm dimensions have been calculated using a coin placed on the patient's forehead as a reference object

with the origin of an orbitofrontal artery arising proximal to the bifurcation, and point upwards, downwards or laterally. The former can be considered as side wall aneurysms and are best managed by endosaccular packing since this is usually successful and technically relatively straight forward. Furthermore, the endovascular approach is less likely to interfere with lenticulostriate perforators than surgical clipping. Aneurysms associated with larger arteries of the distal M1 may be confused with bifurcation aneurysms and pose similar difficulties for endovascular treatment if the neck cannot be clearly visualised. However, M1 aneurysms and early bifurcation aneurysms are generally easier to image, and therefore treat, because they arise at simple bifurcations (Fig. 6.16).

6.4.4 MCA Bifurcation Aneurysms

The MCA bifurcation is by far the commonest site of aneurysms; only three of 96 MCA aneurysms in the Newcastle series arose from the M1 segment [47]. Saccular aneurysms distal to the bifurcation are also uncommon and occur with decreasing frequency in second and third order branches. Bifurcation aneurysms point infero-laterally or supero-laterally and project either anteriorly or posteriorly. They are surrounded by the early MCA branches; the "trifurcation" configuration makes angiographic demonstration of the neck particularly difficult (Fig. 6.15 and Fig 6.17). A careful analysis of the

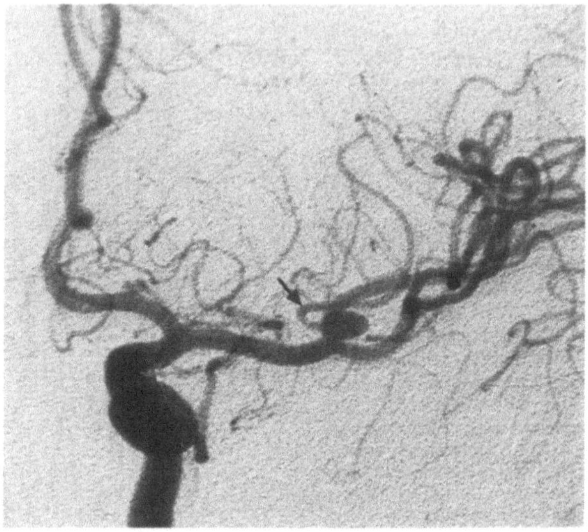

Fig. 6.17.
Left middle cerebral artery aneurysm arising at the bifurcation. The orbitofrontal artery arises from the superior trunk (*arrow*) and its origin is intimately related to the aneurysm neck. An early branch of the M2 arteries such as this may be difficult to separate, on imaging, from the aneurysm neck

angiogram is needed to be sure that early branches of either the superior or inferior trunks are not incorporated in the aneurysm neck. The proximal orbitofrontal branch, arising from the superior trunk, is not infrequently present or this branch may arise from the M1 immediately proximal to the bifurcation (Fig. 6.17). Aneurysms generally grow laterally and larger sacs tend to separate the two trunks, so that their branches are easier to visualise, but they are therefore closely applied to the sac and may be compromised by mechanical distortion during endosaccular packing (Fig. 6.18). The aneurysm sac is to a greater or lesser extent buried in the frontal or temporal lobe.

Aneurysms distal to the bifurcation arise at branch points and can be treated by endosaccular packing with coils (Fig. 6.19) but may require sacrifice of one or more parent arteries (see Chap. 4). Detachable coils are used since a temporary parent artery occlusion can be performed to assess collateral blood flow prior to permanent aneurysm or parent artery occlusion.

6.5 Aneurysms of the Posterior Circulation

6.5.1 Incidences

Posterior fossa aneurysms account for 10–15% of all intracranial saccular aneurysms [11, 15, 41], and those sited at the BA termination are the commonest, representing up to a half of the total, i.e. 5–8% of all intracranial aneurysms.

Fig. 6.18 a–c.
Large middle cerebral artery aneurysm. **a** A large bifurcation aneurysm has been catheterised prior to endosaccular packing with coils. **b** Line drawing of the same aneurysm showing that its long axis parallels that of M1. Enlargement of the aneurysm has separated the M2 (superior and inferior trunks) arteries. **c** A different and larger aneurysm following endosaccular packing with coils. At this stage, the bifurcation is well seen, despite a wide neck to the aneurysm

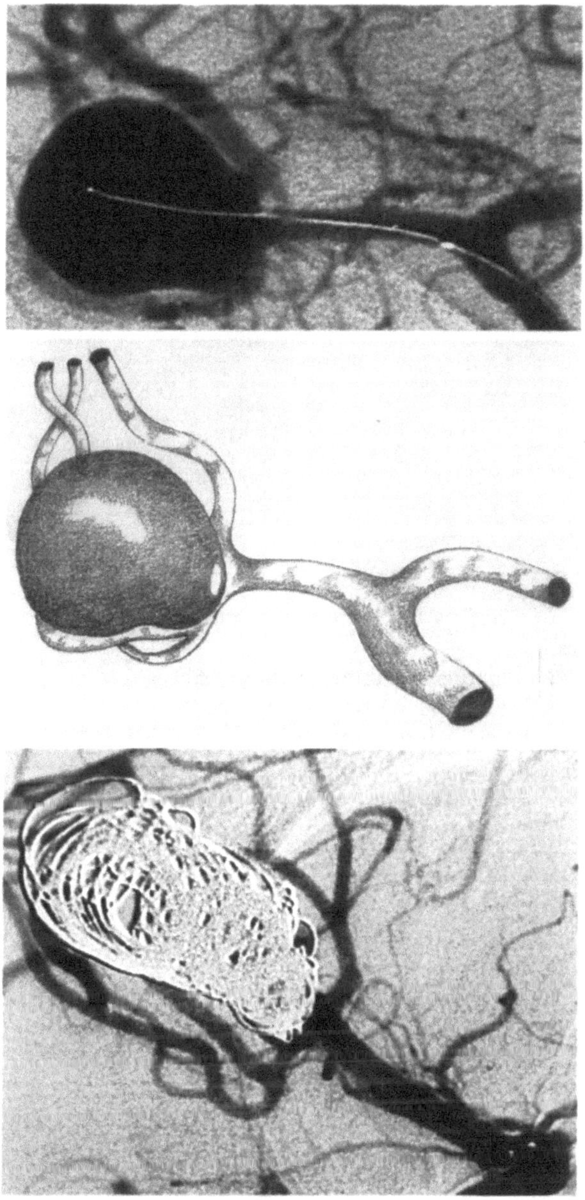

a b c

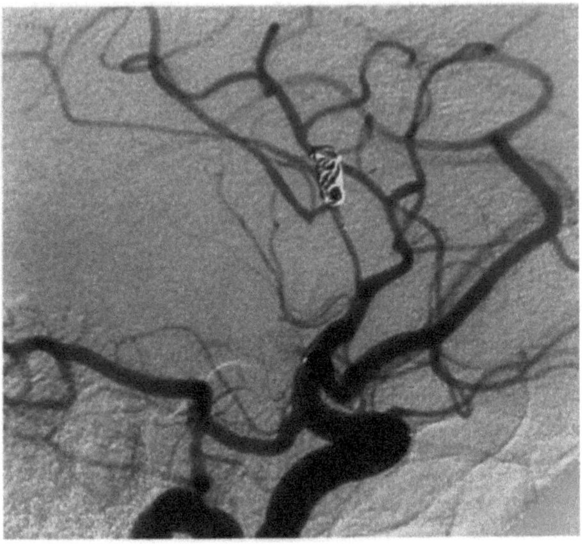

Fig. 6.19.
Oblique lateral intra-arterial digital subtraction angiogram during coil embolisation of a small distal middle cerebral artery aneurysm. The aneurysm arises at the origins of the posterior parietal and angular branches of the M2. Treatment of such aneurysms may require occlusion of one or more of the distal arteries

The relative incidences of aneurysms at sites in the posterior circulation are [41]:

- BA termination aneurysms (50%)
- BA trunk aneurysms, comprising:
  - BA/SCA junction (16%)
  - BA/AICA junction (8%)
  - VA confluence (8%)
- PCA aneurysms, comprising:
  - PCA/PCoA (4%)
  - PCA at P2 (3%)
- VA and PICA aneurysms (11%).

6.5.2 Vascular Anatomy

The VA penetrates the dura in the postero-lateral portion of the foramen magnum, entering the cerebellomedullary cistern to run obliquely and rostrally, across the anterior medulla, to terminate at the basilar artery BA origin. The posterior inferior cerebellar artery (PICA) typically arises 15 mm proximal to the confluence. It is a highly variable vessel, its territory of supply having a reciprocal relationship with the ipsilateral AICA. Classically, the PICA course is separated into five segments: anterior medullary, lateral medullary, tonsillomedullary, telovelotonsillar and cortical [21]. The anterior medullary segment is intimately related to the hypoglossal nerve and the lateral medullary and tonsillomedullary segments to cranial nerves IX, X and XI (Fig. 6.20).

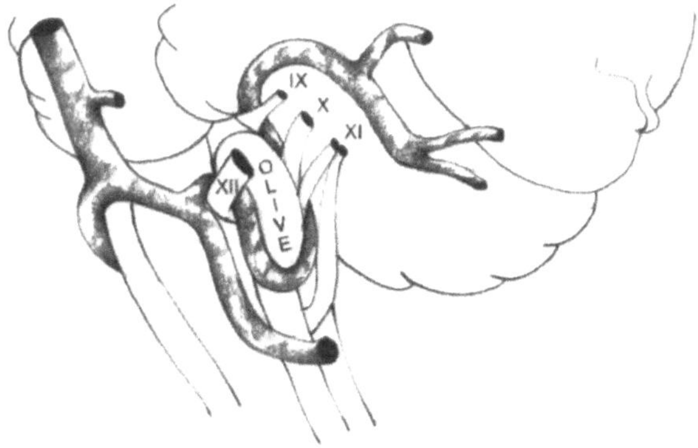

Fig. 6.20. Line drawing of the lateral medulla oblongata showing the origin of the posterior inferior cerebellar artery and its relationship to the lower cranial nerves. Its anterior medullary portion turns behind the emerging hypoglossal nerve (*XII*) and then loops around the lateral medulla (*olive*), passing between the cranial and spinal roots of accessory nerve (*XI*) to run behind the emerging rootlets of the vagus (*X*) and glossopharyngeal nerves (*IX*)

The BA lies between the sixth cranial nerves as they emerge from the brain stem, just below the pontomedullary junction. It runs rostrally, on the anterior surface of the pons, to terminate at a variable level above the pontomesencephalic junction. Its gives bilateral AICA and SCA and multiple small perforating arteries to the pons and mid brain. The AICA usually arises at the junction of the lower one third and upper two thirds of the BA and runs laterally on the anterolateral surface of the pons to the flocculus. It supplies branches to the internal acoustic canal and the inferior cerebellar hemisphere, sharing a territory of supply with PICA. The SCA usually arises 1–3 mm below the termination of BA and parallels the course of the PCA around the cerebral peduncle in the ambiens cistern. It is separated from the PCA by the oculomotor and trochlear nerves. Below the free edge of the tentorium and posterolateral to the midbrain it divides into the superior vermian artery and branches to the superior cerebellar hemisphere. The PCA is the terminal branch of the BA and completes the COW posteriorly. The level of the BA termination is variable; it is usually within 1 cm of the tip of the dorsum sella but in 30% of cases it is above and in 19% below [60]. Furthermore, the level of the termination, and therefore the PCA and SCA origins, varies from a level 1 cm below the pontomesencephalic junction to as far rostrally as the mamillary bodies. A caudal position impedes the anterior extravascular surgical approach, particularly the subtemporal route.

The PCA can be divided in three main segments for description: P1, from origin to PCoA; P2, from PCoA to the posterior aspect of the midbrain; and P3, in the quadrageminal cistern to the termination of PCA at the anterior limit of the calcarine fissure [27]. The anatomy pertinent to aneurysms at specific sites will be considered in more detail below (Fig. 6.21).

6.6 Posterior Cerebral Artery Aneurysms

The most common site for PCA aneurysms is at the PCoA junction, but they may arise adjacent to large perforating arteries of P1 or posterior temporal

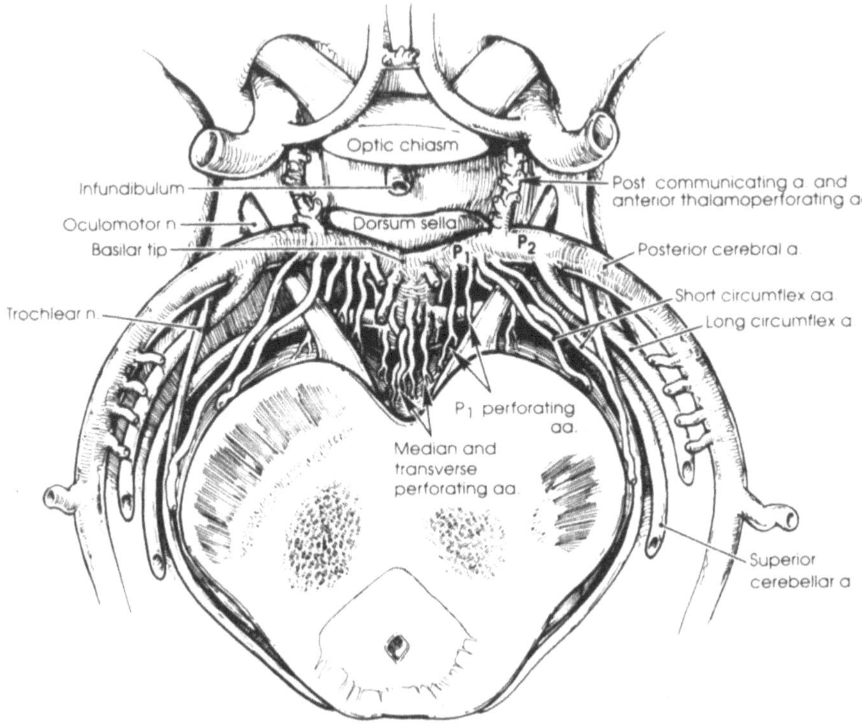

Fig. 6.21. The midbrain and posterior cerebral artery origins, showing the origins of perforater arteries [55] (Reproduced with permission)

branches of P2 and at terminal branches of P3. Clipping or proximal ligation is hazardous when the aneurysm is proximal because of adjacent perforators and parent occlusion is best avoided proximal to the origin of the posterior choroidal arteries.

6.6.1 Vascular Anatomy

The PCA branches can be grouped as follows:

- Central Group
  - Perforating arteries as detailed below from P1 and thalmogeniculate/peduncular branches from P2 (Fig. 6.22)
  - Circumferential arteries
- Choroidal Group
  - Medial posterior choroidal artery, arises as 1–3 branches at P1–P2 junction and supplies the choroid of third and lateral ventricles
  - Lateral posterior choroidal artery, arises as 1–6 branches at P2 and supplies the choroid of the lateral ventricle. Both posterior choroidal artery groups give small branches to supply the midbrain and thalamus

- Cortical Group
  - Inferior temporal arteries from P2 and/or P3 can be considered as four groups: the hippocampal, anterior, middle and posterior from anterior to posterior. They supply part of the uncus, hippocampal gyrus, dentate gyrus, inferior surface of the temporal lobe, occipital pole and lingual gyrus
  - Parietal-occipital artery supplies the cuneus, precuneus, lateral occipital gyrus and potentially the precentral gyrus
  - Calcarine artery, the other terminal branch of PCA supplies the visual cortex.

6.7 Basilar Termination Aneurysms

In a series of 174 small and large bifurcation aneurysms, Drake [8] reported that 63% pointed vertically, 23% projected posteriorly and 14% anteriorly. A third of the aneurysms were larger than 12.5 mm and described as bulbous. Anterior pointing aneurysms are more accessible surgically than posterior projecting aneurysms because the neck can be more easily separated from intimately related perforating arteries. The height of the neck relative to the dorsum sella is also important. For the endovascular approach the width of the neck is the single most important consideration and this is related to the overall size of the lumen (Fig. 6.23). Termination aneurysms, as they enlarge, tend to dilate the distal BA, thus the PCA origins and theoretically per-

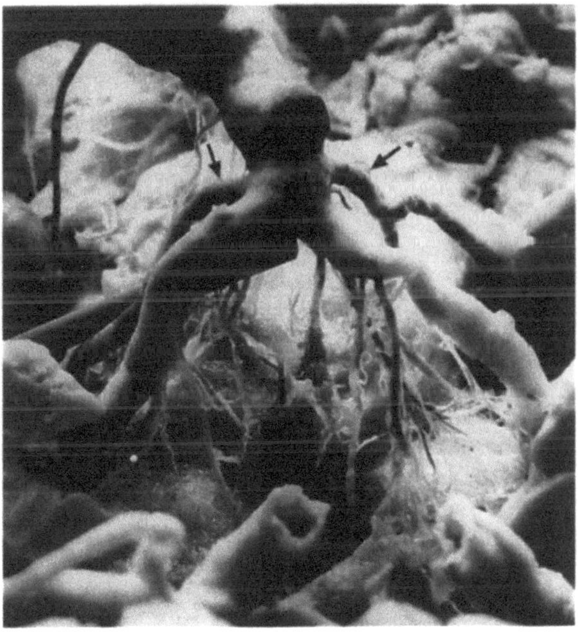

Fig. 6.22. Post mortem specimen photographed upside down to demonstrate the posterior thalmoperforating arteries arising from the proximal posterior cerebral arteries. There is a sessile aneurysm of the basilar artery, just proximal to the origins of the superior cerebellar arteries (*arrows*). (Courtesy of Mr A. Bacchus)

forator arteries arising from the BA become incorporated in the neck and are at risk of occlusion during endosaccular packing.

6.7.1 Vascular Anatomy

The terminal 5 mm of the BA is a rich source of perforating arteries. They arise from its posterior and lateral surfaces; between 3–18 vessels were identified by Saeki and Rhoton [45], most of which enter the posterior perforating substance. In addition, an average of four separate arteries arise from the superior and posterior surfaces of P1, and multiple arteries from PCoAs, even if this vessel is hypoplastic (Fig. 6.22). These vessels can be recognised as forming two groups on lateral angiography: anterior thalmoperforating arteries arising from PCoA and posterior thalmoperforating arteries arising from P1 and BA. Yasargil [58] divides these arteries and those arising from the proximal SCA into groups: an interpeduncular group, a peri-infundibular group, a perimamillary group and a retro-optic group. Such distinctions are less relevant to the endovascular approach. A simpler scheme describes perforators that enter the anterior and posterior parts of the posterior perforating substance as *paramedian thalamic* and *superior paramedian mesencephalic arteries*, respectively. The perforators that supply the brain stem posterior to the posterior substance are the *inferior paramedian mesencephalic arteries* [40]. Together these vessels supply: anterior and posterior parts of the thalamus, the posterior limb of the internal capsule, hypothalamus, subthalamus, substantia nigra, red nucleus and the oculomotor and trochlear nuclei, part of the rostral mesencephalon, with the most anterior arteries supplying the optic chiasm.

Two circumflex arteries (short and long) run parallel to the proximal PCA in the ambiens cistern of both sides (see Fig. 6.21). They arise from the distal P1 or proximal P2 sections. The long circumflex artery extends to the colliculi and supplies the tectum, tegmentum, cerebral peduncle and geniculate body, the short circumflex just the geniculate body, the peduncle and part of the tegmental area.

The perforating vessels of the posterior COW supply:

Site	Functional Substrate
• Optic radiation and tract	Visual loss
• Thalamus/medial lemniscus	Sensory disturbance
• Internal capsule/peduncle	Hemiparesis
• Hypothalamus	Memory disturbance
• Diencephalon	Autonomic disturbance
• Hypothalamus/pituitary	Endocrine disturbance
• Extra ocular motor nuclei	Diplopia
• Cerebello-thalmo-striatal tracts	Movement disorders

Fig. 6.23 a, b.
Basilar artery (BA) termination aneurysm on frontal (**a**) and oblique (**b**) intra-arterial digital subtraction angiogram. This aneurysm points upwards and to the right side. Lateral deviation of the aneurysm sac is due to asymmetry of the inflow. The bifurcation of the BA, in this case, is low relative to the dorsum sella and the P1 arteries are therefore directed vertically. The right P1 is obscured and oblique views (**b**) are used to show the relationship of the aneurysm neck to the posterior cerebral artery origins. Note that both posterior communicating arteries fill and the proximity of P1 and SCA origins

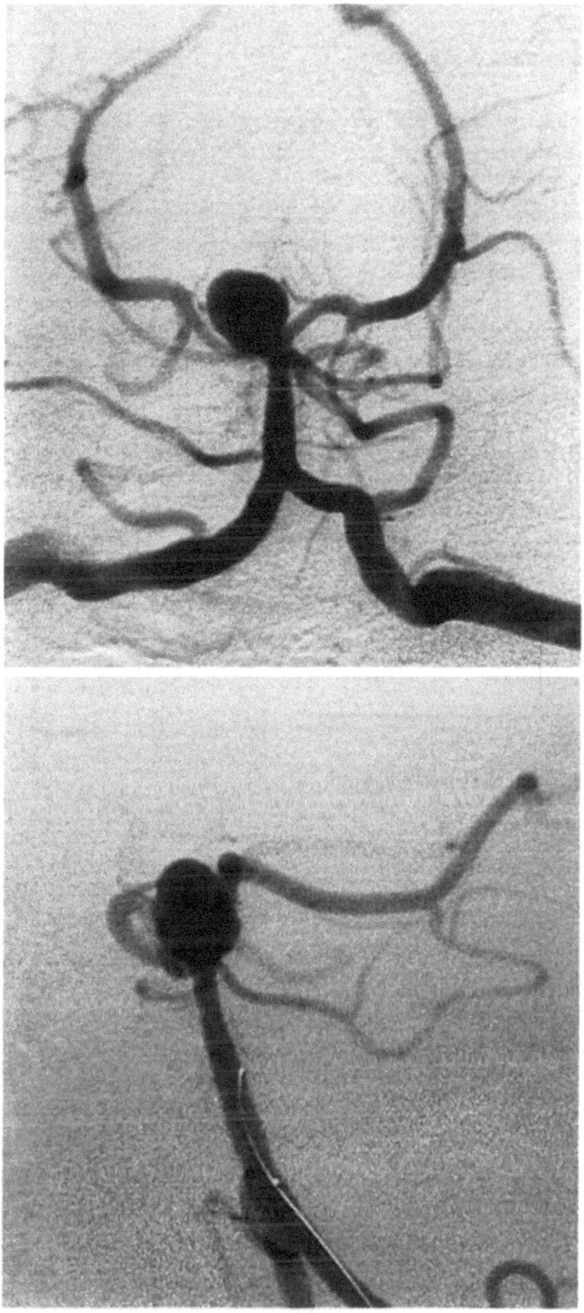

a

b

6.7.2 Anatomic Variations

The terminal BA is a common site for arterial variations, the more common variations being:

Absent P1. The PCA maintains the primitive arrangement being a continuation of PCoA, i.e. the embryological caudal division of ICA. The PCoAs may be symmetrical (16–65.4%) or asymmetrical with one side hypoplastic (22–70%) or absent (0.6–3.6%). The figures in parentheses are the range of reported incidences quoted by Lasjaunias and Berenstein [32]. If the primitive PCA origin is present the ipsilateral P1 is absent in up to 40% of instances [32].

Caudal Fusion of P1. The appearance of a low BA termination with P1 and SCA having a common origin. The incidence of this variation has been reported as 2% by Hardy and Rhoton [19] and as 17% by Yasargil [58] (Fig. 6.23).

Duplication of SCA. Unilateral or bilateral duplications of SCA have an incidence of 8–14% [19, 20]. Rarely this artery may triplicate.

6.8 Basilar Trunk Aneurysms

Saccular and fusiform aneurysms may occur at any level of the BA. The BA is a relatively common site for fusiform aneurysms or dolichoectasia, which is due to degenerative changes in the arterial wall and generally occurs in older patients (see Chap. 1, Sect. 1.6.2). Fusiform aneurysms may cause brain stem compression, cranial nerve compression or occlusion of perforating arteries, but are usually not associated with rupture [49]. They will not be considered further here since they are generally not treatable by endosaccular packing techniques. Saccular aneurysms of the basilar trunk occur at the sites of major arterial branches or fenestrations; these will be considered according to the nearest branch artery.

6.8.1 Superior Cerebellar Artery Aneurysms

Aneurysms at this site develop superior to the SCA origin and point laterally and usually slightly posteriorly. The fundus thus lies close to the oculomotor nerve and, if large, the aneurysm may compress the nerve and cerebral peduncle causing Weber's syndrome. The neck is confined between the PCA and SCA origins and is generally narrow enough to retain coils if the lumen is small, but as aneurysms at this site enlarge, either branch artery may become incorporated in the neck. Small aneurysms are considered relatively straight forward to clip since it is unusual for perforators to arise from the superior surface of the SCA, except when caudal fusion of P1 occurs [58].

6.8.2
Vascular Anatomy of the SCA

The SCA may take its origin for BA or from PCA in 2–20% of cases [32]. It loops initially downwards and then courses around the upper pons below the third and above the fifth cranial nerves. It gives the centerolateral marginal artery which runs downwards over the lateral pons and then hemispheric branches which ramify over the cerebellar hemisphere before terminating as the superior vermian artery. It thereby supplies the: mesencephalon, pons and tectum via perforators; superior and middle cerebellar peduncles; dentate nucleus; superior vermis; and the superior cerebellar hemisphere.

The lateral hemispheric divisions supply the superior cerebellum alone rather than in combination with AICA or PICA in 67% of cases [28]. The superior vermian artery may anastomose with the inferior vermian branch of PICA but the extent of collateral support is variable and can not be assumed to be sufficient to maintain blood flow if the proximal artery is compromised.

6.8.3
Anterior Inferior Cerebellar Artery Aneurysms

Aneurysms typically develop distal to the AICA origin, but may arise proximally and point in any direction. This location is relatively inaccessible for clipping and the feasibility of endovascular packing depends on the relative neck size.

6.8.4
Vascular Anatomy of AICA

The size and distribution of AICA is variable. It arises from BA and runs laterally across the lower pons to the flocculus and the emerging seventh and eighth cranial nerves. It continues in a horizontal course with these nerves, passing behind the internal acoustic canal to enter the cerebellum. At the acoustic canal AICA typically loops into the canal and gives the internal acoustic artery. The internal acoustic artery rarely arises directly from BA [48].

The size of AICA and its territory of supply has a reciprocal relationship with the ipsilateral PICA. There is no relationship in the area of supply between the two sides [57]. AICA rarely arises from VA and its origin is duplicated in approximately 20% of cases [33]. It supplies: the trigeminal nerve, internal acoustic canal, horizontal fissure of cerebellum, and the choroid of the sixth ventricle.

6.8.5 Vertebral Artery Junction Aneurysms

Aneurysms at this site are commonly associated with anomalies such as fenestrations or absent VA. Extravascular access is often difficult. Aneurysms associated with fenestrations typically have broad necks making endosaccular packing with coils difficult [50].

6.8.6 Anatomic Variations

Fenestrations. Formation of the BA is by fusion of the primitive longitudinal neural system in a craniocaudal direction. Fenestration can occur at any BA level and aneurysms, if present, develop at the proximal end of a fenestrated section (Chap. 1, Fig. 1.2) [50].

Persistent Primitive Trigeminal Artery. This and other persistent primitive connections between the carotid and vertebrobasilar systems, i.e. hypoglossal, otic and proatlantic arteries, have been considered above (see Sect. 6.2.2). In a review of 40 aneurysms associated with PPTA, Naruse and Odake found aneurysms at various levels of BA [35].

Asymmetry and Duplications. Distal VA anomalies cause absence or hypoplasia of one vertebral, C1 or C2 origin of PICA, or duplication of VA (Chap. 1, Fig. 1.9).

6.9 Vertebral Artery/Posterior Inferior Cerebellar Artery Aneurysms

The incidence of aneurysms arising from the VA is 3% of all intracranial aneurysms. Fusiform and saccular aneurysms occur and the VA proximal or distal to PICA may be the site of dissections and traumatic aneurysms (see Chap. 5, Fig. 5.6). Saccular aneurysms typically arise just distal to the PICA origin and tend to incorporate this artery in their neck as they enlarge (Fig. 6.24). They are usually small and are directed upwards. Rarely aneurysms occur in the distal PICA, usually at the origins of the vermian or tonsillohemispheric branches. Most aneurysms can be equally well treated by clipping or coil embolisation. For larger and wide-necked aneurysms proximal VA ligation or balloon occlusion should be considered when adequate collateral supply exists.

6.9.1 Vascular Anatomy of the PICA

The course, size and territory of PICA are highly variable. Bilateral symmetric vessels are present in only about 20% of cases [51]. It may arise from

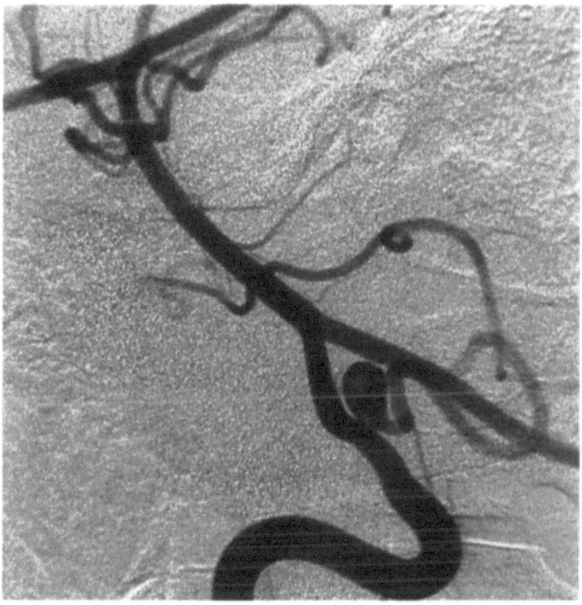

Fig. 6.24.
Oblique lateral intra-arterial digital subtraction angiogram following vertebral artery (VA) injection. There is a small saccular aneurysm arising from the posterior inferior cerebellar artery (PICA). The neck of the aneurysm is clearly separate from VA; arising from the apex of the initial downward turn of the lateral medullary section of PICA. The aneurysm points upwards and medially

the VA above or below the foramen magnum. Origins at the foramen occur in 4% and below the foramen in 18% [32]. It classically makes two loops (the caudal loop lateral to the medulla oblongata and the cranial loop on the medial surface of the tonsil) which are easily identifiable at angiography [18]. The apex of the distal cranial loop marks the inferior limit of the fourth ventricle. In its retromedullary course it divides into vermian and tonsillohemispheric branches. It usually supplies: the tonsil and biventral lobule, the inferior vermis, the choroid plexus, the gracile nucleus, the lateral medulla (with perforators from VA), and the meninges (see also Sect. 6.5.2).

6.9.2 Anatomic Variations

Variants in its course and origins are:
Duplications: Only rarely is the artery duplicated and incidences of only 1–6% have been reported [32].
Anomalous origins: These are associated with persistance of primitive arterial systems, i.e. hypoglossal and proatlantic arteries or with segmental variations causing extracranial PICA origins at C2 or C3 [32].

References

1. Abanou A, Lasjaunias P, Manelfe C, Lopez-Ibor L (1984) The accessory middle cerebral artery (AMCA). Diagnosis and therapeutic consequences. Anat Clin 6:305–309
2. Andrew J, Nathan PW (1964) Lesions of the anterior frontal lobes and disturbances of micturition and defecation. Brain 87:233–262

3. Baptista AG (1963) Studies on the arteries of the brain II. The anterior cerebral artery: some anatomic features and their clinical implications. Neurology (Minn) 13:825–835
4. Bernasconi V, Casinari V (1957) Caratteritische angiografiche die meningiomi del tentorio. Radiol Med 43:1015–1023
5. Carpenter MB, Noback CR, Moss ML (1954) The anterior choroidal artery: its origins, course, distribution, and variations. Arch Neurol Psychiatry 71:714–722
6. Critchley M (1930) The anterior cerebral artery and its syndromes. Brain 53:120
7. Day AL (1990) Aneurysms of the ophthalmic segment. A clinical and anatomical analysis. J Neurosurg 72:677–691
8. Drake CG (1979) The treatment of aneurysms of the posterior circulation. Clin Neurosurg 26:96–144
9. Drake CG, Vanderlinden RG, Amacher AL (1968) Carotid-ophthalmic aneurysms. J Neurosurg 29:24–31
10. Fergurson GG (1985) Carotid-ophthalmic aneurysms. In: Wilkins RG, Rengachary SS (eds) Neurosurgery, vol 2. McGraw-Hill, New York, pp 1385–1393
11. Fergurson GG (1989) Intracranial arterial aneurysms – a surgical perspective. In: Vinken PJ, Bruyn GW, Klawans HL (eds) Handbook of clinical neurology, vol II. Elsevier Science, New York, pp 41–87
12. Fischer E (1938) Die Lageabweichungen der vorderen Hirnarterie im Gefäßbild. Zentralbl Neurchir 3:300–313
13. Flamm ES (1985) Aneurysms of internal carotid and anterior communicating arteries. In: Wilkins RG, Rengachary SS (eds) Neurosurgery, vol 2. McGraw-Hill, New York, pp 1394–1404
14. Fox JH, Boez TC, Jakoby RH (1964) Differentiation of aneurysm from infundibulum of the posterior communicating artery. J Neurosurg 12:135–138
15. Fox JL (1983) Intracranial aneurysms, vol 1. Springer, Berlin Heidelberg New York
16. Fox JL (1988) Microsurgical treatment of ventral (paraclinoid) internal carotid aneurysms. Neurosurgery 22:32–39
17. Gibo H, Carver CC, Rhoton AL et al (1981) Microsurgical anatomy of the middle cerebral artery. J Neurosurg 54:151–169
18. Greitz T, Sjogren SE (1963) The posterior inferior cerebellar artery. Acta Radiol 1:284–297
19. Hardy DG, Rhoton AL (1978) Microsurgical relationships of the superior cerebellar artery and the trigeminal nerve. J Neurosurg 49:669–678
20. Hardy DG, Peace DA, Rhoton AL (1980) Microsurgical anatomy of the superior cerebellar artery. Neurosurgery 6:10–28
21. Hudgins RJ, Day AL, Quisling RG et al (1983) Aneurysms of the posterior inferior cerebellar artery: a clinical and anatomical analysis. J Neurosurg 58:381–387
22. Jain KK (1964) Some observations of the anatomy of the middle cerebral artery. Can J Surg 7:134–139
23. Kassel NF, Torner JC, Haley C, Jane JA et al (1990) The international cooperative study on the timing of aneurysm surgery. Part 1: overall management results. J Neurosurg 73:18–36
24. Kirgis HD, Fisher WL, Llewellyn RC, Peebles EM (1966) Aneurysms of the anterior communicating artery and gross anomalies of the circle of Willis. J Neurosurg 25:73–78
25. Kobayashi S, Kyoshima K, Gibo H et al (1989) Carotid cave aneurysms of the internal carotid artery. J Neurosurg 70:216–221
26. Kothandaram P, Dawson BH, Kruyt RC (1971) Carotid-ophthalmic aneurysms. A study of 19 patients. J Neurosurg 34:544–548
27. Krayenbuhl HA, Yasargil MG (1968) Cerebral angiography. Butterworths, London, pp 54–66
28. Lang J (1983) Clinical anatomy of the head, neurocranium, orbit, craniocervical regions. Springer, Berlin Heidelberg New York
29. Lang J, Dehling U (1980) A. cerebri media. Abgangszonen und Weiten ihrer rámi corticales. Acta Anat 108:419–429
30. Lapayowker MS, Leibman EP, Ronis ML, Safer JN (1971) Presentation of the internal carotid artery as a tumor of the middle ear. Radiology. 98:293–297
31. Lasjaunias P, Berenstein A (1990) Surgical Neuroangiography, vol 1. Functional vascular anatomy of craniofacial arteries. Springer, Berlin Heidelberg New York
32. Lasjaunias P, Berenstein A (1990) Surgical neuroangiography, vol 3: functional vascular anatomy of brain, spinal cord and spine. Springer, Berlin Heidelberg New York

33. Martin RG, Grant JL, Pearce D et al (1980) Microsurgical relationships of the anterior inferior cerebellar artery and the facial-vestibulo-cochlear nerve compex. Neurosurgery 6:483–507
34. McConnell EM (1953) The arterial blood supply of the human hypophysis cerebri. Anat Rec 115:175
35. Naruse S, Odake G (1979) Primitive trigeminal artery with an ipsilateral intracavernous giant aneurysm: a case report. Neuroradiology 17:259–264
36. Nutik S (1978) Carotid paraclinoid aneurysms with intradural origin and intracavernous location. J Neurosurg 48:526–533
37. Ogawa A, Suzuki M, Sakurai Y, Yoshimoto T (1990) Vascular anomalies associated with aneurysms of the anterior communicating artery: microsurgical observations. J Neurosurg 72:706–709
38. Ohno K, Momma S, Suzuki R et al (1990) Saccular aneurysms of the distal anterior cerebral artery. J Neurosurg 27:907–913
39. Parkinson D (1965) A surgical approach to the cavernous portion of the carotid artery: anatomical studies and case report. J Neurosurg 23:474–483
40. Pedroza A, Dujovny M, Ausman JI et al (1986) Microvascular anatomy of the interpeduncular fossa. J Neurosurg 64:484–493
41. Peerless SJ, Drake CG (1990) Management of aneurysms of the posterior circulation. In: Youmanas (ed) Neurological surgery: a comprehensive reference guide to the diagnosis and management of neurological problems, 3rd edn. Saunders, Philadelphia, pp 1764-1806
42. Perlmutter D, Rhoton AL (1976) Microsurgical anatomy of the anterior cerebral anterior communicating recurrent artery complex. J Neurosurg 45:259–272
43. Redekop G, Ferguson G (1994) Intracranial aneurysms. In: Carter LH, Spetzler RF (eds) Neurovascular neurosurgery. McGraw-Hill, New York, pp 625–648
44. Riggs HE, Rupp C (1963) Variation in form of the circle of Willis. Arch Neurol 8:24–30
45. Saeki N, Rhoton AL (1977) Microsurgical anatomy of the upper basilar artery and the posterior circle of Willis. J Neurosurg 46:563–578
46. Saltzman GF (1959) Patent primitive trigeminal artery studied by cerebral angiography. Acta Radiol 51:329–336
47. Sengupta RP, McAlister VL (1986) Subarachnoid haemorrhage. Springer, Berlin Heidelberg New York, pp 119–138
48. Smaltino F, Bernini FP, Elefante R (1971) Normal and pathological findings of the angiographic examination of the internal acoustic artery. Neuroradiology 2:216
49. Stehbens WE (1972) Pathology of the cerebral blood vessels. Mosby, St Louis, p 357
50. Tasker AD, Byrne JV (1997) Basilar artery fenestration in association with aneurysms of the posterior cerebral circulation. Neuroradiology 39:185–189
51. Taveras JM (1996) Neuroradiology, 3rd edn. Williams and Wilkins, Baltimore, pp 909–1044
52. Teal JS, Rumbaugh CL, Bergeron RT et al (1973) Congenital absence of the internal carotid artery associated with cerebral hemiatrophy, absence of the external carotid artery, and persistence of the Stapedial artery. Am J Roentgenol 118:534–545
53. Turnbull I (1962) Agenesis of the internal carotid artery. Neurology 12:588–590
54. Ueda T, Goya T, Wakisaka S, Kinoshita K (1984) Fenestration of the middle cerebral artery associated with aneurysms. AJNR 5:639–640
55. Wascher TM, Spetzler RF (1994) Saccular aneurysms of the basilar bifurcation. In: Carter LH, Spetzler RF (eds) Neurovascular neurosurgery, McGraw-Hill, New York, p 730
56. Wilson G, Riggs HE, Rupp C (1954) The pathologic anatomy of rupture cerebral aneurysms. J Neurosurg 11:128–134
57. Woischneck D, Hussein S (1990) The anterior inferior cerebellar artery (AICA): clinical and radiological significance. Neurosurg Rev 14:293–295
58. Yasargil MG (1984) Microneurosurgery I. Microsurgical anatomy of the basal cisterns and vessels of the brain, diagnostic studies, general operative techniques and pathological considerations of the intracranial aneurysms. Thieme/Stratton, New York
59. Yasargil MG, Fox JL (1974) The microsurgical approach to intracranial aneurysms. Surg Neurol 3:7–14
60. Zeal AA, Rhoton AL (1978) Microsurgical anatomy of the posterior cerebral artery. J Neurosurg 48:534–559

CHAPTER 7

Results of Endovascular Treatment

7.1 Introduction

The results of endovascular treatments by parent artery occlusion techniques and endosaccular packing with Guglielmi detachable coils (GDC) will be presented in this chapter. It is obviously important for those undertaking any medical treatment to be aware of the likelihood of its success. Published results allow us to rationally audit personal performance, provide objective advice to patients about treatment options, and to recognise and anticipate problems. These elements of care are linked to obtaining informed consent for the potentially lethal procedures used to treat intracranial aneurysms. We should also recognise that interventional neuroradiology is a young discipline and that many endovascular techniques currently practised are relatively novel. In this situation, it is a responsibility of those practising to continue the process, pioneered by our predecessors, of developing and refining these treatments in order to improve their efficacy and safety. To this end, audit of outcomes and appropriate follow-up of patients must be good practice. The data obtained will then provide the framework on which the discipline can grow.

Treatment results will be discussed primarily in terms of clinical outcome, i.e. how effective treatments are for the relief of symptoms, their associated morbidity, and the influence they have on the predictable natural history of intracranial aneurysms. These are to a large extent determined by patient interview and physical examination. The technical success (or failure) of treatment, i.e. its effect on the aneurysm size and degree of filling, is generally assessed by imaging. An anatomical cure usually represents the same end point as clinical cure, provided there is no possibility of aneurysm recurrence, nor any long-term or delayed complication of the treatment. An anatomical cure does not, therefore, necessarily mean that aneurysm recurrence or regrowth can never occur, and it is an unfortunate reality that the long-term security of coil embolisation remains unknown.

7.2 Results of Endovascular Treatment by Parent Artery Occlusion

7.2.1 Early Clinical Outcome: Periprocedural Morbidity

The efficacy and safety of endovascular treatment by parent artery occlusion (PAO) depend on the technique being appropriately applied. Selection of patients able to tolerate arterial occlusion is crucial to its safety, as has been discussed previously (see Chap. 4, Sect. 4.3.5). Since anatomic cure and the effectiveness of this form of endovascular treatment are so inter-related, outcomes, as judged by resolution of symptoms and aneurysm regression, will be considered together in Sect. 7.2.2.

Table 7.1. Procedural morbidity after treatments by endovascular parent artery balloon occlusion

Authors	$n=$	Site of occlusion	Transient deficits	Permanent deficits	Mortality
Fox et al. [19]	65	AC + PC	12.3%	1.5%	0%
Higashida [31]	68	AC	10.3%	4.4%	0%
Anon et al. [1]	40	AC	7.5%	2.5%	0%
Higashida [31]	10	PC	10%	0%	0%
Hodes et al. [34]	16	AC + PC	31 %	18%	12.5%
Aymard et al. [3]	21	PC	5%	5%	5%

AC, anterior circulation; PC, posterior circulation; *n*, number.

The morbidity of endovascular balloon PAO in the more recently reported series of patients are presented in Table 7.1. Preliminary temporary balloon occlusion (TBO) was performed in these patients and collateral blood flow support provided by a surgical by-pass procedure, if needed. The rates for procedural complications and their outcomes amongst patients of the three larger series of anterior circulation aneurysms (1, 19, 32) are comparable, i.e. 7.5%–12.5% transient deteriorations, 0%–4.4% permanent deficits and 0% mortality.

Endovascular PAO is generally safer than surgical ligation. For example, Drake et al. [17] reported a series of 160 patients with giant anterior circulation aneurysms treated by PAO since 1961, using both endovascular balloon occlusion and surgical ligation. Amongst this series, which presumably includes some of the same patients reported by Fox et al. [19], were 133 patients treated by carotid artery occlusion for aneurysms of the internal carotid artery (ICA) (21 of which arose at the ICA termination). The artery was occluded proximal to the aneurysm in 40 patients by Selvestone clamp or ligature and in 72 patients by endovascular balloon occlusion. The procedural morbidity and mortality of treatment by surgical ligation was 10% and 5%; and for treatment by endovascular balloon occlusion 2.7% and 0% respectively. The additional surgical morbidity was due to various complications, including surgical trauma to the artery, but the commonest cause of deterioration was cerebral infarction due to thromboembolism or inadequate collateral blood flow. PAO can also be performed with coils but treatment of only a few patients has so far been reported [6, 21, 48,].

The risks of morbidity due to balloon PAO appears to be greater in the posterior cerebral circulation (Fig. 7.1). The report of Hodes et al. [34] details the highest rate of complications of those listed in Table 7.1. Of 16 patients treated for inoperable aneurysms of the anterior (five patients) and posterior circulation (11 patients), two procedure-related deaths occurred – both patients with posterior circulation aneurysms. Furthermore, transient neurological deficits occurred following treatment of five patients, of which four were performed for posterior circulation aneurysms. It is difficult to draw any firm conclusions from such small numbers but it seems probable that part of this additional morbidity is because the adequacy of collateral blood flow is more difficult to predict in the posterior circulation [3]. How-

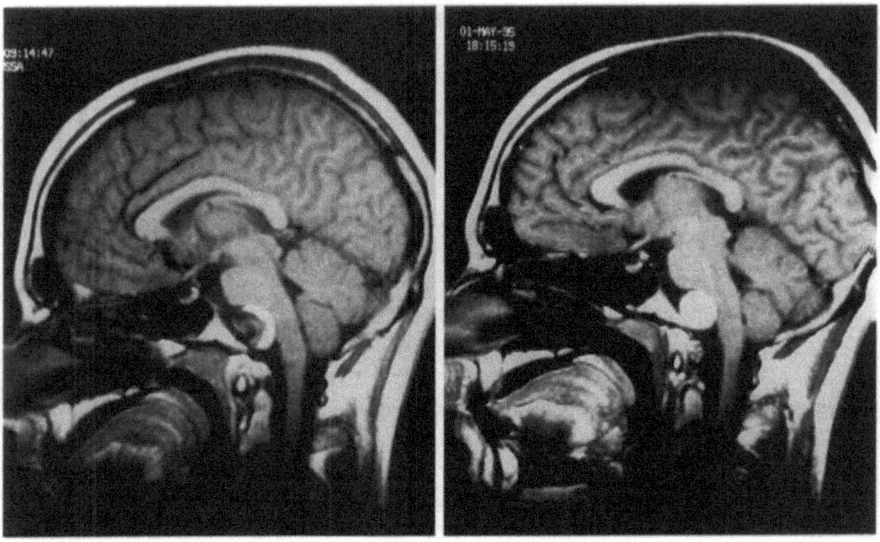

a b

Fig. 7.1 a, b. Sagital T1-weighted magnetic resonance imaging in the mid-line before (**a**) and 3 months after (**b**) bilateral balloon occlusion of the vertebral arteries below the posterior inferior cerebellar artery. There is a large fusiform aneurysm of the proximal basilar artery which is smaller and completely thrombosed after flow reversal was induced in the parent artery. This patient presented following rupture of the aneurysm and made an excellent recovery

ever, the incidence of different types of aneurysms found in anterior and posterior circulations is another factor since dolichoectatic and fusiform aneurysms are more common in the vertebrobasilar arteries and are associated with a particularly high risk of complications. In both the reports of Hodes et al. [34] and Aymard et al. [3], fatal outcomes occurred in patients with fusiform aneurysms of the basilar artery (BA). Anson et al. [2] reported a series of 40 patients with fusiform aneurysms. Good outcomes were achieved in 90% of 20 anterior circulation but only 65% of 21 posterior circulation aneurysms, using a variety of extravascular techniques, including PAO. Conversely, balloon occlusion of the vertebral artery (VA) for dissecting aneurysms is relatively safe and effective [28].

The results of surgical ligation in the posterior circulation are no better than those of endovascular PAO. Steinberg et al. [56] reported the immediate and long-term clinical results in 201 patients treated by occlusion of the VA or BA. All BA occlusions, and all but eight of the VA occlusions, were performed by surgical ligation, usually under general anaesthesia. This series comprised a mixed group of clinical presentations, with 88 patients presenting following subarachnoid haemorrhage (SAH). Symptoms of ischaemia occurred in 35 patients (17.4%), which were transient in nine patients (4.5%) and permanent in 26 (13%). Additional morbidity in the perioperative period was due to rebleeding (12 patients), surgical trauma (seven patients) and vasospasm (five patients). The overall morbidity rate at 1 month was 25%, attributable to surgical trauma in 3.5%, to vertebrobasilar ischaemia resulting in permanent deficits in 13%, early rebleeding after treatment in 6% and vasospasm in 2.5%. Thus procedure-related complications caused major neurological defficts in 22.5% of patients and 24 deaths, i.e. 12% of the whole series. None of the cases of procedural morbidity or mortality occurred in the eight patients treated by VA balloon occlusion. These authors, like others [45], commented that the size of the posterior communicating artery (PCoA) correlated with the patients' tolerance to BA occlusion: 26% of patients were unable to tolerate occlusion when one PCoA was small and 45% when both PCoAs were small. Furthermore, patients with atherosclerotic fusiform BA aneurysms did particularly badly, with four of five dying.

These reports suggest, firstly, that PAO is more hazardous in the posterior circulation and secondly that the additional morbidity (compared with treatments for anterior circulation aneurysms) appears to be partially due to variations in pathology and partially to the extent of collateral blood flow [62]. The criteria for choosing the level for balloon placement in the vertebrobasilar system depends on the need to induce thrombosis of the aneurysm lumen and to maintain collateral blood flow. These are sometimes conflicting, since the former is best achieved by placing the embolus as close as possible to the aneurysm, whilst the latter may demand maintainence of blood flow through or past the aneurysm lumen. Furthermore, this difficulty is compounded by the lack of generally applicable criteria for defining successful test occlusion [3]. Comparing results and drawing firm conclusions is therefore difficult, since the reports of patients treated by endovascular PAO are few and generally include treatment of both saccular and fusiform aneurysms by a variety of techniques, including unilateral or bilateral VA occlusion, performed above or below the posterior inferior cerebellar artery (PICA). Obviously, the site of occlusion has different haemodynamic consequences and chances of success.

The second feature common to most reports is that endovascular occlusion (with balloons or coils) is safer than surgical ligation [17, 19, 28, 32, 56]. The lower procedural morbidity attributable to the adoption of endovascular PAO is largely due to the relative ease of functional testing in the awake patient (see Chap. 4, Sect. 4.3.5). Direct surgical trauma is the cause of some of the morbidity due to extravascular arterial ligation [17, 55]. However, there is no room for complacency amongst endovascular therapists, since the detachment of currently available balloons is not totally reliable and technical complications remain a cause of morbidity [34].

7.2.2
Medium-term Outcome: Anatomical Results

The goal of endovascular treatment by PAO is to induce intra-aneurysmal thrombosis and the subsequent permanent involution of the aneurysm. Organisation and fibrosis of induced thrombosis and the removal of the haemodynamic conditions responsible for the genesis of the aneurysm will then cause the sac to shrink, relieving symptoms due to neural compression and preventing rupture and further aneurysm growth. It may take months or years

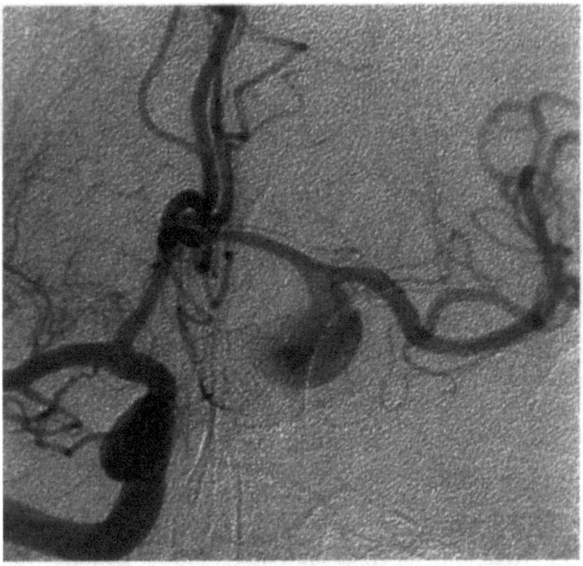

Fig. 7.2.
Frontal intra-arterial digital subtraction angiography following injection of contrast in the right internal carotid artery (ICA). The left ICA has been occluded proximal to a giant carotid-ophthalmic aneurysm; contrast filling of the contralateral middle cerebral artery and retrograde filling of the distal left ICA and aneurysm is evident. Note how the anterior cerebral arteries are displaced by the aneurysm

for large or giant aneurysms to involute, particularly if the walls are very thick and calcified [33, 47]. However, relief of pressure symptoms and signs is usually quicker after either PAO or reversal of flow in the parent artery because pulsation of the sac is immediately reduced and small reductions in the aneurysm size may be sufficient to relieve pressure on adjacent neural structures [29]. However, transient swelling may occur acutely after thrombosis of the sac and exacerbate symptoms, such as cranial nerve palsies or hydrocephalus.

Thus clinical outcome and angiographic outcome are two sides of the same coin. Imaging, in order to assess the degree of luminal thrombosis and sac size, can predict successful outcome though residual aneurysm filling after treatment by PAO may not have the same long-term significance as after treatment by endosaccular packing. In other words, if the flow pattern at the aneurysm neck has been changed by PAO, the impetus for growth and risk of rupture may be reduced and minor degrees of residual lumen filling remain stable. The natural history of unruptured symptomatic aneurysms has been considered in Chap. 2 (see Chap. 2, Sect. 2.4.1); those requiring treatment by PAO are usually large or giant, while those remaining untreated are associated with a very poor prognosis [33]. Bull [8] reported a series of 22 patients with giant aneurysms of the skull base; 13 were treated surgically but only four (30%) improved and three of nine patients treated conservatively died within 1 year of diagnosis. Against this background, parents should be followed by clinical review and assessments performed by planar scanning.

The efficacy of proximal endovascular PAO at inducing complete thrombosis of large and giant aneurysms is related to the likelihood of their continued filling by retrograde blood flow (Fig. 7.2). In the anterior circulation, carotid artery occlusion, below the ophthalmic artery (OphA) origin, is virtually always effective. In the series of Fox et al. [19], all 37 aneurysms of the cavernous carotid region were completely thrombosed following proximal PAO, whilst only 50% of 21 ICA aneurysms, sited above the OphA origin, thrombosed without any additional trapping procedures. Higashida et al. [32] also reported stable complete thrombosis in 100% of 68 cavernous carotid aneurysms and reported that symptoms of local compression caused by giant aneurysms improved, despite no initial evidence of shrinkage on follow-up planar scans. Like Fox et al. [19], few details of the compression symptoms suffered by these patients were given, though Fox et al. [19] noted that transient worsening of cranial nerve palsies occurred acutely in three patients following proximal PAO.

Anon et al. [1] followed 39 patients with aneurysms of the cavernous carotid artery treated by ICA balloon occlusion for a mean of 4.7 years. The presenting symptoms and percentages of patients affected were: cranial nerve palsies (87.5%), headache (47.5%), decreased visual acuity (20%), epistaxis (12.5%), SAH (2.5%) and asymptomatic (5%). Symptoms or signs of compression affected the third cranial nerve in 19 patients (47.5%), the fourth cranial nerve in eight patients (20%), the sixth cranial nerve in 26 patients (65%), the seventh cranial nerve in nine patients (22.5%), and eight patients (20%) had signs of reduced visual acuity. Following PAO, all patients were completely relieved of headache and facial pain. A total of 16 of 19 patients (84%) with third cranial nerve palsies resolved completely and four of the eight patients with decreased visual acuity improved. Complete occlusion of 100% of treated aneurysms was documented by computed tomography (CT), magnetic resonance imaging (MRI) and intra-arterial (IA)-angiography and the mass of these thrombosed aneurysms was shown to gradually reduce during the follow-up period (Fig. 7.3). Thus endovascular PAO is effective at relieving symptoms and inducing regression of intra-cavernous aneurysms [1, 4, 14, 19, 32].

Aneurysms of the distal ICA and those at the level of the circle of Willis are less likely to thrombose completely following proximal ICA occlusion (see Chap. 3, Fig. 3.8), and therefore additional treatment by surgical trapping or endosaccular packing with coils should be considered. In the series of giant anterior circulation aneurysms reported by Drake et al. [17], 21 aneurysms of the carotid termination were treated. Occlusion of the cervical carotid was performed in 11 patients (five by Selverstone clamp and six by endovascular balloon occlusion) and of the distal ICA in ten patients (by combined ICA and A1 occlusion or trapping). Complete thrombosis occurred in only six (55%) of those treated by cervical carotid occlusion but the treatment was effective in preventing continued enlargement or bleeding on prolonged follow-up in all the patients. Occlusion of the cervical carotid artery was also performed for ICA aneurysms at other supraclinoid sites. Complete occlusion was achieved in 11 of 23 (49%) COA aneurysms and four of seven (57%) PCoA aneurysms. Overall clinical outcome amongst patients treated for giant aneurysms of the distal ICA by extravascular and endovascular PAO techniques in this series was excellent or good in 44 of 51 (86%) patients [17].

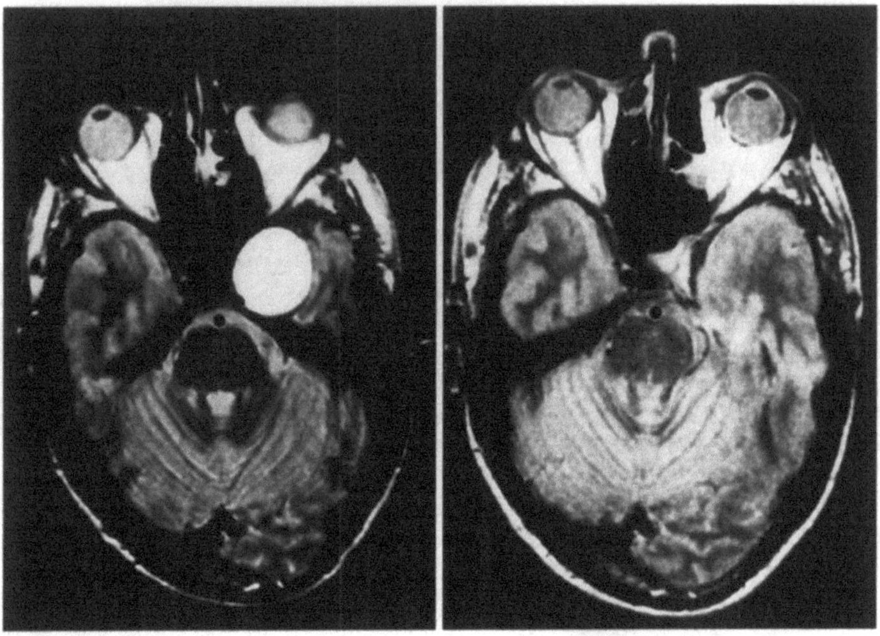

a b

Fig. 7.3. **a** Axial T2-weighted magnetic resonance imaging (MRI) showing a large intracavernous aneurysm of the left internal carotid artery (ICA). This patient presented with pain and ophthalmoplegia; after balloon occlusion of the ICA proximal to the aneurysm, symptoms and signs resolved within 4 weeks. **b** Follow-up MRI performed 3 months later

Similar angiographic and long-term clinical results have been reported for PAO of posterior circulation aneurysms [3, 5, 17, 19, 31, 45, 56]. Aymard et al. [3] established angiographic cure in 13 (62%) and partial thrombosis in six (29%) of 21 patients managed by endovascular balloon occlusion. The clinical outcomes were described as follows: normal in 12 patients, improved in four patients and stable in two patients. Thus, despite complete thrombosis being achieved in only two thirds of aneurysms, clinical improvement occurred in 16 of 18 (88%) patients whose treatment was uncomplicated. The surgical series of Steinberg et al. [56] achieved successful thrombosis in 78% of 201 patients, the majority of whom were treated by surgical ligation. The long-term clinical outcome varied according to aneurysm location. Results were excellent or good in 64% of BA termination aneurysms, 76% of BA trunk aneurysms, 74% of vertebrobasilar junction aneurysms and 78% of VA aneurysms. These results, as detailed above, were achieved with generally higher procedural morbidity rates than in the smaller endovascular series [3, 31]. Therefore, treatment by both surgical and endovascular routes appears to be equally effective in the medium-term, but because of the safety afforded by test occlusion and avoidance of general anaesthesia, the endovascular route offers significant treatment advantages.

7.2.3 Late Outcome: Delayed Complications

Fundamental to the long-term benefit of any intervention to occlude intracranial aneurysms is the need to effectively prevent their regrowth and/or rupture. An additional concern is that PAO, by reducing the capacity of the cerebral arterial system, causes delayed complications due to inadequate cerebral blood flow reserve or by increasing flow in the remaining arteries, cause the formation of new aneurysms.

Late complications reported after endovascular PAO include aneurysm regrowth, rupture and the development of new aneurysms. Anon et al. [1] followed 39 patients treated by ICA balloon occlusion for a mean of 4.7 years, using a protocol of annual imaging by CT, MRI and IA-angiography. None of the aneurysms regrew, despite revascularisation of the carotid syphon in one patient. No aneurysmal bleeding or de novo aneurysms were reported. Aymard et al. [3] described late rebleeding in one patient treated by unilateral vertebral artery occlusion for a basilar termination aneurysm and Hodes et al. [34] the development of a new aneurysm on the MCA proximal to a therapeutic balloon occlusion. In the latter report, recanalisation of previously occluded parent arteries was observed in four of 16 surviving patients, but no rebleeding occurred [34].

Since the numbers of patients in these reports are small it is worth considering the long-term results in patients treated by extravascular surgical ligation. Carotid artery ligation was commonly practised for a variety of anterior circulation aneurysms prior to the introduction of microsurgical clipping. The technique was used in the management of patients with a wide range of aneurysms and, for lack of an alternative, in some inappropriate situations, i.e. ACoA and MCA aneurysms [43], where it is unlikely to be effective in causing permanent occlusion or in protecting patients against rebleeding and regrowth [13]. It is generally accepted that, ligation of the common carotid artery (CCA) or cervical ICA provides some protection against aneurysm rebleeding [42, 58]. However, late rebleeding rates of 3%–10% were reported by a number of authors [52, 58] and Winn et al. [61] showed that CCA ligation did not protect against rehaemorrhage of PCoA aneurysms in the first 12 months. In a more recent surgical series of vertebrobasilar artery aneurysms reported by Steinberg et al. [56], patients were followed for 1–23 years (mean 9.5 years). Aneurysm rebleeding occurred in six patients (3%), 6 months to 2 years after PAO. Haemorrhage was from incompletely thrombosed aneurysms, of which there were 29; the rate of rebleeding amongst patients with incomplete aneurysm thrombosis was therefore 21%. Though symptomatic improvement may occur following incomplete thrombosis, it is hardly surprising that, unless aneurysms are completely thrombosed, patients remain at risk of rebleeding.

Symptoms of cerebral ischaemia are also liable to occur years after therapeutic carotid ligation. Oldershaw and Voris [43] reported hemiplegia developing 1 year and 13 years after ICA ligation in a series of 21 patients. Others have reported incidences of both cerebral infarction and transient ischaemic deficits in patients treated by CCA or ICA ligation [52, 56]. In Roski et al.'s [52] series of 39 patients followed for 1–19.5 years, the incidence of such events was up to 16.6%. It is likely that patients undergoing carotid ligation are at greater risk than the normal population of ischaemic cerebrovascular disease, but the extent of any additional risk caused by PAO is difficult to define from the literature. Delayed symptoms may be due to acute or chronic cerebral hypoperfusion, or thromboemboli arising from the carotid stump or a residual aneurysm lumen [56].

A further possible late complication of PAO by endovascular balloon occlusion [34, 57] or surgical ligation [12, 18] is de novo aneurysm formation. Aneurysms developing on the contralateral carotid artery after carotid ligation have been reported by several authors [12, 18, 53]. It remains a matter of speculation as to whether such aneurysms are due to the same pathological process (e.g. atherosclerosis) that caused the original aneurysm or increased blood flow in the surviving carotid artery [53]. The infrequency of these reports suggest that the risk is small and does not deter us from performing parent artery sacrifice, given that it is often the only therapeutic option available for complex aneurysms.

7.3 Results of Endovascular Treatment by Endosaccular Packing

7.3.1 Clinical Outcome: Factors Influencing Outcome After GDC Treatment

The endovascular management of patients with acutely ruptured intracranial aneurysms has two main goals: prevention of rebleeding and prevention and treatment of symptomatic cerebral vasospasm [41]. Vasospasm, which is the leading cause of death and morbidity in patients admitted to hospital after intracranial aneurysm rupture [60], influences the outcome of GDC embolisation after SAH. Symptomatic vasospasm is diagnosed following delayed deterioration in level of consciousness or a new focal neurological deficit in patients without evidence of aneurysm rebleeding, hydrocephalus, intracerebral haematoma, electrolyte abnormalities or toxic and metabolic causes. Evidence of vasospasm on IA-angiography or transcranial Doppler (TCD) studies are insufficient for diagnosis in the absence of neurological deterioration. Aggressive treatment of symptomatic vasospasm should be instituted only after the putative aneurysm has been treated; initially by so-called triple H therapy (hypertension, hypervolemia, haemodilution) and, if there is no improvement, by chemical or mechanical angioplasty in patients with angiographic evidence of vasospasm appropriately sited to explain their symptoms (Fig. 7.4).

Unlike treatment by craniotomy and surgical clipping, the endovascular approach does not provide the opportunity for subarachnoid clot removal. Surgical lavage of the basal cisterns and other subarachnoid spaces has been reported to prevent cerebral vasospasm. To assess the relevance of this theoretical limitation of the endovascular approach, Murayama [40], in a recent

Fig. 7.4 a–c.
a Frontal intra-arterial digital subtraction angiography of a patient with a small, acutely ruptured fusiform aneurysm (*arrow*) of the right superior cerebellar artery and vasospasm of the basilar artery (*two arrows*). **b** The aneurysm was occluded with Guglielmi detachable coils (GDCs) and balloon angioplasty of the basilar artery performed. Subsequent recanalisation of the aneurysm was treated with two "comma shaped" GDC-10 coils deployed to occlude the superior cerebellar artery (*arrows*). **c** This angiogram was obtained 2 years later and shows exclusion of the aneurysm from the circulation with a normal calibre basilar artery. The patient is neurologically intact (c see p. 218)

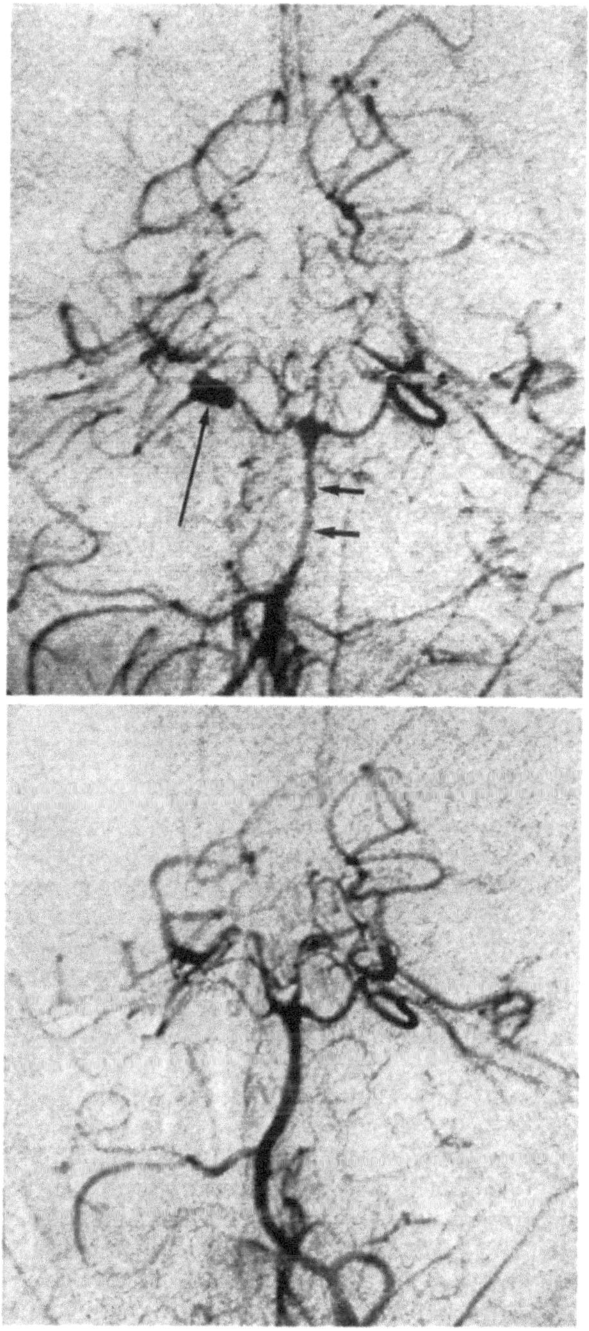

a

b

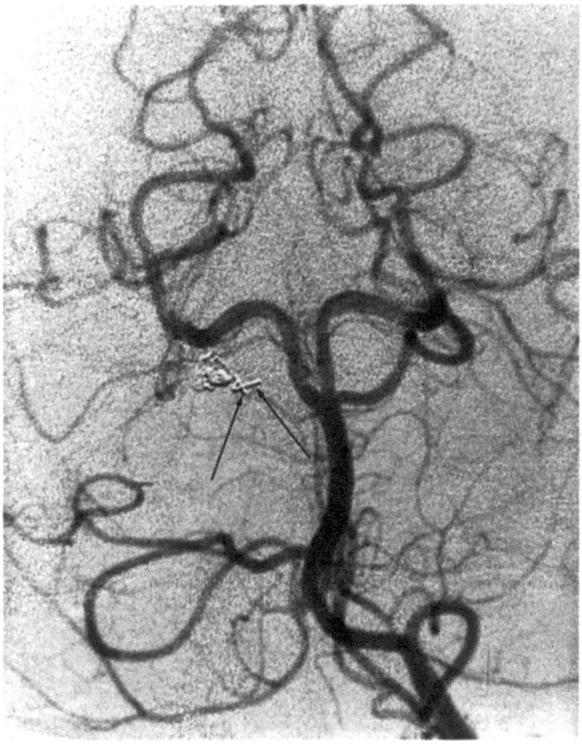

Fig. 7.4c

study on 69 patients presenting with SAH in grade I–III (Hunt and Hess) and treated with GDCs within the first 72 h post-haemorrhage, demonstrated a 23% incidence of symptomatic vasospasm (16 of 69 patients). All 16 patients underwent post-GDC aggressive treatment of vasospasm with hypertensive, hypervolaemic therapy. Twelve patients (75%) were in good clinical condition at the 6-month follow-up, two were moderately disabled, none was severely disabled or in a vegetative state, and two had died from vasospasm. The overall outcome of these 69 patients was good in 87%, moderate disability in 7%, severe disability in 3% and death in 3% (two cases). The 23% incidence of symptomatic vasospasm was lower than that reported in the cooperative aneurysm study without cisternal lavage [30] and similar to that reported in patients undergoing clipping and cisternal drainage [36]. Although definitive conclusions cannot be drawn from this single report, it is conceivable that craniotomy and aneurysm clipping may influence vasospasm by mechanical stimuli such as brain retraction and vessel manipulation, which may counteract the benefit of blood clot removal.

The patient's neurological condition upon admission to hospital is the single most important factor in predicting the final clinical outcome after SAH and can be evaluated according to the Hunt and Hess grading scale (see Chap. 2). Patients with incidental or unruptured aneurysms are classified as grade 0. The clinical presentation of the patient (grading) or the presence of vasospasm does not affect the feasibility of the endovascular treatment of aneurysms with the GDC system. While the timing of surgery is still controversial, there is consensus that endovascular coil embolisation can and should be performed as soon as possible after SAH to prevent rebleeding of the aneurysm and to allow aggressive management of symptomatic vasospasm, should it develop. Established vasospasm can impede endovascular access, but in most instances chemical or mechanical angioplasty are able to provide sufficient vasodilation for catheterisation of the aneurysm. Intense vasospasm may restrict contrast filling of aneurysms and their parent arteries. Endosaccular packing should not be undertaken with poor quality angiography and, although in theory relieving vasospasm proximal to a recently ruptured aneurysm may risk rebleeding, in practice embolisation is safer and more effective when the operator is able to fully visualise the aneurysm and its local anatomy.

7.3.2 Periprocedural Morbidity

The commonest procedural complications associated with endosaccular packing with GDC are stroke due to thromboemboli or inadvertent PAO and aneurysm rupture (see Chap. 5, Sect. 5.4.5). The reported rates of procedural morbidity and mortality for treatments with GDC range from 3.0%–8.9% and 1.5%–3.0%, respectively [8, 26, 49, 59]. There have been three reports concerning patients treated acutely after aneurysm rupture [9, 22, 59]. The largest series [59] concerned 403 patients and reported 84.9% of patients unchanged and 8.9% of patients worse after embolisation and 6.2% of patients dead within 1 week of treatment. However, only just under one third of mortalities were attributed to operative complications. Byrne et al. [9] reported outcomes 6 weeks after the acute treatment of ruptured aneurysms in 69 patients as excellent or good in 87%, fair in 6%, while 7% of patients died. In both reports complications occurred with equal frequency during treatments for anterior or posterior circulation aneurysms.

Thromboembolic complications may also occur in the hours following the GDC procedure (see Chap. 5, Sect. 5.4.5.2). These are due to the progression of thrombosis from the aneurysmal sac to the parent vessel. This complication is more likely when coils impinge on the parent vessel or have been inadvertently placed in the parent vessel (Fig. 7.5). Delayed transient ischaemic events (TIAs) may occur up to 3–4 weeks after GDC treatment [8] and are most often seen after treatment of basilar termination aneurysms [49]. They were observed after GDC embolisation in two of 50 patients with surgically inoperable aneurysms treated by Byrne et al. [8] and resolved following re-prescription of oral aspirin.

Periprocedural results should be interpreted in the context of the patient's condition prior to GDC embolisation. In a series of 100 patients [37], the procedure-related permanent morbidity rate was 2%, and the mortality rate was 2%. The deaths occurred in two patients who were treated while in grade IV or V. Considering only those patients that were treated in grades

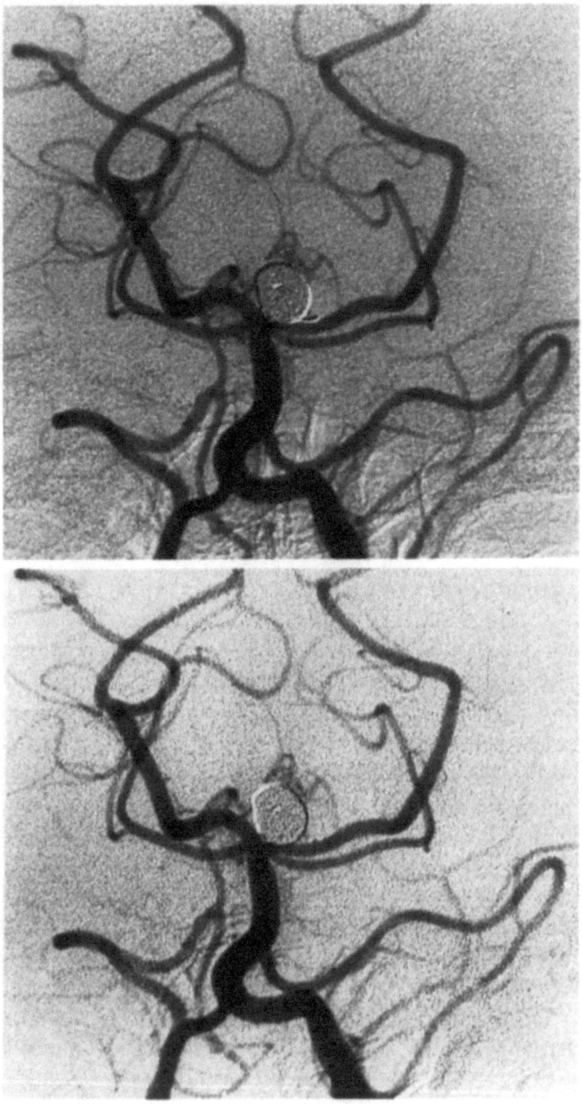

a

b

Fig. 7.5 a, b.
Vertebral intra-arterial digital subtraction angiography (**a**) immediately after treatment and (**b**) 6 months later. **a** The basilar artery termination aneurysm has been densely packed with Guglielmi detachable coils (GDCs) but a short length of coil herniates into the left posterior cerebral artery. **b** On follow-up angiography, this segment of coil has become embedded in the artery wall and is barely visible on this subtracted image. The complication was asymptomatic and managed by prophylactic anticoagulation for 48 h and oral low-dose aspirin for 6 months

0–III, the procedure-related mortality was 0%. The rate of complications is influenced by the experience of the operator, patient selection criteria, and perioperative protocols such as those described for the anticoagulation of patients. In a study of 200 consecutive cases [37], the procedure-related morbidity due to thromboembolic events dropped from 8% in the first 100 patients to 3% in the second 100 patients, and procedure-related deaths from 2% to 1%. The incidence of coil migration also fell from 2% to 0%.

Richling et al. [51] compared outcomes in a consecutive series of 220 patients treated by GDC embolisation or microsurgical clipping. In this retrospective non-randomised study, the percentages of patients achieving excellent or good outcomes were similar after clipping or embolisation in all Hunt and Hess grades, except grade III. For patients in grades I and II, 93% and 95% achieved excellent or good outcomes following treatment by clipping and GDC embolisation, respectively, but in grade III patients 70% of the surgical and 87.5% of the GDC treated patients achieved this result. Results in patients treated in grades IV and V were equally poor with excellent or good outcomes achieved in only 42% of the surgical and 38.5% of the endovascular treated patients). It can be anticipated that results of GDC embolisation will improve in the future as technical problems are resolved and our experience with the technology increases.

7.3.3
Angiographic Results: Complete Occlusion, Subtotal Occlusion, Neck Remnants

Aneurysm rebleeding following partial surgical clipping [15, 16, 20] or GDC embolisation may occur. It is caused by incomplete occlusion or aneurysm regrowth. In a series of 200 patients [24], late bleeding due to rupture of one large and five giant aneurysms occurred; all had been subtotally occluded (see Chap. 5, Sect. 5.5.1 and 5.5.2). To prevent aneurysm (re)bleeding, every effort should be made to achieve a dense aneurysm coil packing at the first session, but multiple sessions may be needed to adequately fill large or giant wide-necked aneurysms.

The degree of aneurysm occlusion attainable by endosaccular packing with coils depends upon many factors. However, the size of the aneurysm and its neck appear to be the most important factors and its in predicting whether an aneurysm can be completely occluded. Aneurysms with a small neck (<4 mm) can be completely occluded since the neck holds coils in place, allowing dense packing with little risk of coil migration or narrowing of the parent artery. Dense coil packing at the aneurysm neck is clearly important for secure occlusion of the sac. Follow-up angiography of 175 patients treated in Oxford showed a higher proportion of regrowth in subtotally occluded aneurysms and a clear correlation between aneurysm size and

Table 7.2. Stability of coil embolisation on follow-up angiography (6-12 months after treatment) in 175 aneurysms according to degree of occlusion (expressed as a percentage of total lumen occluded) at the end of treatment

Aneurysm size		% Occlusion at completion of treatment			
		100	95	<95	Total (*n*) (%)
<10 mm	Stable:	54	14	9	79 (79)
(*n*=100)	Regrowth:	12	5	4	21 (21)
10-25 mm	Stable:	26	16	0	42 (66)
(*n*=64)	Regrowth:	14	6	2	22 (34)
>25 mm	Stable:	1	1	0	2 (18)
(*n*=11)	Regrowth:	5	2	2	9 (82)

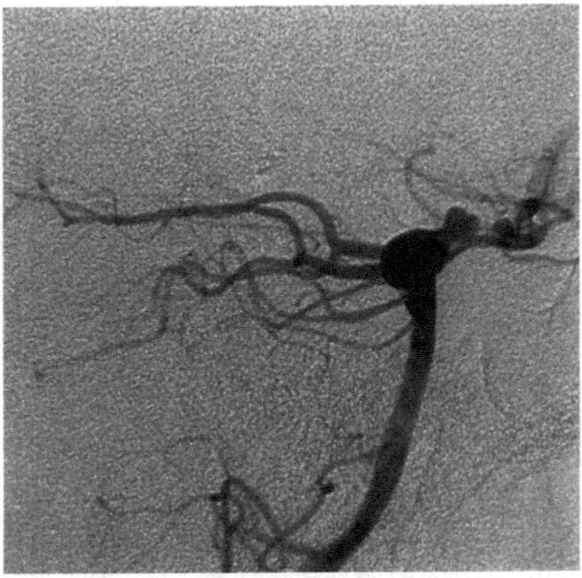

a

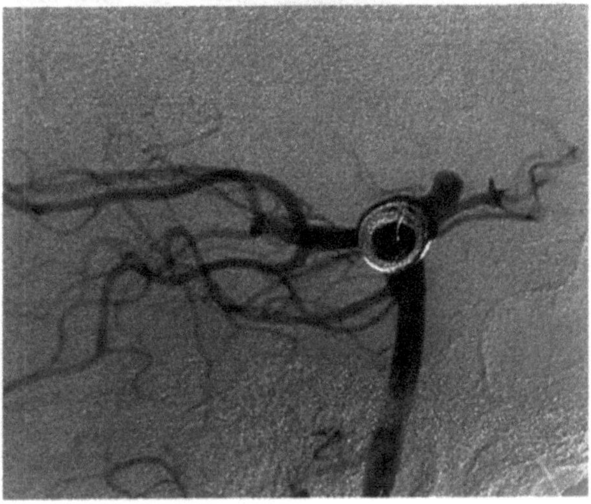

b

Fig. 7.6 a–d.
Vertebral intra-arterial digital subtraction angiography showing a basilar artery termination aneurysm (**a**) before, (**b**, **c**) during and (**d**) after packing with Guglielmi detachable coils (GDCs). The aneurysm was treated 48 h after rupture; there is an anterosuperior lobule to the lumen at the rupture point. **b** Coils are placed to obstruct the aneurysm neck without attempting to pack the lobule. **d** Once an initial "basket" of coils has been placed further coils are delivered to densely pack the lumen. (**c** and **d** see p. 223)

regrowth after GDC embolisation (Table 7.2). Bridging the neck area with a dense meshwork of coils is a determinant factor in preventing their subsequent compaction (Fig. 7.6).

Wide-necked aneurysms (neck size >4 mm) are more difficult to totally occlude because of the risk of coil herniation into the parent artery. This technical difficulty limits the number of coils that can be deployed and may make it impossible to place enough coils to bridge the entire neck area without the use of a helper balloon in the parent artery (see Chap. 8, Fig. 8.3). Only a minority of wide-necked aneurysms can be completely occluded and sometimes the operator has to accept subtotal occlusion of the neck in order

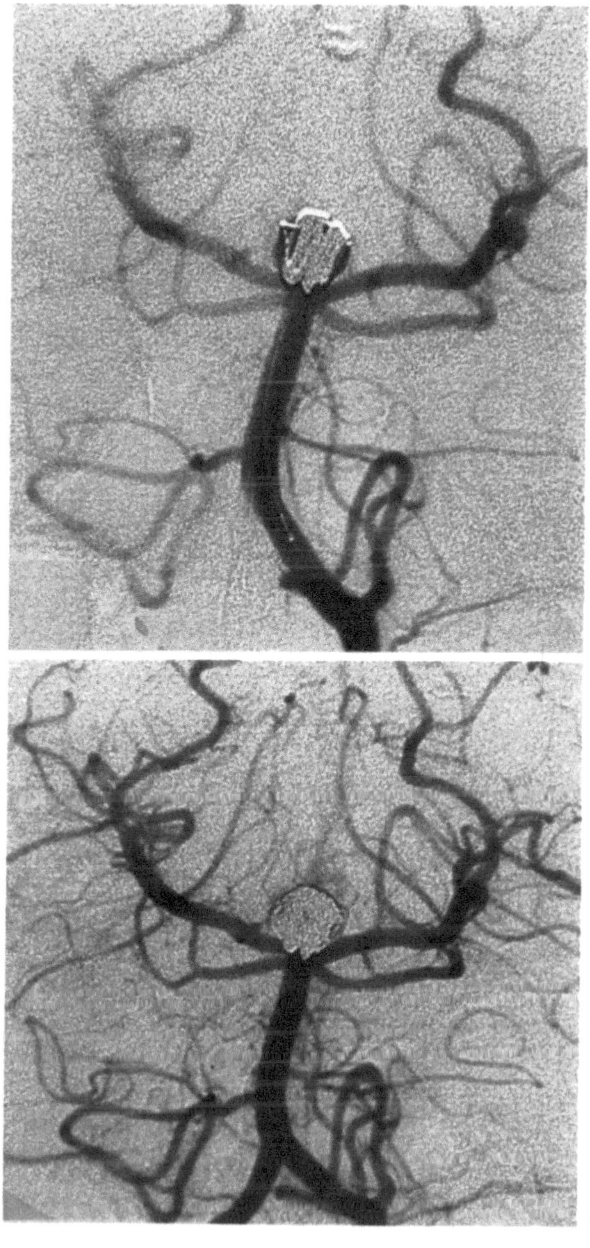

Fig. 7.6 c, d

not to impede blood flow in the parent artery. In such cases coils may compact in the months following the procedure and re-expose portions of the aneurysm lumen to arterial blood flow [35]. Coil compaction and recurrence should be retreated and, faced with incomplete occlusion, further GDC sessions may be necessary and should be anticipated as a part of the treatment protocol [24] (Fig. 7.7).

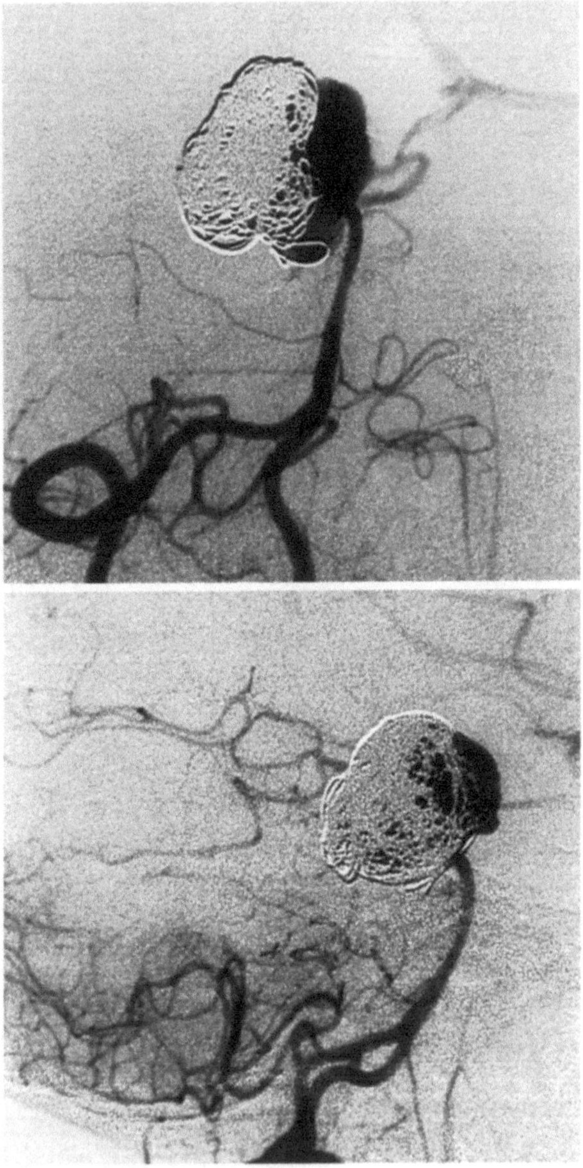

a

b

Fig. 7.7 a–c.
Vertebral intra-arterial digital subtraction angiography showing (**a**) oblique and (**b**, **c**) lateral views of a giant basilar artery termination aneurysm. Coil compaction has caused refilling and enlargement of the aneurysm (**a**, **b**) which was repacked with Guglielmi detachable coils (**c**). (**c** see p. 225)

The timing of follow-up angiography depends partly on the success of the initial treatment. Our protocol is to perform control angiography for patients with completely occluded, small-necked aneurysms 6–8 months and 2 years after embolisation. But for patients with wide-necked larger aneurysms which have been subtotally occluded, the first follow-up angiogram should be performed after 3 months and, at the same session, further treatment may

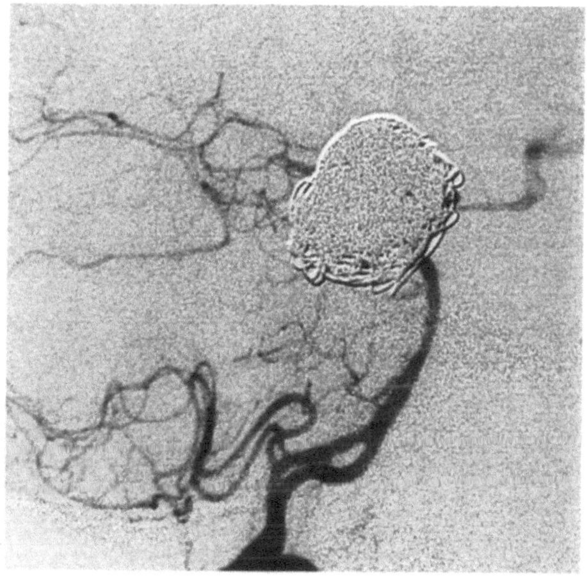
Fig. 7.7 c

be performed. Then, depending on the degree of occlusion achieved, further angiography and possible retreatment is planned (Fig. 7.8).

The reason for coil compaction is not yet been fully established. Three factors, however, may be responsible: (1) Systolic energy, (2) intra-aneurysmal thrombolysis, and (3) return of the coils to their original shape. In wide-necked and larger aneurysms, the orifice of the aneurysm (i.e. its neck) exposes a large area of coil meshwork to the force of arterial blood flow. This, together with possible thrombolysis of the blood clot [10, 50] formed within the meshwork of coils, may cause progressive compaction of coils. However, since it is known from experimental data that the systolic energy is insufficient to permanently deform the mechanical structure of GDCs, it is logical to believe that the coils tend, with time, to return to their original shape. The original shape of a GDC is a series of loops disposed in circles, forming flat rings. When GDCs are delivered into an aneurysm they are often forced to assume different shapes determined by the lumen. Subsequently, because of their mechanical "memory", coils tend to return to their original, circular shape. This tendency may be facilitated by arterial pulsations that, by inducing periodic vibrations of the coils, promote re-adjustment of the loops. As a result, the mass of coils occupy less space and the entire coil mesh becomes compacted.

7.3.4 Management of Recanalisation After Endosaccular Packing

Selecting the most appropriate patients and aneurysms for treatment by endosaccular coil embolisation requires experience and not only influences the chances of primary success, but also the rate of recanalisation and therefore the need for further treatment. At UCLA, the number of patients requiring

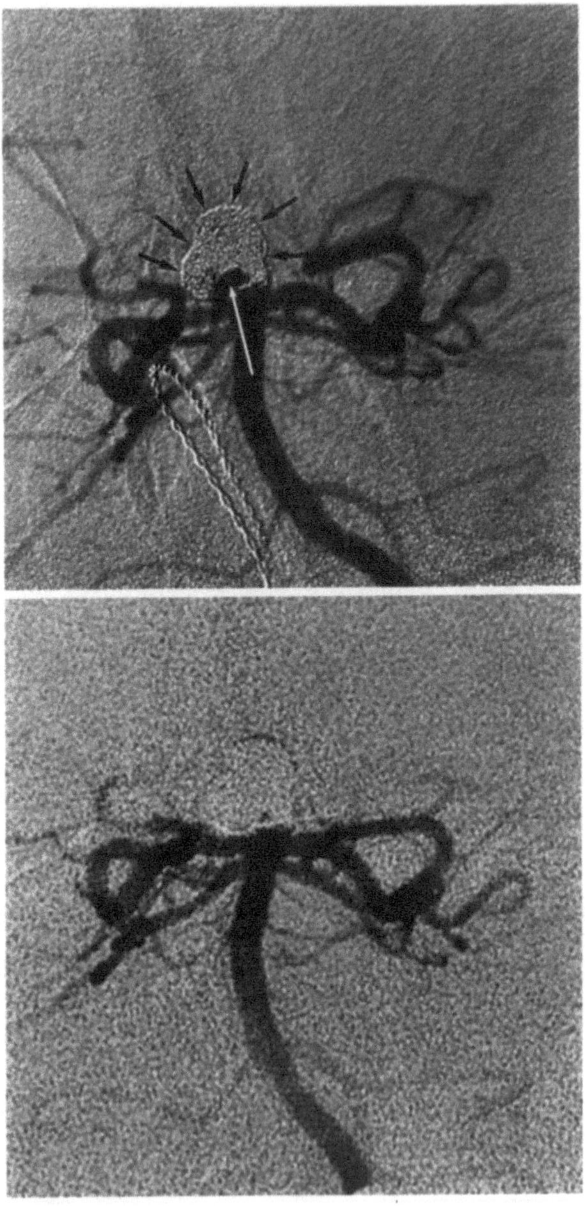

Fig. 7.8 a, b.
a Patient with a ruptured, large, wide-necked aneurysm of the basilar termination (*arrows*). Due to the size of the aneurysm neck, it was not possible to obtain a dense coil packing in one session and the treatment was staged. This follow-up angiogram was obtained after two Guglielmi detachable coil (GDC) sessions. There is still filling of a portion of the base of the aneurysm (*white arrow*).
b Following retreatment with GDCs, complete exclusion of the aneurysm from the circulation was obtained. The patient is neurologically intact

two GDC sessions has dropped from 18% in the first 100 patients, to 9% in the second 100 patients. The number of patients requiring three GDC sessions has dropped from 8% to 1%. The number of patients requiring additional endovascular or surgical treatment has dropped from 20% in the first 100 patients to 6% in the second 100 patients. However, part of this improvement in recurrence rates is due to fewer giant aneurysms being treated;

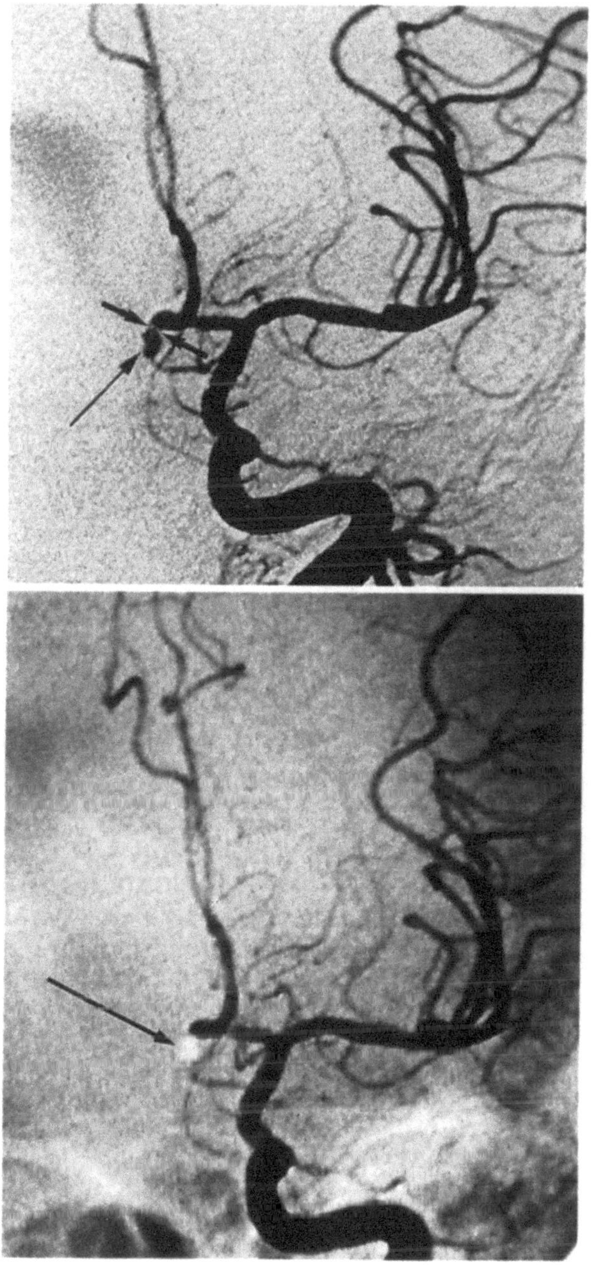

a

b

Fig. 7.9 a, b.
a Frontal intra-arterial digital subtraction angiogram of a patient with a small, acutely ruptured anterior communicating artery aneurysm (*long arrow*). This aneurysm has a small neck (*between arrows*) and was treated via a Tracker-10 Guglielmi detachable coil (GDC) microcatheter positioned in the neck of the aneurysm. **b** It was possible to deliver one GDC-10 "soft", 3 mm in circular memory and 6 cm in length (*arrow*) to completely occlude the aneurysm

amongst the first 100 patients there were 25, and in the second 100 patients 16 giant aneurysms treated [37]. In Casasco et al.'s [11] series of aneurysms treated with fibre coils, 11 of 71 (15.5%) aneurysms were subtotally occluded, of which 37% showed regrowth. Using GDC, Byrne et al. [8] reported regrowth 6 months after treatment in 17% of small, 19% of large and 50% of giant aneurysms (Fig. 7.9)

Aneurysm recanalisation, which usually involves some degree of compaction of endosaccular coils, is an indication for retreatment. In this situation, all methods of aneurysm treatment should be considered, including balloon-assisted repacking, surgical clipping (if feasable), combined endovascular and extravascular surgical approaches, and endovascular treatment by PAO. Patients with recurrant large and giant aneurysms of the anterior circulation can be managed by endovascular balloon or coil occlusion of the ICA, with an extra-intracranial by-pass if TBO is not tolerated (see Chap. 4, Fig. 4.5). If the PCoAs are normally developed, BA or VA occlusion(s) with balloons or coils can be curative for giant lesions of the basilar termination [3].

7.3.5 Clinical Results in the Mid-term Period

In April 1990 the first clinical GDC procedure for the treatment of an intracranial aneurysm was performed at UCLA. At the same institution, the 100th patient was treated in February 1994. There have, since then, been many reports of the device's use in clinical practice [5, 8, 9, 21–27, 37–39, 46, 49, 51, 54, 59, 63]. In early 1996, a campaign of clinical follow-up studies was carried out to assess the mid-term (defined as follow-up greater than 2 years) clinical status of these first 100 consecutive patients [37]. Follow-up information was obtained by clinical examination, from reports of the referring physician and from telephone interviews with the patient or their relatives.

In six patients the follow-up is still pending. The average follow-up period in the 94 remaining patients was 3.5 years (range: 2 years–5.5 years). Patients were classified according to a modified Glasgow Outcome Scale, using the following categories: excellent (neurologically intact, without any detectable neurologic deficit), good (mild hemiparesis, cranial nerve palsy or other deficit that does not interfere with daily functions or work), fair (significant hemiparesis, aphasia, confusion or other deficit which interferes with daily activities or prevents a return to work), poor (coma or severe neurologic deficit rendering the patient totally dependent upon family or nursing staff), and dead. Outcomes were considered relative to the patients' neurological condition prior to treatment and classified as improved, unchanged or worsened at the follow-up date.

Six patients died of unrelated causes (three of myocardial infarction, one of AIDS, one of marantic endocarditis and one due to moyamoya disease) prior to reaching 2-year survival. Nine patients were treated in Hunt and Hess grades IV or V; one had a fair outcome, two had poor outcomes, and six died from the consequences of the initial haemorrhage, with no rebleeding.

A total of 18 patients underwent additional aneurysm treatment after GDC (clipping in eight cases and parent vessel sacrifice in ten cases). None of these 18 patients experienced post-GDC haemorrhage in the time period between the GDC procedure and the additional treatment. The mid-term clinical outcome of these 18 patients did not show any significant difference from the outcome of the patients that had endosaccular embolisation with GDC as their definitive treatment.

Clinical mid-term outcomes of the remaining 61 patients who had GDC as their definitive treatment were classified as excellent in 75% (46 cases), good in 11% (seven cases), fair in 5% (three cases), poor in 2% (one case), and dead in 7% (four cases). All four deaths occurred in patients with giant lesions. The mid-term post-GDC haemorrhage rate was 0% for small aneurysms, 4% (one patient) for large aneurysms, and 33% (five patients) for giant aneurysms.

These results indicate that, in small and large aneurysms, the GDC system is safe and effective in preventing rebleeding in the mid-term period (2–5.5 years, average 3.5 years). The efficacy of acute GDC embolisation in preventing aneurysm rerupture was considered by Graves et al. [22] in 13 patients and Byrne et al. [9] in 69 patients. Both reported lower early rebleeding rates that would be anticipated from our knowledge of the natural history of ruptured aneurysms. Giant aneurysms still constitute a formidable challenge and, in this subset of patients, results are less satisfying, although with significant exceptions (Fig. 7.10). The benefits of recent refinements of the GDC technique (new GDC sizes and shapes, new microcatheters, "soft" GDCs, shorter detachment time) are already apparent in practice, and these should lead to future improvements in clinical and angiographic results. Longer-term clinical follow-up studies (which will be conducted on the same group of patients) are needed to determine the long-term efficacy of treatment with the GDC system.

7.4 Conclusions

The technique of endovascular occlusion of intracranial aneurysms with GDC coils has generally been applied, so far, in patients with high surgical risk or inoperable aneurysms. This selected population of patients can be divided into two categories: patients that were considered difficult to treat by surgical clipping because of the anatomical configuration of the aneurysm (giant or large, wide-necked aneurysms), and patients with technically operable lesions (small, narrow-necked aneurysms) but with coincidental medical problems or poor neurological grading that contraindicated surgery. The best angiographic-anatomical results were obtained in the second category, since the size of the aneurysm neck is the most important factor determining treatment success using the GDC technique.

Coil embolisation appears to be a safe option in the acute period after SAH and, since complication rates are simular for treatment of anterior or posterior circulation aneurysms, it is usually safer than surgical clipping in

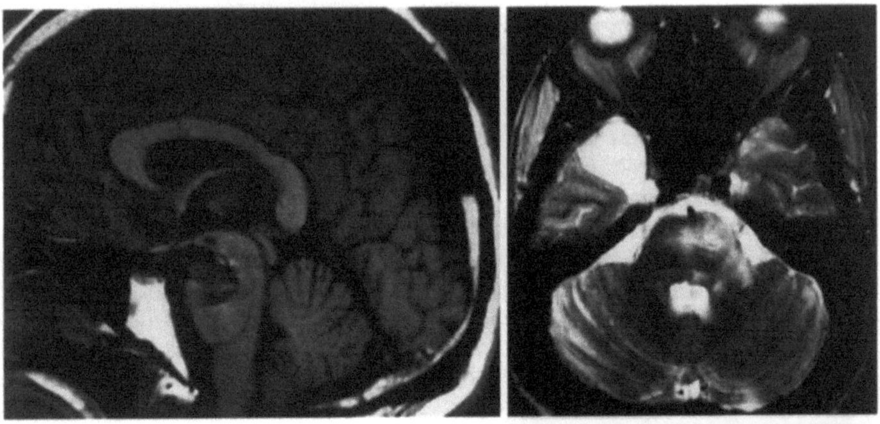

a b

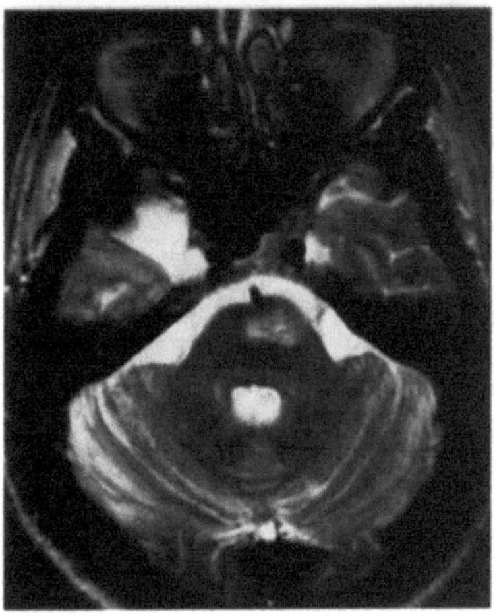

c

Fig. 7.10a–c.
Sagital T1-weighted (**a**) and axial T2-weighted magnetic resonance images (**b, c**) showing a large basilar artery aneurysm embedded in the midbrain and pons. The aneurysm has been treated by endosaccular packing with Guglielmi detachable coils (GDCs). **a, b** Signal change is evident in the brainstem immediately after coil embolisation. **c** It has substantially resolved concurrent with the relief of compression symptoms on follow-up scanning 12 months later

the latter, where the best surgical results for treatment of ruptured aneurysms report morbidity rates of 8.5% and mortality rates of 6.5% [44].

The results of short- and mid-term clinical and angiographic follow-up studies indicate that small-necked aneurysms (neck <4 mm) can be completely occluded. In these cases, follow-up angiograms (up to 5 years) show that the GDC system is capable of permanently occluding intracranial aneurysms and protecting patients from rebleeding. Wide-necked aneurysms (neck >4 mm), on the other hand, commonly develop post-treatment remnants and follow-up angiograms may show coil compaction with re-exposure of part of the aneurysm lumen to blood flow. In these cases further GDC treatment and/or a combined approach (endovascular-surgical) should be considered since unoccluded portions of aneurysms may rupture.

Continued angiographic and clinical monitoring of the initial groups of treated patients will help determine the longer-term durability of endovascular coil embolisation for the treatment of intracranial aneurysms.

References

1. Anon VV, Aymard A, Gobin YP et al (1992) Balloon occlusion of the internal carotid artery in 40 cases of giant intracavernous aneurysm: technical aspects, cerebral monitoring and results. Neuroradiology 34:245–251
2. Anson JA, Lawton MT, Spetzler RF (1996) Characteristics and surgical treatment of dolichoectatic and fusiform aneurysms. J Neurosurg 84:185–193
3. Aymard A, Govin YP, Hodes JE et al (1991) Endovascular occlusion of vertebral arteries in the treatment of unclippable vertebrobasilar aneurysms. J Neurosurg 74: 393–398
4. Berenstein A, Ransohoff J, Kuppersmith M et al (1984) Transvascular treatment of giant aneurysms of the cavernous carotid and vertebral arteries. Surg Neurol 21:3–12
5. Bradac GB, Riva A, Berguli M et al (1995) Endovascular coil embolisation of cerebral aneurysms. Riv Neuroradiol 8:637–644
6. Braun IS, Hoffman JC Jr, Casarella WJ, Davis PC (1985) Use of coils for transcatheter carotid occlusion. AJNR 6:953–956
7. Bull J (1969) Massive aneurysms at the base of the brain. Brain 92:535–570
8. Byrne JV, Adams CBT, Kerr RSC et al (1995) Endosaccular treatment of inoperable intracranial aneurysms with platinum coils. Br J Neurosurg 9:585–592
9. Byrne JV, Molyneux AJ, Brennen RP, Renowden SR (1995) Embolisation of recently ruptured intracranial aneurysms. J Neurol Neurosurg Psychiatry 59:616–620
10. Byrne JV, Hope JKA, Hubbard N, Morris JH (1997) The nature of thrombosis induced by platinum and tungsten coils in saccular aneurysms. AJNR Am J Neuroradiol 18:29–33
11. Casasco AE, Aymard A, Gobin P et al (1993) Selective endovascular treatment of 71 intracranial aneurysms with platinum coils. J Neurosurg 73:3–10
12. Clark WC, Ray MW (1982) Contralateral intracranial aneurysm formation as a late complication of carotid ligation. Surg Neurol 18:455–462
13. Cuatico W, Cook AW, Tyshchenko V et al (1967) Massive enlargement of intracranial aneurysms following carotid ligation. Arch Neurol 17:609–613
14. Debrun G, Fox A, Drake C et al (1981) Giant unclippable âneurysms: treatment with detachable balloons. AJNR 2:167–173
15. Drake CG, Vanderlinden RG (1967) The late consequences of incomplete surgical treatment of cerebral aneurysms. J Neurosurg 27:226–238
16. Drake CG, Friedman AH, Peerless SJ (1984) Failed aneurysm surgery. Reoperation in 115 cases. J Neurosurg 61:848–856
17. Drake CG, Peerless SJ, Ferguson GG (1994) Hunterian proximal arterial occlusion for giant aneurysms of the carotid circulation. J Neurosurg 81:656–665
18. Dyste GW, Beck DW (1989) De novo aneurysm formation following carotid ligation: case report and review of the literature. Neurosurg 24:88–92
19. Fox AJ, Viñuela F, Pelz DM et al (1987) Use of detachable balloons for proximal artery occlusion in the treatment of unclippable cerebral aneurysms. J Neurosurg 66:40–46
20. Giannotta SL, Litofsky NS (1995) Reoperative management of intracranial aneurysms. J Neurosurg 83:387–393
21. Gobin P, Viñuela F, Gurian J et al (1996) Treatment of large and giant fusiform intracranial aneurysms with Guglielmi detachable coils. J Neurosurg 84:53–62
22. Graves V, Strother C, Duff T et al. (1995) Early treatment of ruptured aneurysms with Guglielmi Detachable Coils: effects on subsequent bleeding. Neurosurgery 37:640–648
23. Graves VB, Strother CM, Weir B, Duff TA (1996) Vertebrobasilar junction aneurysms associated with fenestration: treatment with Guglielmi detachable coils. AJNR 17:35–40
24. Guglielmi G (in press) The interventional neuroradiological treatment of intracranial aneurysms. In: Cahadon F (ed) Advances and technical standards in neurosurgery. Springer, Berlin Heidelberg New York
25. Guglielmi G, Viñuela F, Dion J et al (1991) Electrothrombosis of saccular aneurysms via endovascular approach. Part II. Preliminary clinical experience. J Neurosurg 75:8–14
26. Guglielmi G, Viñuela F, Duckwiler G et al (1992) Endovascular treatment of posterior circulation aneurysms by electrothrombosis using electrically detachable coils. J Neurosurg 77:515–524
27. Gurian J, Martin N, King W et al (1995) Neurosurgical management of cerebral aneurysms following unsuccessful or incomplete endovascular embolization. J Neurosurg 83:843–853

28. Halbach VV, Higashida RT, Dowd CF et al (1993) Endovascular treatment of vertebral artery dissections and pseudoaneurysms. J Neurosurg 79:183–191
29. Halbach VV, Higashida RT, Dowd CF et al (1994) The efficacy of endosaccular aneurysm occlusion in alleviating neurological deficits produced by mass effect. J Neurosurg 80:659–666
30. Haley EC Jr, Kassel NF, Torner JC et al (1994) A randomized trial of two doses of nicardipine in aneurysmal subarachnoid hemorrhage. A report of the cooperative aneurysm study. J Neurosurg 80:788–796
31. Higashida RT, Halbach VV, Cahan LD et al (1989) Detachable balloon embolisation therapy of posterior circulation intracranial aneurysms. J Neurosurg 71:512–519
32. Higashida RT, Halbach VV, Dowd C et al (1990) Endovascular detachable balloon embolization therapy of cavernous carotid artery aneurysms: results in 87 cases. J Neurosurg 72:857–863
33. Hisobuchi Y (1979) Direct surgical treatment of giant intracranial aneurysms. J Neurosurg 51:743–756
34. Hodes JE, Aymard A, Gobin YP et al (1991) Endovascular occlusion of the intracranial vessels for curative treatment of unclippable aneurysms: report of 16 cases. J Neurosurg 75:694–701
35. Hope JKA, Byrne JV, Molyneux AJ (submitted for publication) Factors influencing successful angiographic occlusion of aneurysms treated by coil embolisation
36. Kawakami Y, Shimamura Y (1987) Cisternal drainage after early operation of ruptured intracranial aneurysms. Neurosurgery 20:8–14
37. Malisch T, Guglielmi G, Viñuela F et al (1997) Intracranial aneurysms treated with the Guglielmi detachable coil: midterm clinical results in 100 consecutive patients. J Neurosurg 87:176–183
38. Massoud TF, Guglielmi G, Viñuela F, Duckwiler GR (1996) Endovascular treatment of multiple aneurysms involving the posterior intracranial circulation. AJNR 17:549–554
39. McDougall CG, Halbach VV, Dowd CF et al (1996) Endovascular treatment of basilar tip aneurysms using electrolytically detachable coils. J Neurosurg 84:393–399
40. Murayama Y, Malisch T, Guglielmi G et al (in press) Early endovascular treatment of acutely ruptured aneurysms with GDC coils: the incidence of cerebral vasospasm. J Neurosurg
41. Norlen G, Olivecrona H (1953) The treatment of intracranial aneurysms of the circle of Willis. J Neurosurg 10:404–415
42. Odom GL, Tindall GT (1968) Carotid ligation in the treatment of certain intracranial aneurymsm. Clin Neurosurg 15:101–106
43. Oldershaw JB, Voris HC (1966) Internal carotid artery ligation. A follow-up study. Neurology 16:937–938
44. Peerless SJ, Hernesniemi JA, Gutman FB et al (1994) Early surgery for ruptured vertebrobasilar aneurysms. J Neurosurg 80:643–649
45. Pelz DM, Viñuela F, Fox AJ et al (1984) Vertebrobasilar occlusion therapy of giant aneurysms. Significance of angiographic morphology of the posterior communicating arteries. J Neurosurg 60:560–565
46. Pierot L, Boulin A, Castaings L et al (1996) Selective occlusion of basilar artery aneurysms using controlled detachable coils: report of 35 cases. Neurosurgery 38:948–954
47. Polin RS, Shaffrey ME, Jensen ME et al (1996) Medical management in the endovascular treatment of cavernous-carotid aneurysms. J Neurosurg 84:755–761
48. Quintana F, Diez C, Gutierrez A et al. (1996) Traumatic aneurysm of the basilar artery. AJNR 17:283–285
49. Raymond J, Roy D, Bojanowski M et al (1997) Endovascular treatment of acutely ruptured and unruptured aneurysms of the basilar bifurcation. J Neurosurg. 86:211–219
50. Reul J, Weis J, Spetzger U et al (1997) Long-term angiographic and histopathologic findings in experimental aneurysms of the carotid bifurcation embolized with platinum and tungsten coils. AJNR 18:35–42
51. Richling B, Bavinzski G, Gross C et al (1995) Early clinical outcome of patients with ruptured cerebral aneurysms treated by endovascular (GDC) or microsurgical techniques. Intervent Neuroradiol 1:19–27
52. Roski RA, Spetzler RF, Nulsen FE (1981) Late complications of carotid ligation in the treatment of intracranial aneurysms. J Neurosurg 54:583–587
53. Salar G, Mingrino S (1981) Development of intracranial saccular aneurysms: report of two cases. Neurosurgery 8:462–465
54. Scotti G, Righi C, Simionato F, Hua Li M (1944) Endovascular therapy of intracranial aneurysms with Guglielmi detachable coils (GDC). Riv Neuroradiol 7:723–733

55. Solomon RA, Matthew EF, Pile-Spelman J (1994) Surgical management of unruptured intracranial aneurysms. J Neurosurg 80:440–446
56. Steinberg GK, Drake CG, Peerless SJ (1993) Deliberate basilar or vertebral artery occlusion in the treatment of intracranial aneurysms. J Neurosurg 79:161–173
57. Timperman PE, Tomsick TA, Tew JM et al (1995) Aneurysm formation after carotid occlusion. AJNR 16:329–331
58. Vijay KK, Taylor AR, Gordon DS (1973) Proximal carotid ligation for internal carotid aneurysms. A long-term follow-up study. J Neurosurg 39:503–513
59. Viñuela F, Duckwiler G, Mawad M (1997) Guglielmi detachable coil embolisation of acute intracranial aneurysm: perioperative anatomical and clinical outcome in 403 patients. J Neurosurg 86:475–482
60. Weir B (1985) Intracranial aneurysms and subarachnoid hemorrhage: an overview. In: Wilkins RH, Rengachary SS (eds) Neurosurgery, vol 2. McGraw-Hill, New York, pp 1308–1329
61. Winn HR, Richardson AE, Jane JA (1977) Late morbidity and mortality of common carotid ligation for posterior communicating aneurysms. A comparison to conservative treatment. J Neurosurg 47:727–736
62. Yamada K, Hayakawa T, Ushido Y et al (1984) Therapeutic occlusion of the vertebral artery for unclippable vertebral aneurysm: relationship between site of occlusion and clinical outcome. Neurosurgery 15:834–838
63. Zubillaga A, Guglielmi G, Viñuela F et al (1994) Endovascular occlusion of intracranial aneurysms with electrically detachable coils: correlation of aneurysm neck size and treatment results. AJNR 15:815–820

Chapter 8

Future Developments

8.1 Current Development of the GDC Technique

The technique of endovascular occlusion of intracranial aneurysms with Guglielmi detachable coils (GDCs) was conceived in the late seventies and developed in a research programme that started in 1989 [4]. As part of this programme a new technique for the surgical construction of experimental saccular aneurysms on the carotid artery of swine was developed [6]. This technique involved end-to-side anastomosis of an isolated segment of vein to the artery. The artery was briefly clamped and an elliptic arteriotomy fashioned through the open end of the vein which was then closed, thus creating a lateral vein pouch aneurysm. The size of the aneurysm neck could be varied in order to create either small- or wide-necked aneurysms. This model was then used to develop the technique of endovascular occlusion of saccular aneurysms with electrolytically detachable coils and to test types of coils [1] and embolisation techniques (see Chap. 4). Recently, Cawley et al. [2] reported on the creation of saccular aneurysms by injection of porcine pancreatic elastase into the stump of the ligated external carotid artery of rabbits. In this model, histological examination revealed complete loss of the elastic lamina, which thus more closely simulates clinical aneurysms.

Although the GDC system was first used to treat patients more than 7 years ago (March 6, 1990), laboratory based research is still ongoing to improve and perfect the technique. In vitro studies of electrothrombosis using GDC, for example, are performed to assess the relationship between heparin concentration and the amount of thrombus formed by electrothrombosis.

New GDC sizes, shapes and designs are continuously being tested and evaluated. Available GDCs have a third generation junction; this junction allows faster detachment times (2–3 min) than previous designs, and a fourth generation of GDC is currently being tested.

Further improvements to the GDC system may be possible by increasing the applied electric current. A 1-mA current (in clinical use at present) causes only a thin layer of proteins to be deposited on the surface of the GDC [13]. Higher currents (up to 5 mA) may enhance electrothrombosis without producing unwanted side effects. It is already known that 2 mA is well tolerated in clinical use.

An acoustic signal determines when electrolytic detachment has occurred in the latest version of the GDC power supply. A further refinement of this system is proposed with a new version of the power supply capable of determining correct placement of the platinum–stainless steel junction electronically (Fig. 8.1). This would make the platinum markers on the microcatheter unnecessary and simplify aneurysm treatment.

The hydrophilic Fastracker-GDC (Target Therapeutic, Fremont, California) variable stiffness microcatheter is now available. This catheter should be utilised in patients with difficult and tortuous vascular anatomy. It is also useful for accessing distal aneurysms. Kink resistant microcatheters are also available. They are indicated in the treatment of patients with tortuous vessels to reduce friction between microcatheter and coil caused by kinking.

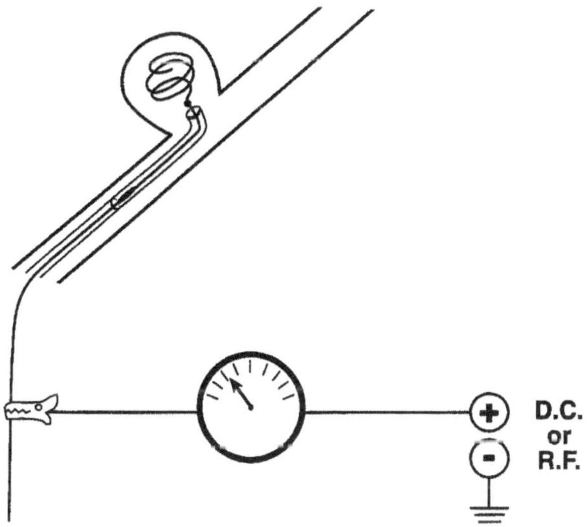

Fig. 8.1.
The positioning of the Guglielmi detachable coil platinum–steel junction could be determined, in the future, with electronic devices rather than with the currently utilised platinum markers. *DC*, direct current; *RF*, radio frequency

Two-diameter GDCs (2D-GDC) and a softer version of the GDC-10 for the treatment of small, acutely ruptured aneurysms are now being used in the clinical setting with excellent initial results. The 2D-GDC has been developed to cope with the problem of the first loops of a coil herniating into the parent artery during the treatment of aneurysms with wider necks or poor neck-to-sac ratios.

Stretch resistent GDCs are being developed and designs are currently undergoing clinical trials. They have a strengthening thread within the platinum coil in order to reduce the risk of stretching, particularly when retrieving soft coils. Three-dimensional GDCs (3D-GDC) are also planned. The concept of 3D-GDCs is that their more complex memory will be less susceptible to the phenomenon of coil compaction and, therefore, prevent aneurysm recurrence after coil embolisation.

8.2
Alternative and Combination Methods of Endosaccular Embolisation

There has been considerable interest in the possible use of endovascular stents to reinforce the aneurysm bearing artery and bridge its neck or ostum. Stents have been deployed in the parent artery across the necks of experimental aneurysms, constructed with especially wide necks. Turjman et al. [14] used a microcatheter introduced through the mesh of a stent to deliver GDCs into the aneurysm sac. This technique allowed tighter packing of the coils without the danger of them herniating into the parent artery or their endovascular migration. When an endovascular stent, suitable for intracranial use, becomes available, this technique may become an alternative method for endosaccular packing of some wide-necked aneurysms.

Fig. 8.2.
Follow-up angiogram of an experimental side-wall aneurysm. The aneurysm contains Guglielmi detachable coils and cellulose acetate polymer. The latter is poorly opaque and only visible at the aneurysm fundus (*arrow*). The parent artery is only slightly narrowed at the level of the occluded aneurysm neck

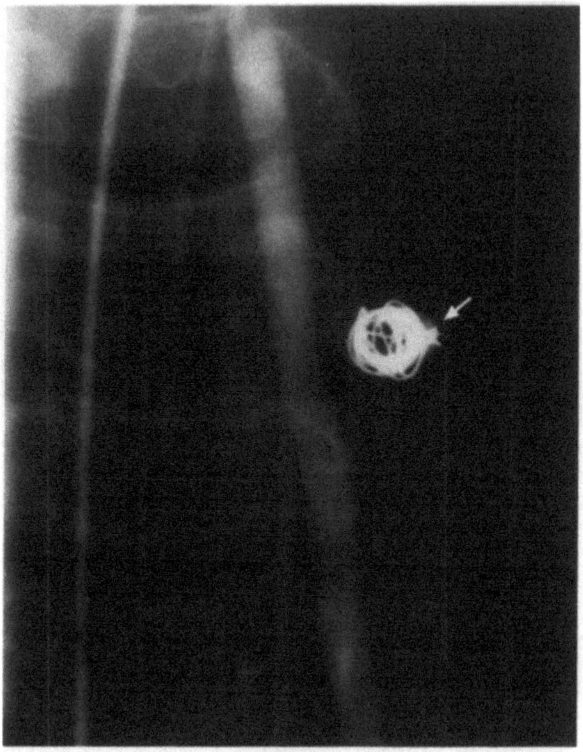

In Japan, a polymerising plastic material has been recently tested in experimental aneurysms and used for endosaccular packing in a small number of selected patients [8, 9]. The material is a viscous liquid composed of cellulose acetate polymer (CAP) and bismuth trioxide dissolved in dimethyl sulphoxide (DMSO). It can be injected through microcatheters to fill the lumen of intracranial aneurysms. The polymer solidifies in approximately 5 min. Temporary occlusion of the parent vessel (with a balloon) is necessary during the time it takes for the material to polymerise. The risk of distal embolisation of the liquid and the toxicity of the solvent DMSO are concerns. An embolic agent such as CAP, which is delivered as a liquid and sets to form a solid embolus within the aneurysm sac has some theoretical advantages since it could fill aneurysms of different sizes and shapes. CAP hardens on contact with blood and can be delivered in a single coherent mass. In order to ensure that the material remained in the aneurysm, Kinugasa et al. [8] placed a balloon at the aneurysm neck, whilst Higgins et al. [7] used coils to reduce blood flow in the aneurysm lumen and stop CAP being washed into the parent artery (Fig. 8.2). The longer term stability of the material and ways of reducing the toxic effects of DMSO (which causes angionecrosis in high concentrations), are currently being studied.

Several other possible methods for improving the results of endosaccular coil embolisation for wide-necked aneurysms have been proposed, including

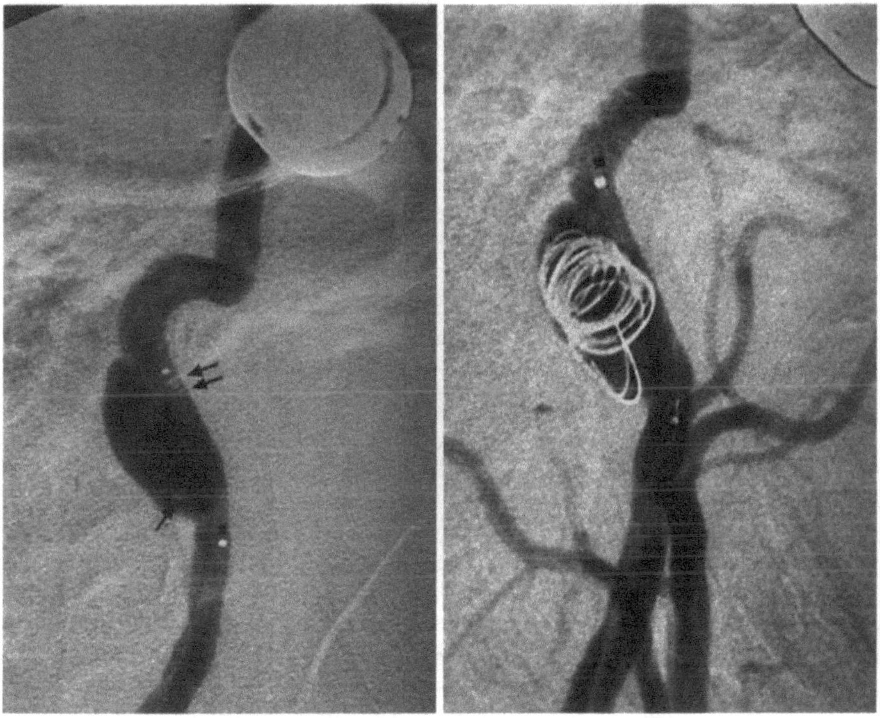

a b

Fig. 8.3 a, b. Wide-necked aneurysm of the cervical internal carotid artery. **a** A balloon catheter has been positioned across the aneurysm neck (*double arrow*) and a microcatheter (*single arrow*) in the aneurysm lumen. **b** During coil placement the balloon was inflated so that coils remained in the aneurysm lumen

partial extravascular clipping, and the use of a non-detachable balloon to protect the parent artery during packing with coils (Fig. 8.3).

The use of a helper balloon in the parent artery has been described as "neckplasty" or "remodelling" and potentially allows the operator to mould the coil mass at the neck of wide-necked aneurysms [5, 10, 12]. The balloon is briefly inflated across the aneurysm neck during GDC deployment, and is then deflated prior to GDC detachment so that the stability of the coils can be assessed. This technique allows treatment of otherwise untreatable aneurysms and may reduce the incidence of aneurysm recurrence. It should be reserved for selected cases of high risk lesions and should be utilised only by operators with considerable experience in the use of endovascular balloons. Moret et al. [10] have reported its use with minimal additional procedural morbidity despite more frequent aneurysm rupture during coil deployment.

8.3
Future Developments

The therapeutic challenges still posed by intracranial aneurysm have been discussed in the previous chapters of this book. The issues that remain unresolved, and which future management will have to address, are the following:

- The identification of patients at risk of developing intracranial aneurysms
- The pre-emptive treatment or prevention of aneurysms, before they cause symptoms or pose a risk of rupture
- Earlier and celeritous diagnosis, admission and treatment of patients presenting with subarachnoid haemorrhage, to prevent lethal rebleeding
- Prevention (or improved treatment) of cerebral ischemia due to vasospasm.

From the standpoint of the endovascular therapist, the goal is to protect the fragile aneurysmal wall from the hemodynamic stress of pulsatile blood flow and subsequent structural fatigue. To achieve this goal and modify the pre-existing condition it is necessary to apply some form of energy. In surgical clipping, for instance, the neurosurgeon's hand physically carries the clip near the aneurysm, opens and positions the clip; the mechanical energy stored in the clip then re-approximates the walls of the aneurysm neck [11]. In GDC treatment, the coil is physically pushed by the mechanical energy of the operator's hands towards the aneurysm. Then, the mechanical energy stored in the coil causes it to deform to the shape of the aneurysm lumen. Energies such as the electricity to detach GDCs or the removal ("detachment") of the clip applicator, are not directly involved in the aneurysm treatment.

One or more forms of energy will be utilised for aneurysm treatment in the future: mechanical, electromagnetic, magnetic, electrical, thermal, sound, light, chemical, nuclear, atomic, biochemical. The energy can be applied directly into the aneurysm (as with balloons or coils), outside the aneurysm (as with clips or stents), or at a distance from the aneurysm (i.e. surgical or endovascular trapping). The source of energy can be outside the aneurysm and delivered via a microcatheter or generated and then focused within the aneurysm, or a combination of both. Figure. 8.4 shows examples of the possible combinations of such energies [3].

The direction of therapeutic efforts are now firmly set on a less invasive approach and the endovascular route currently offers the best means of achieving that objective. The future will no doubt bring novel ideas and methods to the process of reducing the morbidity caused by intracranial aneurysms and their safer and more effective treatment. Some of these im-

Fig. 8.4 a–d. Different forms of energy, or a combination of energies, could be utilised for future endovascular aneurysm treatment by excluding the aneurysm from the blood circulation or by sealing the aneurysmal wall. **a** Electromagnetic (laser) energy, **b** ultrasonic energy, **c** crystallization energy, **d** biochemical energy

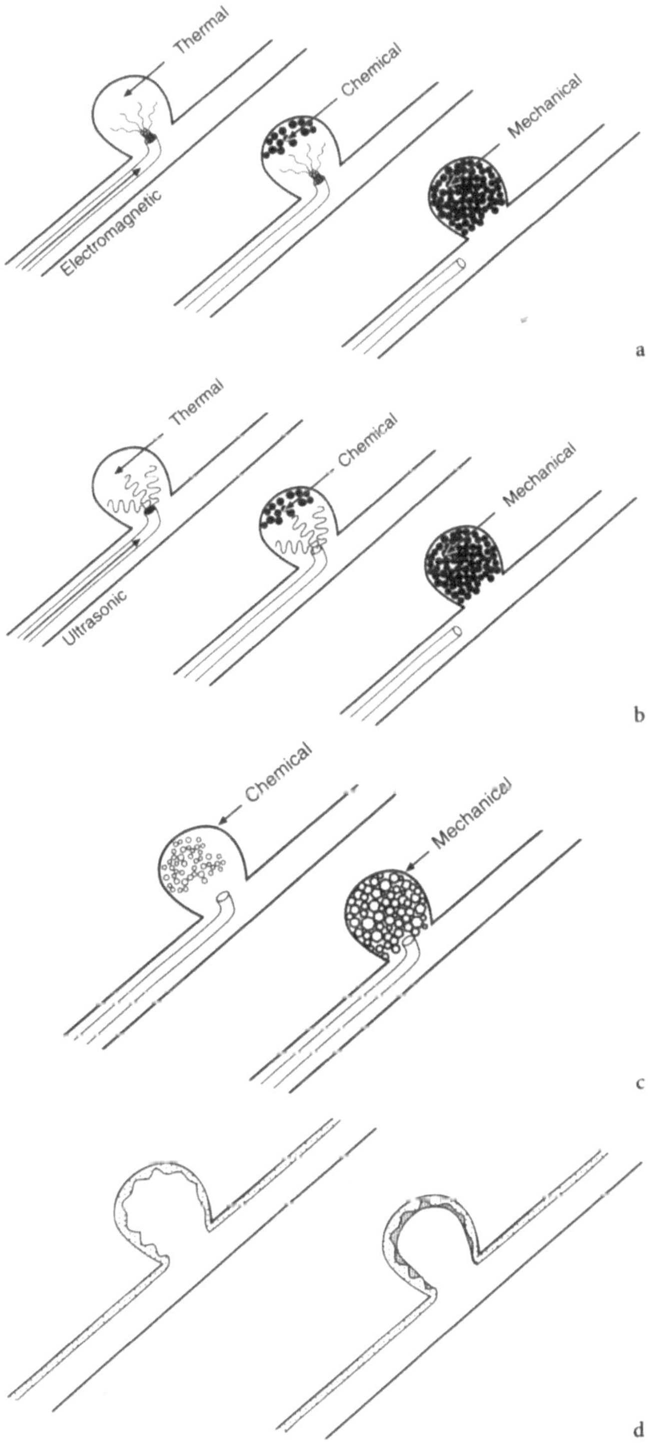
Thermal
Chemical
Mechanical
Electromagnetic
a
Thermal
Chemical
Mechanical
Ultrasonic
b
Chemical
Mechanical
c
d

provements will involve the engineering of more sophisticated endovascular devices, while others will come from allied disciplines such as imaging (e.g. interactive three-dimensional imaging) and anaesthesia. All one can be certain of is that the future will bring change.

References

1. Byrne JV, Hope RKA, Hubbard N, Morris JH (1997) The nature of thrombosis induced by platinum and tungsten coils in saccular aneurysms. AJNR 18:29–33
2. Cawley CM, Dawson RC, Shengelaia G et al. (1996) Arterial saccular aneurysm model in the rabbit. AJNR 17:1761–1766
3. Guglielmi G (1995) Present and future development in the endovascular management of intracranial aneurysms. Interventional Companion Course of the American Society of Interventional and Therapeutic Neuroradiology, Chicago, 21–22 April
4. Guglielmi G, Viñuela F, Sepetka I, Macellari V (1991) Electrothrothrombosis of saccular aneurysms via endovascular approach. Part 1. Electrochemical basis, technique, and experimental results. J Neurosurg 75:1–7 (special article)
5. Guglielmi G, Viñuela F, Briganti F, Duckwiler G (1992) Carotid-cavernous fistula due to a ruptured intracavernous aneurysm: endovascular treatment by electrothrombosis with detachable coils. Neurosurgery 31:591–597
6. Guglielmi G, Ji C, Massoud T, Kurata A, Lownie S, Viñuela F, Robert J (1994) Experimental saccular aneurysms. II. A new model in swine. Neuroradiology 36:547–550
7. Higgins JNP, Byrne JV, Krulle TM, Fleet GWJ (1997) Capping the coil. Neuroradiology 39:146
8. Kinugasa K, Mandai S, Terai Y, Kamata I, Sugiu K, Ohmoto T, Nishimoto A (1992) Direct thrombosis of aneurysms with cellulose acetate polymer. Part II. Preliminary clinical experience. J Neurosurg 77:501–507
9. Mandai S, Kinugasa K, Ohmoto T (1992) Direct thrombosis of aneurysms with cellulose acetate polymer. Part 1. Results of thrombosis in experimental aneurysms. J Neurosurg 77:497–500
10. Moret J, Cognard C, Weill A, Castaings L, Rey A (1997) The "remodeling technique" in the treatment of wide neck intracranial aneurysms. Angiographic results and clinical follow-up in 56 cases. Intervent Neuroradiol, 3:21–35
11. Ooka K, Shibuya M, Suzuki Y (1997) A comparative study of intracranial aneurysms clips: closing and opening forces and physical endurance. Neurosurgery 40:318–323
12. Takahashi A, Ezara M, Yoshimoto (1997) Broad neck basilar tip aneurysm treated by neck plastic intra-aneurysmal GDC embolisation with protective balloon. Intervent Neuroradiol 3:167–170
13. Tenjin H, Fushiki S, Nakahara Y et al. (1995) Effect of Guglielmi detachable coils on experimental carotid artery aneurysms in primates. Stroke 26:2075–2080
14. Turjman F, Massoud T, Ji C, Guglielmi G, Viñuela F, Robert J (1994) Combined stent implantation and endosaccular coil placement for treatment of experimental wide-necked aneurysms: a feasibility study in swine. AJNR Am J Neuroradiol 15:1087–1090

Subject Index

SPRINGER NATURE

GPSR Compliance

The European Union's (EU) General Product Safety Regulation (GPSR) is a set of rules that requires consumer products to be safe and our obligations to ensure this.

If you have any concerns about our products, you can contact us on ProductSafety@springernature.com

In case Publisher is established outside the EU, the EU authorized representative is:

Springer Nature Customer Service Center GmbH
Europaplatz 3
69115 Heidelberg, Germany

Kolibri 360 GmbH
Ferdinand-Jühlke-Straße 7
99095 Erfurt, Deutschland
produktsicherheit@kolibri360.de